Faculty Development in the l

MW00837531

Innovation and Change in Professional Education

VOLUME 11

Series Editor:
W.H. Gijselaers, *School of Business and Economics, Maastricht University, The Netherlands*

Associate Editors:
L.A. Wilkerson, *David Geffen School of Medicine, University of California, Los Angeles, CA, USA*
H.P.A. Boshuizen, *Center for Learning Sciences and Technologies, Open Universiteit Nederland, Heerlen, The Netherlands*

Editorial Board:
T. Duffy, *School of Education, Indiana University, Bloomington, IN, USA*
K. Eva, *UBC Faculty of Medicine, Center for Health Education Scholarship, Vancouver, BC, Canada*
H. Gruber, *Institute of Educational Science, University of Regensburg, Germany*
R. Milter, *Carey Business School, Johns Hopkins University, Baltimore, MD, USA*

SCOPE OF THE SERIES

The primary aim of this book series is to provide a platform for exchanging experiences and knowledge about educational innovation and change in professional education and post-secondary education (engineering, law, medicine, management, health sciences, etc.). The series provides an opportunity to publish reviews, issues of general significance to theory development and research in professional education, and critical analysis of professional practice to the enhancement of educational innovation in the professions.

The series promotes publications that deal with pedagogical issues that arise in the context of innovation and change of professional education. It publishes work from leading practitioners in the field, and cutting edge researchers. Each volume is dedicated to a specific theme in professional education, providing a convenient resource of publications dedicated to further development of professional education.

For further volumes:
http://www.springer.com/series/6087

Yvonne Steinert
Editor

Faculty Development in the Health Professions

A Focus on Research and Practice

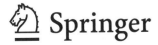 Springer

Editor
Yvonne Steinert
Centre for Medical Education
   and Department of Family Medicine
Faculty of Medicine
McGill University
Montreal, QC, Canada

ISBN 978-94-007-7611-1   ISBN 978-94-007-7612-8 (eBook)
DOI 10.1007/978-94-007-7612-8
Springer Dordrecht Heidelberg New York London

Library of Congress Control Number: 2014930985

© Springer Science+Business Media Dordrecht 2014
This work is subject to copyright. All rights are reserved by the Publisher, whether the whole or part of
the material is concerned, specifically the rights of translation, reprinting, reuse of illustrations, recitation,
broadcasting, reproduction on microfilms or in any other physical way, and transmission or information
storage and retrieval, electronic adaptation, computer software, or by similar or dissimilar methodology
now known or hereafter developed. Exempted from this legal reservation are brief excerpts in connection
with reviews or scholarly analysis or material supplied specifically for the purpose of being entered and
executed on a computer system, for exclusive use by the purchaser of the work. Duplication of this
publication or parts thereof is permitted only under the provisions of the Copyright Law of the Publisher's
location, in its current version, and permission for use must always be obtained from Springer.
Permissions for use may be obtained through RightsLink at the Copyright Clearance Center. Violations
are liable to prosecution under the respective Copyright Law.
The use of general descriptive names, registered names, trademarks, service marks, etc. in this publication
does not imply, even in the absence of a specific statement, that such names are exempt from the relevant
protective laws and regulations and therefore free for general use.
While the advice and information in this book are believed to be true and accurate at the date of
publication, neither the authors nor the editors nor the publisher can accept any legal responsibility for
any errors or omissions that may be made. The publisher makes no warranty, express or implied, with
respect to the material contained herein.

Printed on acid-free paper

Springer is part of Springer Science+Business Media (www.springer.com)

Preface

In May 2011, educators from around the world gathered in Toronto for the 1st International Conference on Faculty Development. Organized by McGill University and the University of Toronto, this conference was designed to encourage the exchange of best practices and research findings, and to build a global community of leaders dedicated to the professional development of faculty members in a variety of settings. Convinced of the importance of faculty development to achieve the goals of medical education in a global context, international faculty development leaders and educators in the health professions came together to explore how faculty development can prepare health professionals for their multiple roles as teachers and educators, leaders and managers, and researchers and scholars.

This book, which is a natural outgrowth of this conference and the deliberations that took place in large group plenaries, workshops, research presentations, and social events, aims to continue the dialogue that took place in 2011. By exploring the scope and practice of faculty development in the health professions, we hope to stimulate discussion about the current status of faculty development, ensure that research (and evidence) informs ongoing practice, and highlight future directions for research and practice.

Palmer (1998)[1] has said that the 'growth of any craft depends on shared practice and honest dialogue among the people who do it' (p. 144). In multiple ways, that is the goal of this book: to make sense of the practical experience and research findings that have accumulated in this community of practice in order to help move the field of faculty development forward.

Faculty development has become an increasingly common enterprise in health professions faculties and schools (and their affiliated hospitals), specialty societies, regulatory bodies, and national and international associations. As a result, this book

---

[1] Palmer, P. J. (1998). *The Courage to Teach*. San Francisco, CA: Jossey-Bass.

marks a moment in time where we can look back at past accomplishments and begin to chart future directions. While there is still much to be accomplished, it is hoped that the ideas and concepts in this book will help to inform future growth and development.

This book is divided into six parts. Following a discussion of what we mean by 'faculty development' and the core concepts and principles that underlie the design and implementation of diverse faculty development initiatives, we will describe the capacity of faculty development programs and activities to enhance teaching and education, leadership and management, research and scholarship, academic career development, and organizational change. Based on the available literature and experience in the field, we will then discuss a number of approaches to faculty development, including work-based learning and communities of practice, peer coaching and mentorship, workshops and seminars, fellowships and other longitudinal programs, and online learning, In addition, we will highlight practical applications and describe how faculty development initiatives can be used to promote role modeling and reflective practice, competency-based teaching and assessment, interprofessional education and practice, and international collaboration and partnerships. The design and development of a comprehensive faculty development program will also be addressed, as will the role of research, scholarship, and knowledge translation in faculty development. The final part of this book will draw upon lessons learned in each chapter and try to develop a road map for the future.

It is hoped that this portrait of faculty development will be of interest to different stakeholders, including faculty developers, educational leaders and administrators, teachers, students, researchers, and policy makers in all of the health professions who are interested in pursuing their own professional learning and that of their colleagues. Although many of the examples in this book are drawn from medicine, the general principles and strategies apply to the professional development of all health professionals. Similarly, although this book is designed for health professionals in particular, many of its concepts and insights are relevant to individuals interested in faculty development in other fields.

Each chapter in this volume is meant to review what we know about faculty development in a designated area, discuss avenues for further development and innovation, and where appropriate, provide a case example. Those who read the book from cover to cover will obtain a comprehensive overview of what faculty development can achieve. However, each chapter can also stand alone and appeal to readers with specific interests.

This book represents the collective efforts of a team of international scholars and educators who accepted the challenge of forging new territory and pushing the boundaries in their thinking and writing about faculty development. Synthesizing the current 'state of the art' and extending the reach of faculty development is no easy feat; however, each of the authors, who represent a broad range of clinical and educational backgrounds, has risen to this challenge, bringing meaningful insights to faculty development based on their experiences in a variety of interprofessional and international contexts.

This Springer Series focuses on innovation and change in professional education. In this case, it is the professional development of faculty members that we are addressing. We hope that this collection, which includes content that is not otherwise available, will facilitate program planning, implementation, and evaluation, move the scholarly agenda forward, and promote dialogue and debate in this important field of practice and scholarship.

Montreal, QC, Canada   Yvonne Steinert, Ph.D.
April 2013

Editor's Bio

Yvonne Steinert is a clinical psychologist and Professor of Family Medicine in the Faculty of Medicine at McGill University, Montreal, Quebec, Canada. She is the Director of the Centre for Medical Education, the Richard and Sylvia Cruess Chair in Medical Education, and the founding Associate Dean for Faculty Development in the Faculty of Medicine (1993–2011). Dr. Steinert has been engaged in medical education and faculty development for over 25 years in a variety of settings and is actively involved in undergraduate and postgraduate medical education, educational research, and the design and delivery of interprofessional faculty development programs and activities. Her research interests focus on teaching and learning in the health professions, curriculum development and program evaluation, the impact of faculty development on the individual and the organization, and the continuing professional development of faculty members. She has written extensively on the topic of faculty development and medical education, is frequently invited to address health professionals and medical educators in academic and scientific settings, and has been a driving force in promoting faculty development in local, national, and international contexts. Dr. Steinert is a Past-President of the Canadian Association for Medical Education and the recipient of several honors and awards in recognition of her contributions to faculty development and health professions education.

Acknowledgements

It has been said that medical education is a team sport. So is faculty development and writing a book. I am deeply grateful to each and every one of the authors for their commitment to this project and for their understanding of the centrality of faculty development in promoting excellence in the health professions.

I would also like to acknowledge Ivan Silver, co-chair of the 1st International Conference on Faculty Development in the Health Professions. I remain indebted to him for his vision, his wisdom, and his friendship. I am also grateful to both series editors, Wim Gijselaers and LuAnn Wilkerson, for having invited me to edit this book and for having recognized the importance of faculty development in the health professions.

Peer review is one of the hallmarks of academic writing, and this book is no exception. Each chapter was reviewed by two of the book's authors, or colleagues in the field, and I would like to acknowledge the following individuals for their constructive feedback on specific chapters: Miriam Boillat, Diana Dolmans, Michelle Elizov, Stacey Friedman, Carol Hodgson, David Irby, Brian Jolly, Karen Leslie, Karen Mann, Judy McKimm, Peter McLeod, Willemina Molenaar, Clare Morris, Catherine O'Keeffe, Patricia O'Sullivan, Ivan Silver, Linda Snell, John Spencer, Tim Swanwick, and Aliki Thomas. The accuracy of references is another challenge in academic writing, and I am indebted to Robert Zhu, Monika Krzywania, and Cristina Torchia, for their help with reference checking, formatting, and making sure that we all cited our colleagues correctly.

Each of us works with a community of teachers, educators, leaders, and scholars. I am deeply grateful to mine: the leadership of the Faculty of Medicine at McGill University, who provided me with a professional home to explore new ideas, take risks, and develop a faculty development program that evolved over 18 years; the academic and administrative members of the Faculty Development Team at McGill, who value learning and professional development and embarked on this journey with me; the faculty members who participated in our faculty development offerings and are committed to excellence in all that they do; and the members of the Centre for Medical Education (another venue for faculty development), who have stimulated my curiosity, challenged my thinking, and engaged in our joint pursuit of innovation, scholarship, and excellence. Without this 'community of practice', my own understanding of this complex process would not have been possible.

Lastly, I would like to acknowledge and thank my family for their ongoing support and encouragement. My husband, Ron, and my daughters, Elana, Shelley, and Danna, have been my best teachers and coaches, educating me about the joys of teaching and learning and inspiring me to pursue my dreams.

Contents

Contributors

Liz Anderson Department of Medical and Social Care Education, University of Leicester, Leicester, UK

Miriam Boillat Centre for Medical Education and Department of Family Medicine, Faculty of Medicine, McGill University, Montreal, QC, Canada

Francois Cilliers Education Development Unit, Faculty of Health Sciences, University of Cape Town, Cape Town, South Africa

David A. Cook Division of General Internal Medicine and Office of Education Research, College of Medicine, Mayo Clinic, Rochester, MN, USA

Willem de Grave Department of Educational Development and Research, Faculty of Health, Medicine and Life Sciences, University of Maastricht, Maastricht, The Netherlands

Michelle Elizov Centre for Medical Education and Department of Medicine, Faculty of Medicine, McGill University, Montreal, QC, Canada

Stacey Friedman Foundation for Advancement of International Medical Education and Research (FAIMER), Philadelphia, PA, USA

Larry D. Gruppen Department of Medical Education, University of Michigan Medical School, Ann Arbor, MI, USA

Marilyn Hammick The Best Evidence Medical Education Collaboration, Dundee, Scotland, UK

Sarah Hean In-2-Theory: Interprofessional Theory and Scholarship Network, School of Health and Social Care, Bournemouth University, Bournemouth, Dorset, UK

Brian Hodges Department of Psychiatry, University of Toronto, Toronto, ON, Canada

University Health Network, Toronto, ON, Canada

Wilson Centre for Research in Education, Health Professions Education Research, University of Toronto, Toronto, ON, Canada

Carol S. Hodgson Faculty of Medicine and Dentistry, Division of Studies in Medical Education, University of Alberta, Edmonton, AB, Canada

David M. Irby Department of Medicine and Office of Research and Development in Medical Education, University of California San Francisco School of Medicine, San Francisco, CA, USA

Brian Jolly Medical Education, School of Medicine and Public Health, Faculty of Health, The University of Newcastle, Callaghan, NSW, Australia

Australian Society for Simulation in Healthcare and Health Division of Simulation Australia, Adelaide, SA, Australia

Karen Leslie Department of Paediatrics and Centre for Faculty Development, Li Ka Shing International Health Education Centre, University of Toronto, Toronto, ON, Canada

Karen V. Mann Division of Medical Education, Faculty of Medicine, Dalhousie University, Halifax, NS, Canada

Désirée D. Mansvelder-Longayroux Faculty Development Programmes, Centre for Innovation in Medical Education, Leiden University Medical Centre, Leiden, The Netherlands

Judy McKimm College of Medicine, Swansea University, Swansea, West Glamorgan, UK

Willemina M. Molenaar Institute for Medical Education, University of Groningen and University Medical Center Groningen, Groningen, The Netherlands

John Norcini Foundation for Advancement of International Medical Education and Research (FAIMER), Philadelphia, PA, USA

Cath O'Halloran Department of Health Sciences, School of Human and Health Sciences, University of Huddersfield, Queensgate, Huddersfield, UK

Patricia S. O'Sullivan Department of Medicine and Office of Research and Development in Medical Education, University of California San Francisco School of Medicine, San Francisco, CA, USA

Richard Pitt Interprofessional Learning, Law and Ethics Interest Group for Health and Social Care, School of Nursing, Midwifery and Physiotherapy, Queens Medical Centre Campus, University of Nottingham, Nottingham, UK

Ivan Silver Department of Psychiatry, Centre for Addiction and Mental Health, Faculty of Medicine, University of Toronto, Toronto, ON, Canada

Linda Snell Centre for Medical Education and Department of Medicine, Faculty of Medicine, McGill University, Montreal, QC, Canada

Royal College of Physicians and Surgeons of Canada, Ottawa, ON, Canada

John Spencer Primary Care and Clinical Education, School of Medical Sciences Education Development, Faculty of Medical Sciences, Newcastle University, Newcastle upon Tyne, UK

Yvonne Steinert Centre for Medical Education and Department of Family Medicine, Faculty of Medicine, McGill University, Montreal, QC, Canada

Tim Swanwick Postgraduate Medical Education, Health Education North Central and East London, London, UK

Ara Tekian Department of Medical Education, College of Medicine, University of Illinois at Chicago, Chicago, IL, USA

Aliki Thomas Occupational Therapy Program, School of Physical and Occupational Therapy and Centre for Medical Education, Faculty of Medicine, McGill University, Montreal, QC, Canada

LuAnn Wilkerson Center for Educational Development and Research, David Geffen School of Medicine at University of California Los Angeles, Los Angeles, CA, USA

Anneke Zanting Centre for Education and Training, Ikazia Hospital Rotterdam, Rotterdam, The Netherlands

Part I
Introduction

Chapter 1
Faculty Development: Core Concepts and Principles

Yvonne Steinert

1.1 Introduction

Faculty development has become an increasingly important component of health professions education, and most faculties and schools (and their affiliated hospitals), specialty societies, regulatory bodies, and health professions organizations now offer formal faculty development programs and activities. In fact, diverse faculty development initiatives have been reported in the health professions (Alteen et al. 2009; Hendricson et al. 2007; McLean et al. 2008; McNamara et al. 2012; Mitcham et al. 2002; Rothman and Rinehart 1990; Scudder et al. 2010), and there is a burgeoning interest in both research and practice. The goal of this chapter is to highlight common goals and definitions, the rationale for faculty development, and the context in which faculty development occurs. We will also address the scope of faculty development, common approaches and practical applications that respond to educational and health care priorities, and the need for research, scholarship, and knowledge translation in this emerging field. Whitcomb (2003) observed that 'the medical school's faculty is its most important asset' (p. 117). Although this observation was made over a decade ago, this belief still underscores much of what we do in faculty development, as we try to nurture and sustain faculty members' curiosity, creativity and commitment.

Y. Steinert, Ph.D. (✉)
Centre for Medical Education and Department of Family Medicine,
Faculty of Medicine, McGill University, Montreal, QC, Canada
e-mail: yvonne.steinert@mcgill.ca

Y. Steinert (ed.), *Faculty Development in the Health Professions: A Focus on Research and Practice*, Innovation and Change in Professional Education 11, DOI 10.1007/978-94-007-7612-8_1, © Springer Science+Business Media Dordrecht 2014

1.2   Common Goals and Definitions

Faculty development, or staff development as it is often called, refers to that broad range of activities that institutions use to *renew* or *assist* faculty in their multiple roles (Centra 1978). In the past, faculty development has traditionally been defined as a planned program designed to *prepare* institutions and faculty members for their various roles (Bland et al. 1990) and *improve* an individual's knowledge and skills in the areas of teaching, research, and administration (Sheets and Schwenk 1990). However, although faculty development has historically been linked with planned programs, we have recently observed that health professionals engage in both *formal* and *informal* faculty development to enhance their knowledge and skills (Steinert 2010a, c) and that much of their professional development is self-directed and linked to experiential and workplace learning. As a result, and for the purpose of this book, **faculty development will refer to all activities health professionals pursue to improve their knowledge, skills, and behaviors as teachers and educators, leaders and managers, and researchers and scholars, in both individual and group settings.**

It has been said that the goal of faculty development is 'to teach faculty members the skills relevant to their institutional and faculty position and to sustain their vitality, both now and in the future' (Steinert 2009, p. 391). With this goal in mind, faculty development can provide individuals with knowledge and skills about teaching and learning, curriculum design and delivery, learner assessment and program evaluation, leadership and administration, and research and scholarship. It can also reinforce or alter attitudes or beliefs about multiple aspects of faculty members' roles and responsibilities, provide a conceptual framework for what is often performed on an intuitive basis, and introduce health professionals to a community of individuals interested in common goals and pursuits (Steinert 2009). In its broadest sense, faculty development should target *all* faculty members' roles (as outlined above) and not be limited to a focus on teaching and education, as is often the case.

It is also important to note that faculty development can serve as a useful instrument in the promotion of organizational change (Jolly Chap. 6; Steinert et al. 2007). For example, faculty development can try to influence the institutional culture by addressing the formal, informal, and hidden curriculum (Hafferty 1998), setting policy, or enhancing organizational capacities (Bligh 2005). In addition, by building consensus, generating support, transmitting core content, and promoting skill acquisition, faculty development can help to support curricular change (Snell Chap. 13) and build educational capacity for the future (Swanwick 2008).

As the reader will note, the literature is replete with diverse definitions of faculty development (McLean et al. 2008; Jolly Chap. 6; Silver Chap. 16). The meaning of this term also differs across cultures and languages. For example, the Dutch term, *docentprofessionalisering*, loosely translates as the professionalization of teaching (Steinert 2012, p. 32). This emphasis on professionalization, of both teachers and teaching, is appealing and aligns well with the more recent proliferation of standards for teaching (Purcell and Lloyd-Jones 2003). The term is limited, however, in its emphasis on teaching at the exclusion of other roles and responsibilities. In some ways, the French expression, *formation professorale*, is more inclusive by referring to the formation of the 'professorial' role, as is the German phrase, *personal- und organisationsentwickelung*, which highlights both individual and organizational development. However, irrespective of the nomenclature used, it is important to be aware of the meaning that faculty development conveys in different languages and how this form of professional development unfolds in different contexts and cultures.

Another question that arises from careful scrutiny of the term faculty development relates to the meaning of 'faculty'. Although the notion of faculty is often considered to be synonymous with 'academic faculty', in this book, **faculty refers to all individuals who are involved in the teaching and education of learners at all levels of the continuum (e.g. undergraduate; graduate; postgraduate; continuing professional development), leadership and management in the university, the hospital, and the community, and research and scholarship, across the health professions (e.g. communication sciences; dentistry; nursing; rehabilitation sciences).** In some ways, the UK term, staff development, avoids a potential bias towards the academic environment. However, it does not distinguish between professional and administrative staff. Importantly, and in the context of this discussion, the term faculty is meant to be inclusive of *all* health professionals working in a variety of settings.

Health professionals frequently question the difference between faculty development and continuing professional development (also known as continuing medical education [CME] in some settings). This potential distinction can become even more confusing as faculty development *is* a form of continuing professional development. However, the distinction that we make, both in practice and for the purpose of this book, is that faculty development refers to the enhancement and reinforcement of faculty roles, which include education, leadership, and research, whereas continuing professional development (or CME) refers to the maintenance and improvement of health professionals' clinical expertise (i.e. as health care providers).

Lastly, it is important to note that in some jurisdictions, faculty development is closely aligned with undergraduate health professions education; in other countries and settings, it is often embedded within postgraduate medical education (Swanwick 2008). For the purpose of this book, **faculty development is seen as integral to all levels of the educational enterprise – across all disciplines.**

1.3   The Rationale for Faculty Development

In the last decade, we have witnessed a significant growth in faculty development activities world-wide (e.g. Adkoli et al. 2009; Anshu et al. 2010; Cornes and Mokoena 2004; Wong and Agisheva 2007). This increase in activity is due, in part, to the realization that health professionals are often not prepared for their faculty roles. As Westberg and Jason (1981) have said:

> The one task that is distinctively related to being a faculty member is teaching; all the others can be pursued in other settings. Paradoxically, the central responsibility of faculty members is typically the one for which they tend to be least prepared (p. 100).

The proliferation of formal faculty development programs is also linked to a growing sense of public accountability, the changing nature of healthcare delivery, an ongoing pursuit of excellence, and the professionalization of teaching and medical education (Gruppen et al. 2006; Swanwick 2008). An emphasis on quality assurance in healthcare, and a desire to offer quality training programs for students and residents (Schofield et al. 2010), also drives the need for faculty development, as do many emerging educational priorities (e.g. the teaching and learning of professionalism; cultural awareness and humility; interprofessional education and practice). At the same time, we cannot ignore the influence of regulatory and international bodies that have started to pay attention to the accreditation of teachers and teaching (General Medical Council 2006; World Federation for Medical Education 2007), and in so doing, have highlighted the importance of faculty development in the certification of educators (Eitel et al. 2000). As McLean et al. (2008) have stated, referring specifically to the role of teacher and educator, 'with demands on medical faculties to be socially responsible and accountable, there is increasing pressure for the professionalization of teaching practice' (p. 555). In the UK, for example, the General Medical Council (2006) states that 'if you are involved in teaching, you must develop the skills, attitudes and practices of a competent teacher' (p. 14), and the role of teacher is increasingly recognized as a core professional activity for all doctors that 'cannot be left to chance, aptitude or inclination' (Purcell and Lloyd-Jones 2003, p. 149). In North America, the Liaison Committee on Medical Education (2012) requires that members of a medical school have the ability to be effective teachers, and in Canada, the Maintenance of Certification Program recognizes faculty development as a critical element in maintaining professional standards (Royal College of Physicians and Surgeons of Canada 2011). Interestingly, although faculty members' roles as leaders and researchers have not yet come under the same scrutiny, it would not be surprising if standards for all faculty roles will emerge in the next decade, and not only in the health professions.

1.4   The Context in Which Faculty Development Occurs

Faculty development in the health professions takes place in an ever-changing (and complex) environment, including universities and health professions schools, teaching hospitals and community sites, and national and international associations and organizations (Hueppchen et al. 2011). In all of these contexts, faculty development programs and activities must be responsive to changes in health care delivery, educational practice, and the ever-changing roles of health professionals. It has been said that medical education needs to align its goals and objectives with societal needs (Nora 2010); faculty development must do the same.

1.4.1 Healthcare Delivery

Health care, and the context in which it is delivered, has changed dramatically in the last decade. We have witnessed significant changes in disease profiles (e.g. an aging population; more complex illnesses; a shift from acute to chronic disease), sites of health care delivery (e.g. from single institutions to networks of care), and health care providers (e.g. from a single professional to teams of health professionals). Patients' (and families') knowledge and expectations have also changed, as has their involvement in health care. Technological developments have created new hopes and expectations, leading to the potential of personalized medicine and increasing costs. In fact, preoccupations with rising costs and performance have led to increased government intervention and reform in much of the Western world, and it is in this environment, of increased complexity and uncertainty, interdependency and change (Mamede and Schmidt 2004), that faculty development must unfold.

1.4.2 Clinical and Academic Environments

The clinical and academic environments in which faculty development occurs are also changing. For example, Swanwick and McKimm (2010) describe a number of challenges in the clinical environment that affect all health professionals: the need to balance busy clinical, teaching, and research workloads; a perpetual lack of time; feelings of isolation; increasing numbers of patients and students at all levels of the continuum; and the stress of keeping up-to-date. The academic setting is also marked by changing structures and growing interdependence (Nora 2010), an increase in workload, greater competition for grant funding, and new demands for scholarly productivity. How then do health professionals find the time to engage in faculty development? Steinert et al. (2010b) explored the reasons why faculty members participate in structured faculty development activities and identified four factors: the perception that faculty development enables personal and professional growth; the value that is placed on learning and self-improvement; the opportunity to network with colleagues; and initial positive experiences that encourage ongoing involvement. Awareness of these and other motivators can be very helpful in the design and delivery of faculty development initiatives.

1.4.3 Educational Trends and Opportunities

Emerging educational trends and innovations also create new challenges – and opportunities – for faculty members. On the one hand, we are experiencing a changing student body, marked by increased diversity and high expectations, and greater calls for institutional accountability (Dankoski et al. 2012). On the other hand, we are exploring new (and renewed) educational frameworks (e.g. competency-based education; interprofessional education and practice), alternative venues for learning (e.g. community-based education), and novel pedagogical methods (e.g. simulation and other advanced technologies). All of these developments require a different skill set, as do growing demands from regulatory bodies (as described above). The globalization of health care, as described by Friedman et al. (Chap. 15), also poses new opportunities, and it is in this context that educational leaders and faculty developers must remain responsive and flexible, helping faculty members to balance competing demands and priorities.

1.4.4   The Role of Context

As is evident in this section, no discussion of faculty development would be complete without addressing the role of the environment in which faculty members learn and practice. The context in which faculty members work, and the institutional norms and policies that reward and regulate their behavior, clearly influence their professional growth (Lieff 2010). For example, some health professions schools and organizations provide professional development opportunities and encourage experimentation with new ideas. Others may discourage such behaviors and may not lend administrative support to innovation and scholarship. It is surprising how little has been written about the role of context – and the institutional environment – in reports on faculty development. However, as highlighted by Silver (Chap. 16), faculty developers must be sensitive to institutional and environmental needs and priorities, especially as they will influence the form and focus of various programs and activities. The culture in which faculty development occurs must also be recognized and acknowledged, and we must remain cognizant of the fact that what we do is shaped by the cultures in which we work.

1.5   The Scope of Faculty Development

As stated earlier, faculty development can promote change at the individual and organizational level. Moreover, although faculty development initiatives tend to primarily focus on teaching and instructional effectiveness (Steinert et al. 2006), there is a critical need for these activities to address *all* faculty members' roles, including that of leader and manager and research and scholar (Steinert 2011). Faculty development's role in career development and organizational change can also not be ignored, and each of these areas will be discussed in Part II.

1.5.1 Teaching Effectiveness

As outlined by Hodgson and Wilkerson (Chap. 2), the birth of faculty development can be traced to early efforts to enhance instructional effectiveness in higher education and the health professions. In fact, the desire 'to teach teachers to teach' has been at the root of this movement, which came to the fore in the early 1990's. Activities and programs in this area have been designed for all health professionals teaching in the university, the hospital, and the community setting, at undergraduate, graduate, and postgraduate levels of education. Common areas of focus have included large and small group instruction, feedback and assessment, and enhanced teaching and learning in the clinical setting. More recently, specific content areas (e.g. alcoholism and substance abuse; medical errors) have become part of the faculty development agenda (Skeff et al. 2007). Surprisingly, however, the majority of faculty development programs have not grounded their work in a theoretical (or conceptual) framework (Steinert 2011) or framed their initiatives around expected outcomes or competencies for teachers. However, Hodgson and Wilkerson (Chap. 2) do just that, situating the literature on faculty development for teaching improvement in the context of the Academy of Medical Educators' (2012) professional standards. Irrespective of whether we adopt this teaching framework, or those of other colleagues (e.g. Milner et al. 2011; Molenaar et al. 2009; Srinivasan et al. 2011), it remains important to have a working blueprint. As Purcell and Lloyd-Jones (2003) have observed, in many countries 'there is a plethora of teacher training programmes for medical teachers. But what is good medical teaching? Unless we know what it is, how can we develop it?' (p. 149). Outcomes-based education for faculty members seems as important as it is for students at all levels of training, as long as we attend to personal goals, priorities, and passions.

1.5.2 Leadership Development

As mentioned previously, health care delivery, clinical practice, and medical education are all in a state of flux. To deal with the rapid changes and shifting paradigms that are occurring in all three domains, health professionals need to demonstrate diverse – and effective – leadership and management skills. As Swanwick and McKimm (Chap. 3) highlight, 'effective leadership is considered a pre-requisite for the delivery of high quality health care and professional practice'. Leadership development can also be a critical factor in assuring educational innovation and excellence, scholarly output, and a successful research career. Although the possibilities are vast (Steinert et al. 2012), faculty development initiatives addressing leadership and management can address a number of topics, including personal and interpersonal effectiveness, leadership styles and change management, conflict resolution and negotiation, team building and collaboration, and organizational change and development. To date, the faculty development literature has primarily focused on educational leadership (Spencer and Jordan 2001). However, we need to think more broadly and equip ourselves and our colleagues with leadership capabilities that will enable us to cope with complexity and change at multiple levels (Steinert 2011).

1.5.3 Research and Scholarship

Frontera et al. (2006) have stated that, 'the advancement of medical science depends on the production, availability and use of new information generated by research' (p. 70). As these colleagues suggest, 'a successful research enterprise not only depends on a carefully designed agenda that responds to clinical and societal needs but also on the research capacity necessary to perform the work' (Frontera et al. 2006, p. 70). Faculty development has a critical role to play in developing research capacity, as outlined by Hodges (Chap. 4). We therefore need to ask ourselves to what extent we are preparing health professionals to be scholarly. Boyer (1990) identified four categories of scholarship: the scholarship of discovery; the scholarship of integration; the scholarship of application; and the scholarship of teaching. Although many faculty members will agree that the promotion of scholarship is an important aspect of the professional development of health professionals, this area has not been fully developed. Programs designed to promote scholarship can focus on definitions of scholarship, ways of promoting scholarship among colleagues and peers, methods of disseminating scholarly work, and 'moving from innovation to scholarship' (Steinert 2011). Programs designed to build research capacity can focus on asking good research questions, developing knowledge or skills in a focal area (e.g. developing a research team; grantsmanship), understanding principles of research design, data collection and analysis, and academic writing (Hodges Chap. 4). In addition, a wide range of modalities, including workshops or other modular programs, longitudinal programs and graduate degrees, can achieve these objectives.

1.5.4 Career Development

The academic environment is increasingly complex. As Leslie (Chap. 5) points out, faculty development for academic and career development includes the:

> … explicit provision of guidance, learning opportunities and resources that enable individuals to reflect on their careers and those of others, to identify goals and required resources, to implement appropriate plans and activities and to assess the processes and outcomes of their work. The goal is for faculty to experience success and fulfillment within their contexts and cultures of practice.

Other authors have described faculty development as an 'organized, goal-directed process to achieve career progression and growth' (Hamilton and Brown 2003, p. 1334). From this perspective, faculty development represents a conscious effort to help faculty members succeed in their career path, often (but not exclusively) in the academic setting (Duda 2004; Hamilton and Brown 2003). Faculty development for career development can address a wide range of topics, including the alignment of values between individuals and their organizations, the processes, structures, and resources within institutions that relate to academic roles and responsibilities, and career planning. It can also consist of formal programs (including workshops and seminars), informal approaches (including coaching and mentoring), or the provision of materials and resources that can guide and advance career development. It is surprising that faculty development programs to support career development have not been more frequently described, especially in light of Kanter's (2011) view that career progression can be seen as an overarching framework for faculty development.

1.5.5 Organizational Change

As stated earlier, faculty development can play an important role in promoting organizational change and development. For example, faculty development can promote a culture of change by helping to develop institutional policies that support and reward excellence, encourage a re-examination of criteria for academic promotion, recognize innovation and scholarship, and provide learning opportunities and resources for junior and senior faculty members (Steinert 2011). In the educational arena, faculty development can serve as a useful instrument in the promotion of curricular change (e.g. Snell Chap. 13; Steinert et al. 2007), the acknowledgement of excellence in teaching (Brawer et al. 2006), and the overall profile of teaching and learning. It can also help to promote an environment that fosters critical inquiry and play a role in post-change accommodation, adaptation and growth (Jolly Chap. 6). That is, faculty development can help to move organizations into more post-modern frameworks (and demonstrate a greater diversity of institutional goals and structures), promote leadership and management (and encourage team development and role identification), and assist in culture change in the workplace (with an emphasis on professional rewards and incentives). In many ways, it is time for us to capitalize on the benefits of faculty development in producing organizational change and remember that the institution (as well as the individual faculty member) can be the 'client'.

1.6 Approaches to Faculty Development

Health professionals develop their competence as faculty members in a number of ways. For some, this development includes participation in formal workshops or courses; for others, learning occurs in informal ways, often through role modeling and practical experiences in the work place. Figure 1.1 illustrates this perspective on

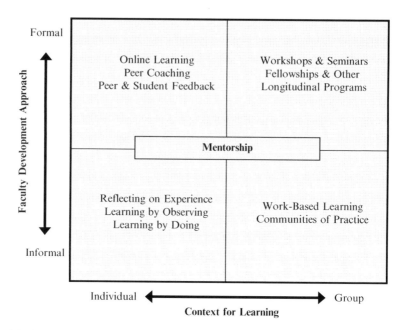

Fig. 1.1 Approaches to faculty development (This figure was originally prepared for a chapter on 'Becoming a Better Teacher: From Intuition to Intent' (Steinert 2010a); it also appeared in *Medical Teacher* (Steinert 2010c) and *Academic Medicine* (Steinert 2011). Re-printed with permission by the American College of Physicians © 2010)

faculty development and provides a pictorial description of how faculty development can move along two dimensions: from individual (independent) experiences to group (collective) learning, and from informal approaches to more formal ones (Steinert 2010a, c). Individual approaches to faculty development include: learning from experience, which includes learning by doing, by observing, and by reflecting on experience; learning from peers and students (at all levels of the continuum); and online learning. Group learning includes structured activities such as workshops and seminars, fellowships and other longitudinal programs, as well as workplace learning and learning in a community of practice. As can be noted in Fig. 1.1, mentorship (which can be both formal or informal) has been placed in the center, as any strategy for self-improvement can benefit from the support and challenge that an effective mentor can provide (Steinert 2010a). These, and other approaches to faculty development, are described in Part III.

1.6.1 Learning from Experience

Health professionals often become adept at what they do by the 'nature of their responsibilities' and 'learning on the job' (Steinert 2010b; Chap. 7). Although most of the published literature in the health professions focuses on formal (structured) faculty development activities (Steinert et al. 2006), informal learning, often in the workplace, is equally important. This form of learning, which incorporates role modeling, reflection, and learning from peers, can also lead to a community of practice (Wenger 1998). O'Sullivan and Irby (Chap. 18) consider the role of work-based learning and communities of practice in proposing new ways to investigate the effectiveness of faculty development programs and activities. Clearly, these approaches to learning should be considered in the design and delivery of faculty development activities, for learning at work is critical in the development of all health professionals. We should also strive to render this learning as visible as possible so that it can become recognized as a legitimate form of professional development.

1.6.2 Peer Coaching and Mentorship

Peer coaching and mentorship are two additionally powerful approaches in the development of faculty members. As Boillat and Elizov (Chap. 8) describe, they are both highly personalized, learner-centered approaches that require a safe environment, mutual trust and collegiality, and reflection. Peer coaching has particular appeal in the health professions because it can occur in the practice setting and fosters collaboration (Steinert 2009). Mentorship builds on these same principles and is often used to facilitate the socialization and career development of faculty members. Given the ability of mentors to provide guidance, support, direction, and expertise, it is surprising that this approach to faculty development has not been described more frequently (Morzinski et al. 1996).

1.6.3 Workshops and Seminars

Workshops and seminars (or short series of seminars) are popular because of their inherent flexibility and provision of active learning. Moreover, although they are most commonly used to promote skill acquisition related to educational roles and responsibilities, they can be equally effective for leadership development and research capacity building. As outlined by de Grave et al. (Chap. 9), the challenge in using this approach to faculty development is articulating the principles underlying their design, incorporating theories of learning into their construction, and integrating strategies to promote transfer to the workplace. Varying in duration, content, and instructional methods, workshops and seminars represent an important aspect of modular learning that can be incorporated into other approaches such as fellowships and other longitudinal programs.

1.6.4 Intensive Longitudinal Programs

Fellowships and other longitudinal programs, which vary in length, format, and emphasis, are most frequently used to develop educational skills (in teaching, assessment, and curriculum design), leadership, and scholarship. However, this format is also effective in developing more generic leadership and research skills. As Gruppen (Chap. 10) points out, intensive longitudinal programs are not just an investment in individual faculty members; they are an investment in the health of the institution. These programs, which have demonstrated the ability to achieve their educational objectives, promote educational leadership and scholarly productivity, and build a sense of community, have been seen as a critical factor in buttressing education as a scientific discipline. Other approaches that complement longitudinal programs include certificate programs and advanced degrees (Hodges Chap. 6; Tekian and Harris 2012).

1.6.5 Online Learning

An underutilized approach to learning in faculty development is online learning. Although interaction and social networks are highly valued by faculty members, faculty development online offers a number of benefits that should not be overlooked. As Cook (Chap. 11) suggests, online learning enables flexible access and opportunities for individualized learning, assessment and feedback, and when blended with more traditional approaches, can capitalize on the strengths of both. Online learning can also be accomplished in a variety of ways (e.g. through online tutorials, computer-supported collaborative learning or computer simulations), and keys to success (beyond adherence to fundamental principles of instructional design and use of multi-media) include focusing on a perceived need, careful planning, clear communication, and creating a sense of community.

   In considering the different approaches to faculty development outlined in this book, it is important to remember that faculty development can provide health professionals with knowledge and skills about teaching and learning, leadership and management, research and scholarship, and career development. Faculty development can also be a powerful tool in developing a community of practice, at the same time as a community of practice can lead to the growth and development of faculty members (Steinert et al. 2010a).

1.7 Re-conceptualizing Faculty Development

In an interesting study of teachers' professional growth, Clarke and Hollingsworth (2002) observed that 'models of teacher professional development have not matched the complexity of the process we seek to promote' (p. 947). This observation can apply equally to faculty development in the health professions, as most of the literature has described formal programs and activities, continuing to reinforce an event-based approach to faculty development when, in fact, we know that much of our development occurs in informal (and unstructured) ways. As Clarke and Hollingsworth (2002) have noted, it is time to shift our focus 'from earlier conceptions of change as something that is done to teachers ... to change as a complex process that involves learning' (p. 948). A similar sentiment has been expressed by Webster-Wright (2009), who argues for a reconceptualization of professional development that moves us away from learning that occurs in 'discrete, finite episodes' to a focus on continuous and authentic professional learning. More specifically, she suggests that we move towards the notion of *promoting learning* that occurs in authentic contexts rather than the *development* of colleagues, which in many ways implies a deficit model, reinforces the notion that we 'do something to' our colleagues, and ignores a critical venue for skill acquisition.

In further describing the process of 'teacher change', Clarke and Hollingsworth (1994, p. 948) identify six inter-related perspectives on how teachers change, all of which could apply to the professional growth of faculty members in the health professions. These interrelated perspectives include:

- Change as training – i.e. change is something that is done to teachers…
- Change as adaptation – i.e. teachers change (or adapt) in response to changed conditions…
- Change as personal development – i.e. teachers seek to change in an attempt to improve performance or develop new skills.
- Change as local reform – i.e. teachers change something for reasons of personal growth.
- Change as systemic restructuring – i.e. teachers enact the change policies of the system.
- Change as growth or learning – i.e. teachers change through professional activity.

Interestingly, the current view of faculty development activities in the health professions seems to align primarily with the notion of change as 'training' and 'personal development'. However, the other perspectives highlighted above should be examined and considered in the design and delivery of faculty development in the health professions.

This discussion also brings to the fore the importance of using theoretical frameworks in faculty development. Silver (Chap. 16) summarizes a number of conceptual approaches that can be used in the design and delivery of faculty development programs, including principles of adult learning, self-directed learning, and reflective practice. Sociocultural and constructivist theories are also described (Cobb and Yackel 1996; Rogoff 1990; Steffe and Gale 1995). Central to this perspective is the view that individuals construct knowledge and meaning through their experiences and interaction with others. In many ways, this frame, and that of situated learning (Brown et al. 1989; McLellan 1996), which views learning as a socially mediated and constructive process, is particularly helpful in understanding the process of faculty development. Situated learning is based on the notion that knowledge is *contextually situated* and fundamentally influenced by the *activity*, *context*, and *culture* in which it is used (Brown et al. 1989). This view of knowledge has important implications for our understanding of faculty development and the design and delivery of instructional activities for faculty members. Some of the key components of situated learning include: cognitive apprenticeship, collaborative learning, reflection, practice, and articulation of learning skills (McLellan 1996), elements that will be discussed further in Chap. 7.

1.8   Practical Applications That Respond to Educational and Health Care Priorities

As stated earlier, faculty development must address educational and health care needs in order to remain relevant and responsive. Faculty development also has a significant role to play in many spheres, including change at the level of the individual (e.g. increased awareness and explicit modeling of appropriate behaviors), the curriculum (e.g. the teaching and assessment of core competencies), clinical practice (e.g. interprofessional education and practice), and international collaboration. Part IV addresses each of these areas as well as the critical question of how to start a faculty development program.

1.8.1   Promoting Role Modeling and Reflective Practice

Role modeling and reflective practice have been increasingly recognized as important elements in teaching and learning (Kenny et al. 2003; Schön 1983). Although both elements are equally important in all faculty roles, the literature to date has primarily focused on their importance in the educational realm. As Mann (Chap. 12) suggests, faculty development for role modeling necessitates an awareness of the power of this teaching and learning strategy, attention to personal and professional behaviors, and a focus on the environment in which professional practice unfolds. Reflective practice is closely tied to role modeling and incorporates the ability to think critically about what we do. It is encouraging to know that reflective skills can be learned, that reflective practice can take many forms, and that increased reflection enhances role modeling in all faculty roles (Mann Chap. 12). It is also not surprising that brief, one-time interventions are unlikely to significantly influence role modeling or reflective practice. However, both formal and informal approaches that promote authentic and meaningful learning can promote change.

1.8.2   Enhancing Curriculum Change

Faculty development can both support and drive curricular change and renewal, and in fact, the two processes are inextricably linked. As Snell (Chap. 13) points out, faculty development has a critical role to play in promoting buy-in, addressing resistance to change, enabling knowledge acquisition and skill development, and attending to the organizational culture in which curricula unfold. Faculty development for educational leadership and management, educational scholarship, and outcomes evaluation is also needed. Problem-based learning and competency-based education are examples of curricular initiatives that require faculty development to ensure that faculty members are prepared to lead educational reform. These experiences also demonstrate that different approaches to professional development can help faculty members to master new content areas as well as methods of teaching and assessment.

1.8.3   Advancing Interprofessional Education and Practice

Anderson et al. (Chap. 14) state that interprofessional education and practice is a response to specific changes in health care delivery that aim to promote integrated, patient-centered care. Moreover, as these authors suggest, the development of interprofessional curricula (which aim to foster interprofessional practice) face a number of significant challenges: the crossing of professional boundaries; integrating interprofessional curricula into each profession's existing curricula; paying attention to the theoretical rigor and evidence base of interprofessional education; and recognizing the fact that interprofessional learning is complex and different (Anderson et al. Chap. 14). For faculty development to be effective in this arena, formal approaches must address existing barriers to teaching and learning, at both the individual and organizational level, and prepare faculty members to design and facilitate interprofessional experiences in both the classroom and the clinical environment.

1.8.4   Creating International Faculty Development Partnerships

The need to extend beyond national borders in faculty development is increasingly apparent in the health professions. In fact, as Friedman et al. (Chap. 15) demonstrate, international faculty development partnerships arise in response to a range of needs and opportunities, including issues related to health care priorities, educational imperatives, and the professional development of faculty members globally. As these authors illustrate, international partnerships differ in structure and purpose as well as the degree of organizational independence and interdependence. However, different models can achieve similar goals, and the benefits of these relationships can be experienced at many levels, including that of the individual, the institution, and the system at large. The relationship itself can also be a source of pride and accomplishment, leading to new initiatives and collaborations (Friedman et al. Chap. 15). Well-functioning partnerships allow for exposure to methods, materials, opportunities, and networks that may not otherwise be available, and cultural bridging, effective communication, and mutual goal-setting are critical ingredients for sustainability.

1.8.5 Starting a Faculty Development Program

The design and development of a faculty development program is no easy feat. Moreover, once the challenge to undertake such an enterprise is accepted, it involves a number of steps, as outlined by Silver (Chap. 16): understanding the institutional and organizational culture; developing a change strategy; forming a guiding coalition; conducting an environmental scan; establishing the vision and values of the program; and defining clear goals and objectives. Determining the faculty development curriculum and method of delivery, based on available evidence and pertinent conceptual frameworks, forms the next important step, to be followed by the development of an evaluation rubric as well as a plan for sustainability. The old adage that 'one size does not fit all' must also be remembered in this context, as each setting and culture will determine its own pathway to success.

1.9 Faculty Development Research, Scholarship and Knowledge Translation

Research, scholarship, and knowledge translation are vitally important in moving the field of faculty development forward. Although each chapter in this book is based on the current literature and available evidence, we need to continue to expand the research base in this area by systematically evaluating our diverse programs and activities, assessing outcomes at multiple levels, and examining how faculty members develop. We must also ensure that research informs practice – and that practice informs research – as highlighted in Part V.

1.9.1 The 'State of the Art'

Research on the impact of faculty development activities designed to improve teaching effectiveness has shown that overall satisfaction with programs is high and that participants recommend these activities to colleagues (Steinert et al. 2006). More specifically, health professionals report a positive change in attitudes towards teaching as well as self-reported changes in knowledge about educational principles and specific teaching behaviors. Other benefits include increased personal interest and enthusiasm, improved self-confidence, a greater sense of belonging to a community, and educational leadership and innovation. In a more recent review of faculty development initiatives designed to enhance leadership (Steinert et al. 2012), very similar results were found. Participants reported a positive change in attitudes toward their own organizations, leadership abilities and leadership roles, positive gains in knowledge and skill related to leadership concepts, principles and strategies, and changes in leadership behavior, including new roles and responsibilities.

In examining these and other systematic reviews of faculty development in higher education (Amundsen and Wilson 2012; Stes et al. 2010), Spencer (Chap. 17) concludes that although we have a preliminary understanding that faculty development 'works', we still need to understand 'how and why change occurs'. In addition, despite numerous program descriptions, few programs have conducted rigorous evaluations to ascertain what effect the program is having on faculty members, and conclusive data to support the efficacy of these initiatives, on both the individual and the organization, have been lacking. Of the studies that have been conducted in this area, most have relied on the assessment of participant satisfaction; some have evaluated changes in cognitive learning or performance, whereas others have examined the long-term impact of these interventions. However, most research studies have relied on self-report rather than objective outcome measures or observations of change. There is clearly a need for more rigorous research designs and a greater use of qualitative and mixed methods to capture the complexity of faculty development interventions. The use of newer methods of performance-based assessment, incorporating diverse data sources, as well as process-oriented studies comparing different faculty development strategies and the maintenance of change over time, is also needed (Spencer Chap. 17; Steinert et al. 2006).

1.9.2   Research Paradigms and Methodologies

Building on the available evidence, O'Sullivan and Irby (Chap. 18) suggest that this area of scholarship has been over-reliant on a positivist research paradigm and recommend a consideration of post-positivist, interpretivist, and critical theory paradigms. These authors also propose the use of alternative research methods, including design research (Collins et al. 2004), success cases (Brinkerhoff and Dressler 2003), and sustainability narratives (Swart et al. 2004). Each of these methods can provide new insights into the process and value of faculty development. O'Sullivan and Irby (2011, Chap. 18) also put forth a new conceptual framework for conducting faculty development research, locating faculty development within two separate but related communities: (1) the faculty development community and (2) the community of teaching practice in the workplace. As the authors suggest, the faculty development community refers to the real and virtual environments where faculty members discuss their concerns and challenges as educators, and learn new roles and skills; the second community is situated in the workplace, be it in the classroom or the clinical setting, where teaching, research or leadership takes place. For the faculty development community, four key elements include: the participants; the faculty development program; the facilitator; and the context in which the program occurs. For the workplace community, there are four additional components: the relationships and networks of associations that participants have with colleagues and learners; the educational tasks and activities that must be completed in the work setting; the mentoring that is available to help accomplish specific goals and objectives; and the organization and culture of the workplace. Given the social nature of faculty development (D'Eon et al. 2000) and an increasing emphasis on communities of practice (Wenger 1998), we believe that this conceptual framework offers a rich menu of possibilities to advance scholarship in the field.

1.9.3   Knowledge Translation and Faculty Development

The creation of knowledge – and the transfer of knowledge to practice – remains a challenge for faculty development. As a result, Part V concludes with a discussion of knowledge translation and its applications to faculty development. Knowledge translation has been defined as an iterative, interdisciplinary process used to move knowledge into practice, primarily in the clinical setting (Graham et al. 2006). However, as Thomas and Steinert (Chap. 19) postulate, the implications of knowledge translation for faculty development can include a number of options:

> ... (1) basing faculty development programs on the best available knowledge and/or scientific evidence; (2) using educational and other knowledge translation strategies that are known to be effective; (3) recognizing that, in the absence of scientific evidence to support faculty development activities or when scientific knowledge is not congruent with existing practices or values, alternative sources of knowledge are needed; and (4) conceptualizing faculty development activities as knowledge translation interventions in their own right.

It is hoped that applying a lens of knowledge translation to faculty development will help to accomplish two objectives: a more systematic use of evidence in the design, delivery, and evaluation of both formal and informal approaches to faculty development, and a more concerted effort in creating new knowledge in the field.

1.10   Conclusion

The chapters in this book represent the work of a scholarly community of international health professions educators, leaders, and researchers. They also portray the scope, diversity of approaches, practical applications, and research opportunities that this aspect of professional development encompasses.

The discussions in this book touch on a number of themes that will need greater attention in the future. For example, although this book is entitled *Faculty Development in the Health Professions*, the majority of examples are drawn from medicine due to the current 'state of the art'. Moreover, although there is a growing consensus that faculty development is meant to target *all* faculty roles, most of the literature to date focuses on faculty development for educational improvement, often in an academic setting. Shifting our focus to include faculty members as leaders and managers and researchers and scholars, and conceptualizing the breadth of faculty development outside of the academic milieu, remains a challenge. So does the recommendation that we re-orient our emphasis from faculty *development* to faculty *learning*. Part VI summarizes future directions for faculty development, based on what has been presented in the preceding pages.

Faculty vitality has been defined as 'those essential, yet intangible positive qualities of individuals and institutions that enable purposeful production' (Clark et al. 1985, p. 3). The goal of faculty development is to nurture, promote, and reinforce the vitality of faculty members and the institutions in which they work (within and outside the academic setting), so that we can facilitate the development of future health professionals and, ultimately, improve patient care.

1.11 Key Messages

- Faculty development includes both formal and informal activities that address the multiple roles and responsibilities of faculty members in a variety of settings.
- Faculty development has a role to play in nurturing and sustaining health professionals as teachers and educators, leaders and managers, and researchers and scholars. It can also help to enhance academic and career development as well as organizational change.
- Common approaches to faculty development include experiential learning in the workplace, peer coaching and mentoring, workshops and seminars, longitudinal programs, and online learning.
- Practical applications of faculty development can include change at the level of the individual (e.g. role modeling and reflective practice), the curriculum, clinical practice (e.g. interprofessional education and practice), and international collaboration.
- Research, scholarship, and knowledge translation are needed to move the field of faculty development forward in the health professions.

References

Academy of Medical Educators. (2012). *Professional standards*. London, UK: Academy of Medical Educators. Available from: http://www.medicaleducators.org/index.cfm/linkservid/180C46A6-B0E9-B09B-02599E43F9C2FDA9/showMeta/0/

Adkoli, B. V., Gupta, V., Sood, R., & Pandav, C. S. (2009). From reorientation of medical education to development of medical educators. *Indian Journal of Public Health, 53*(4), 218–222.

Alteen, A. M., Didham, P., & Stratton, C. (2009). Reflecting, refueling, and reframing: A 10-year retrospective model for faculty development and its implications for nursing scholarship. *The Journal of Continuing Education in Nursing, 40*(6), 267–272.

Amundsen, C., & Wilson, M. (2012). Are we asking the right questions? A conceptual review of the educational development literature in higher education. *Review of Educational Research, 82*(1), 90–126.

Anshu, Sharma, M., Burdick, W. P., & Singh, T. (2010). Group dynamics and social interaction in a South Asian online learning forum for faculty development of medical teachers. *Education for Health, 23*(1), 311.

Bland, C. J., Schmitz, C., Stritter, F., Henry, R., & Aluise, J. (1990). *Successful faculty in academic medicine: Essential skills and how to acquire them.* New York, NY: Springer Publishing.

Bligh, J. (2005). Faculty development. *Medical Education, 39*(2), 120–121.

Boyer, E. L. (1990). *Scholarship reconsidered: Priorities of the professoriate.* Princeton, NJ: Carnegie Foundation.

Brawer, J., Steinert, Y., St-Cyr, J., Watters, K., & Wood-Dauphinee, S. (2006). The significance and impact of a faculty teaching award: Disparate perceptions of department chairs and award recipients. *Medical Teacher, 28*(7), 614–617.

Brinkerhoff, R. O., & Dressler, D. E. (2003). *Using the success case impact evaluation method to enhance training value & impact.* San Diego, CA: American Society for Training and Development International Conference and Exhibition.

Brown, J. S., Collins, A., & Duguid, P. (1989). Situated cognition and the culture of learning. *Educational Researcher, 18*(1), 32–42.

Centra, J. A. (1978). Types of faculty development programs. *Journal of Higher Education, 49*(2), 151–162.

Clark, S. M., Boyer, C. M., & Corcoran, M. (1985). Faculty and institutional vitality. In S. M. Clark & D. R. Lewis (Eds.), *Faculty vitality and institutional productivity: Critical perspectives for higher education* (pp. 3–24). New York, NY: Teachers College Press.

Clarke, D., & Hollingsworth, H. (1994). Reconceptualising teacher change. In G. Bell, B. Wright, N. Leeson, & J. Geake (Eds.), *Challenges in mathematics education: Constraints on construction: Vol. 1. Proceedings of the 17th annual conference of the Mathematics Education Research Group of Australasia* (pp. 153–164). Lismore, NSW: Southern Cross University.

Clarke, D., & Hollingsworth, H. (2002). Elaborating a model of teacher professional growth. *Teaching and Teacher Education, 18*(8), 947–967.

Cobb, P., & Yackel, E. (1996). Constructivist, emergent, and sociocultural perspectives in the context of developmental research. *Educational Psychologist, 31*(3/4), 175–190.

Collins, A., Joseph, D., & Bielaczyc, K. (2004). Design research: Theoretical and methodological issues. *Journal of the Learning Sciences, 13*(1), 15–42.

Cornes, D., & Mokoena, J. D. (2004). Capacity building: The enhancement of leadership and scholarship skills for nurse educators in South Africa. *Nursing Update, 28*(3), 32–33.

Dankoski, M. E., Palmer, M. M., Nelson Laird, T. F., Ribera, A. K., & Bogdewic, S. P. (2012). An expanded model of faculty vitality in academic medicine. *Advances in Health Sciences Education, 17*(5), 633–649.

D'Eon, M., Overgaard, V., & Harding, S. R. (2000). Teaching as a social practice: Implications for faculty development. *Advances in Health Sciences Education, 5*(2), 151–162.

Duda, R. B. (2004). Faculty development programs promote the academic advancement of the faculty. *Current Surgery, 61*(1), 93–95.

Eitel, F., Kanz, K. G., & Tesche, A. (2000). Training and certification of teachers and trainers: The professionalization of medical education. *Medical Teacher, 22*(5), 517–526.

Frontera, W. R., Fuhrer, M. J., Jette, A. M., Chan, L., Cooper, R. A., Duncan, P. W., et al. (2006). Rehabilitation medicine summit: Building research capacity. *Journal of Spinal Cord Medicine, 29*(1), 70–81.

General Medical Council. (2006). *Good medical practice.* Retrieved November 18, 2011, from http://www.gmc-uk.org

Graham, I. D., Logan, J., Harrison, M. B., Straus, S. E., Tetroe, J., Caswell, W., et al. (2006). Lost in knowledge translation: Time for a map? *Journal of Continuing Education in the Health Professions, 26*(1), 13–24.

Gruppen, L. D., Simpson, D., Searle, N. S., Robins, L., Irby, D. M., & Mullan, P. B. (2006). Educational fellowship programs: Common themes and overarching issues. *Academic Medicine, 81*(11), 990–994.

Hafferty, F. W. (1998). Beyond curriculum reform: Confronting medicine's hidden curriculum. *Academic Medicine, 73*(4), 403–407.

Hamilton, G. C., & Brown, J. E. (2003). Faculty development: What is faculty development? *Academic Emergency Medicine, 10*(12), 1334–1336.

Hendricson, W. D., Anderson, E., Andrieu, S. C., Chadwick, D. G., Cole, J. R., George, M. C., et al. (2007). Does faculty development enhance teaching effectiveness? *Journal of Dental Education, 71*(12), 1513–1533.

Hueppchen, N., Dalrymple, J. L., Hammoud, M. M., Abbott, J. F., Casey, P. M., Chuang, A. W., et al. (2011). To the point: Medical education reviews – Ongoing call for faculty development. *American Journal of Obstetrics and Gynecology, 205*(3), 171–176.

Kanter, S. L. (2011). Faculty career progression. *Academic Medicine, 86*(8), 919.

Kenny, N. P., Mann, K. V., & MacLeod, H. (2003). Role-modeling in physicians' professional formation: Reconsidering an essential but untapped educational strategy. *Academic Medicine, 78*(12), 1203–1210.

Liaison Committee on Medical Education. (2012). *Functions and structure of a medical school: Standards for accreditation of medical education programs leading to the M.D. degree.* Available from: http://www.lcme.org/publications/functions2012may.pdf

Lieff, S. J. (2010). Faculty development: Yesterday, today and tomorrow: Guide supplement 33.2 – Viewpoint. *Medical Teacher, 32*(5), 429–431.

Mamede, S., & Schmidt, H. G. (2004). The structure of reflective practice in medicine. *Medical Education, 38*(12), 1302–1308.

McLean, M., Cilliers, F., & Van Wyk, J. M. (2008). Faculty development: Yesterday, today and tomorrow. *Medical Teacher, 30*(6), 555–584.

McLellan, H. (1996). *Situated learning perspectives.* Englewood Cliffs, NJ: Educational Technology.

McNamara, A., Roat, C., & Kemper, M. (2012). Preparing nurses for the new world order: A faculty development focus. *Nursing Administration Quarterly, 36*(3), 253–259.

Milner, R. J., Gusic, M. E., & Thorndyke, L. E. (2011). Perspective: Toward a competency framework for faculty. *Academic Medicine, 86*(10), 1204–1210.

Mitcham, M. D., Lancaster, C. J., & Stone, B. M. (2002). Evaluating the effectiveness of occupational therapy faculty development workshops. *American Journal of Occupational Therapy, 56*(3), 335–339.

Molenaar, W. M., Zanting, A., van Beukelen, P., de Grave, W., Baane, J. A., Bustraan, J. A., et al. (2009). A framework of teaching competencies across the medical education continuum. *Medical Teacher, 31*(5), 390–396.

Morzinski, J. A., Diehr, S., Bower, D. J., & Simpson, D. E. (1996). A descriptive, cross-sectional study of formal mentoring for faculty. *Family Medicine, 28*(6), 434–438.

Nora, L. M. (2010). The 21st century faculty member in the educational process – What should be on the horizon? *Academic Medicine, 85*(9 Suppl.), S45–S55.

O'Sullivan, P. S., & Irby, D. M. (2011). Reframing research on faculty development. *Academic Medicine, 86*(4), 421–428.

Purcell, N., & Lloyd-Jones, G. (2003). Standards for medical educators. *Medical Education, 37*(2), 149–154.

Rogoff, B. (1990). *Apprenticeship in thinking: Cognitive development in social context.* New York, NY: Oxford University Press.

Rothman, J., & Rinehart, M. E. (1990). A profile of faculty development in physical therapy education programs. *Physical Therapy, 70*(5), 310–313.

Royal College of Physicians and Surgeons of Canada. (2011). *A continuing commitment to lifelong learning: A concise guide to maintenance of certification.* Retrieved August, 2012, from http://www.royalcollege.ca/portal/page/portal/rc/common/documents/moc_program/moc_short_guide_e.pdf

Schofield, S. J., Bradley, S., Macrae, C., Nathwani, D., & Dent, J. (2010). How we encourage faculty development. *Medical Teacher, 32*(11), 883–886.

Schön, D. A. (1983). *The reflective practitioner: How professionals think in action.* New York, NY: Basic Books.

Scudder, R., Self, T., & Cohen, P. A. (2010). The leadership academy: A new approach for changing times in communication sciences and disorders programs. *Perspectives on Issues in Higher Education, 13*(1), 32–37.

Sheets, K. J., & Schwenk, T. L. (1990). Faculty development for family medicine educators: An agenda for future activities. *Teaching and Learning in Medicine, 2*(3), 141–148.

Skeff, K. M., Stratos, G. A., & Mount, J. F. S. (2007). Faculty development in medicine: A field in evolution. *Teaching and Teacher Education, 23*(3), 280–285.

Spencer, J., & Jordan, R. (2001). Educational outcome and leadership to meet the needs of modern health care. *Quality in Health Care, 10*(Suppl 2), ii38–ii45.

Srinivasan, M., Li, S. T., Meyers, F. J., Pratt, D. D., Collins, J. B., Braddock, C., et al. (2011). 'Teaching as a competency': Competencies for medical educators. *Academic Medicine, 86*(10), 1211–1220.

Steffe, L. P., & Gale, J. (Eds.). (1995). *Constructivism in education.* Mahwah, NJ: Lawrence Erlbaum.

Steinert, Y. (2009). Staff development. In J. A. Dent & R. M. Harden (Eds.), *A practical guide for medical teachers* (3rd ed. pp. 391–397). Edinburgh, UK: Elsevier Churchill Livingstone.

Steinert, Y. (2010a). Becoming a better teacher: From intuition to intent. In J. Ende (Ed.), *Theory and practice of teaching medicine* (pp. 73–93). Philadelphia, PA: American College of Physicians.

Steinert, Y. (2010b). Developing medical educators: A journey not a destination. In T. Swanwick (Ed.), *Understanding medical education: Evidence, theory and practice* (pp. 403–418). Edinburgh, UK: Association for the Study of Medical Education.

Steinert, Y. (2010c). Faculty development: From workshops to communities of practice. *Medical Teacher, 32*(5), 425–428.

Steinert, Y. (2011). Commentary: Faculty development: The road less traveled. *Academic Medicine, 86*(4), 409–411.

Steinert, Y. (2012). Perspectives on faculty development: Aiming for 6/6 by 2020. *Perspectives on Medical Education, 1*(1), 31–42.

Steinert, Y., Mann, K., Centeno, A., Dolmans, D., Spencer, J., Gelula, M., et al. (2006). A systematic review of faculty development initiatives designed to improve teaching effectiveness in medical education: BEME Guide No. 8. *Medical Teacher, 28*(6), 497–526.

Steinert, Y., Cruess, R. L., Cruess, S. R., Boudreau, J. D., & Fuks, A. (2007). Faculty development as an instrument of change: A case study on teaching professionalism. *Academic Medicine, 82*(11), 1057–1064.

Steinert, Y., Boudreau, J. D., Boillat, M., Slapcoff, B., Dawson, D., Briggs, A., et al. (2010a). The Osler Fellowship: An apprenticeship for medical educators. *Academic Medicine, 85*(7), 1242–1249.

Steinert, Y., Macdonald, M. E., Boillat, M., Elizov, M., Meterissian, S., Razack, S., et al. (2010b). Faculty development: If you build it, they will come. *Medical Education, 44*(9), 900–907.

Steinert, Y., Naismith, L., & Mann, K. (2012). Faculty development initiatives designed to promote leadership in medical education. A BEME systematic review: BEME Guide No. 19. *Medical Teacher, 34*(6), 483–503.

Stes, A., Min-Leliveld, M., Gijbels, D., & Van Petegem, P. (2010). The impact of instructional development in higher education: The state-of-the-art of the research. *Educational Research Review, 5*(1), 25–49.

Swanwick, T. (2008). See one, do one, then what? Faculty development in postgraduate medical education. *Postgraduate Medical Journal, 84*(993), 339–343.

Swanwick, T., & McKimm, J. (2010). Professional development of medical educators. *British Journal of Hospital Medicine, 71*(3), 164–168.

Swart, R. J., Raskin, P., & Robinson, J. (2004). The problem of the future: Sustainability science and scenario analysis. *Global Environmental Change, 14*(2), 137–146.

Tekian, A., & Harris, I. (2012). Preparing health professions education leaders worldwide: A description of masters-level programs. *Medical Teacher, 34*(1), 52–58.

Webster-Wright, A. (2009). Reframing professional development through understanding authentic professional learning. *Review of Educational Research, 79*(2), 702–739.

Wenger, E. (1998). *Communities of practice: Learning, meaning, and identity.* New York, NY: Cambridge University Press.

Westberg, J., & Jason, H. (1981). The enhancement of teaching skills in US medical schools: An overview and some recommendations. *Medical Teacher, 3*(3), 100–104.

Whitcomb, M. E. (2003). The medical school's faculty is its most important asset. *Academic Medicine, 78*(2), 117–118.

Wong, J. G., & Agisheva, K. (2007). Developing teaching skills for medical educators in Russia: A cross-cultural faculty development project. *Medical Education, 41*(3), 318–324.

World Federation for Medical Education. (2007). *Global standards programme.* Retrieved December 10, 2012, from http://www.wfme.org

Part II
The Scope of Faculty Development

Chapter 2
Faculty Development for Teaching Improvement

Carol S. Hodgson and LuAnn Wilkerson

2.1   Introduction

Faculty development to improve teaching is the most common type of faculty development activity reported in the health professions literature. Although its North American roots can be traced back to the 1950s, it is now an ongoing activity in medical schools around the world and is growing in importance in other health professions schools. In this chapter, we will consider the emergence of teaching improvement programs in health professions education and then review several competency frameworks, each designed to identify what teachers in the health professions need to know and be able to do in order to promote learning. Several best practice examples demonstrate how these teaching competencies might be developed and illustrate essential features of teaching improvement programs.

2.2   Historical Perspective

The birth of faculty development as a critical tool for improving teaching in the United States has been tracked to the Project in Medical Education. This collaborative venture, funded by the Commonwealth Foundation at the University of Buffalo in 1955 under the collaborative leadership of George Miller, MD, from the School

C.S. Hodgson, Ph.D. (✉)
Faculty of Medicine and Dentistry, Division of Studies in Medical Education,
University of Alberta, Edmonton, AB, Canada
e-mail: carol.hodgson@ualberta.ca

L. Wilkerson, Ed.D.
Center for Educational Development and Research, David Geffen School
of Medicine at University of California Los Angeles, Los Angeles, CA, USA
e-mail: lwilkerson@mednet.ucla.edu

Y. Steinert (ed.), *Faculty Development in the Health Professions: A Focus
on Research and Practice*, Innovation and Change in Professional Education 11,
DOI 10.1007/978-94-007-7612-8_2, © Springer Science+Business Media Dordrecht 2014

of Medicine, and Stephen Abrahamson, PhD, from the School of Education, was focused on bringing the findings of research in education to bear on the design and delivery of teaching in the medical school (Miller 1980). A medical student who joined the Project and completed both an M.D. and an Ed.D. in education, Hilliard Jason (1962), is credited by many as the founder of teaching improvement programs in medical education (Wilkerson and Anderson 2004). A seminal report of the results of a survey of faculty members from medical schools from across the United States published in 1977 indicated that most faculty members felt ill-prepared for their roles as teachers and welcomed opportunities to learn more about how to teach (Association of American Medical Colleges 1977; Jason and Westberg 1982). Through the Association of American Medical Colleges (AAMC), Jason subsequently developed workshops, videos, and reading materials on learning to teach, with a particular emphasis on small group discussion and clinical teaching opportunities.

At this same time in higher education in the United States, the increasing use of student evaluations of teachers led to the emergence of programs to improve the teaching of college and university faculty members (Centra 1976). Similarly, in the Netherlands during the 1970s, the first faculty development programs to improve teaching in higher education began (Metz et al. 1996). Prior to the 1970s, sabbaticals and professional conferences in specific disciplinary fields were the usual approach to the improvement of teaching, reflecting the assumption that content expertise was the critical requirement for university teachers. Stimulated by the work of Allen and his colleagues at the University of Massachusetts in the Clinic to Improve University Teaching, the *Handbook for Faculty Development* by Bergquist and Phillips (1975) and *Toward Faculty Renewal* by Gaff (1975), a focus on the improvement of teaching skills and methods was born (Sorcinelli et al. 2006). The Professional and Organizational Development Network (http://www. podnetwork.org/) was created in 1975 to provide training in and support for faculty development professionals, many of whom were engaged in providing workshops and conducting individual consultations to faculty members interested in teaching improvement.

The focus of teaching improvement programs in higher education has changed as the understanding of how students learn has evolved over the years (Wilkerson and Irby 1998). Behaviorist theories of learning guided the earliest days of teaching improvement programming, creating an emphasis on observable teacher behaviors and discrete teaching skills, often using faculty development approaches such as individual consultation and video-recorded microteaching sessions. For example, typical faculty development sessions addressed setting the objectives of a lecture, asking questions, and responding to students' answers. In the 1980s, a growing interest in cognitive theories of learning was associated with the creation of teaching improvement programs focused on the design of courses and the use of learning methods that stressed students' cognition and information processing, including a growing emphasis on the teacher's ability to translate his or her content expertise in ways to meet the identified needs of learners (Shulman 1986) and the ability to 'reflect in practice,' described by Schön (1987). In the 1990s, concurrent with a growing interest in social constructivist theories of learning, teaching improvement activities included the use of extended seminars and longitudinal workshops in which faculty members would learn from and with one another, using interactive exercises, peer coaching, and the formation of 'learning communities' composed of teachers with common interests and concerns for the purpose of learning from one another. In Great Britain during the 1990s, Peyton (1998) introduced a 'teach-the-teacher' program for clinical teachers using a train-the-trainer model to extend the reach of typical teaching improvement programs to include physicians who teach in the workplace rather than in the academy. All of these types of teaching improvement topics and activities continue to be offered today as part of comprehensive teaching improvement programs in both higher education and health professions education. To this mix, the use of online interactive modules and social media have been added to further increase accessibility of teaching improvement programming.

2.3   A Competency Framework for Teaching

Central to the design of teaching improvement programs is the question of what knowledge, skills, and attitudes are needed by the well-prepared faculty member engaged in health professions education (Irby 1994). Medical education for students and residents depends on the readiness of faculty members to execute their role as teachers. For example, in 2012, at the two medical schools of this chapter's authors, more than 200 new faculty members (primarily clinical) and more than 200 new residents and fellows began teaching trainees. The relatively large number of new faculty and residents entering medical schools each year makes it imperative that we develop a faculty development strategy for training new faculty and residents for their role as teachers in addition to maintaining and updating teacher competencies for our established teachers. What competencies are needed for new faculty members? Once initially prepared, how do we continue to help teachers continue to improve as they progress from instructor to professor? For decades, much has been written about competency-based education for learners in health professions education. Are there competencies we should consider or require of our teachers? A number of competency frameworks have been proposed for educators in higher education and specifically in the health professions that can be used to answer the question of what teachers in the health professions need to know and be able to do.

In 2004, a national quality assurance system for teaching was implemented at all 14 research-intensive universities in the Netherlands (van Keulen 2006). As one example, at Utrecht University both junior and senior teachers are required to document their attainment of a series of qualifications (written as objectives) using a portfolio system. Staff development is offered at Utrecht, but not required as part of the quality assurance system. What is required is evidence of having attained the desired teaching competency. Medical education in the Netherlands followed suit.

Deans at the eight Dutch medical schools joined with the Netherlands Association for Medical Education and formed a taskforce to develop a set of competencies for medical teachers that would constitute a similar teacher qualification system (Molenaar et al. 2009). The taskforce grew to encompass dentistry and veterinary medicine as well. The description of each teaching competency and the overall framework were published online for feedback and discussion by stakeholders nationally.

The resulting framework included six teaching domains that cover the continuum of education with five sub-domains at three teaching levels ('micro,' 'meso,' and 'macro'). The three levels constitute increasing responsibility from (1) 'micro,' the level of the individual teacher, to (2) 'meso,' the faculty member coordinating part of a curriculum, to (3) 'macro' leadership of a course or program. The three levels of the framework ('micro,' 'meso,' and 'macro') allow for assessing faculty members' level of responsibility and providing distinctions between 'teacher' and 'master teacher' and 'educator' and 'master educator' (i.e. teacher vs. educational leader) (Molenaar et al. 2009). The framework, domains, and sub-domains were adopted nationally, but institutions were left to develop specific local descriptors of those teaching domains. This very systematic process, that allowed vetting by all stakeholders at multiple points in time, helped to develop a national climate for buy-in of the process and expectation that teachers across professions would meet a set of core competencies.

Around the same time in the United States, Hand (2006) used a modified Delphi method to query dental schools deans, faculty developers in dentistry, and members of the American Dental Education Association on the competencies needed for dental teachers – both continuing and new. The underlying framework for this set of competencies used the redefinition of teaching as a form of scholarship (Boyer 1990) as its foundation.

In 2009, the Academy of Medical Educators (AoME) in Great Britain established a set of professional standards for clinical and non-clinical medical (i.e. dental, veterinary, and medical) educators (Academy of Medical Educators 2012). The overall goal underpinning the development of the Professional Standards and the educator assessment system was to improve patient-centered care through medical training and practice. A 'key performance target' was to 'assure greater recognition of the central role of medical educators in the delivery of high quality patient care.' (Academy of Medical Educators 2008, p. 5). Members of the Professional Standards Committee consulted a wide range of stakeholders and engaged numerous national organizations in the development of the standards and domains. All of these groups were invited to comment on the proposed standards and more than 100 responses were received. (Academy of Medical Educators 2012).

Central to the AoME Professional Standards are seven core values: (1) professional integrity; (2) educational scholarship; (3) equality of opportunity and diversity; (4) respect for the public; (5) respect for patients; (6) respect for learners; and (7) respect for colleagues. Each medical educator who wishes to apply for membership must first demonstrate a commitment to the core values. Along with these core values are five competency domains central to medical education:

(1) design and planning of learning activities; (2) teaching and support of learners; (3) assessment and feedback to learners; (4) educational research and evidence-based practice; and (5) educational management and leadership (Academy of Medical Educators 2012). Each domain is further broken down into a list of elements and standards (see Appendix A). Just as with the competencies developed in the Netherlands, there are three levels, again very similar to those described by Molenaar et al. (2009). Attainment of the Standards at a particular level provides evidence for membership in the AoME at the level of 'Member' (evidence at levels 1–2) or as a 'Fellow' (evidence at level 3) (Academy of Medical Educators 2012, p. 11). These standards are now part of the United Kingdom's General Medical Council Framework for the Accreditation of Educational Supervisors (Academy of Medical Educators n.d.).

In the United States, several specialties have worked to define teaching competencies relevant to their particular fields. The Alliance for Academic Internal Medicine (AAIM) has put forward a set of skills for internal medicine. Hueppchen et al. (2011) proposed 'seven habits of highly effective medical educators' in obstetrics and gynecology, and Harris et al. (2007), using the Faculty Future Initiative in Family Medicine, developed a broad range of competencies meant for all faculty members, ranging from clinical teachers to education deans.

The work to describe a set of teacher competencies builds on the early work to define and evaluate effective clinical teaching (Harden and Crosby 2000; Irby 1978; Price and Mitchell 1993; Skeff et al. 1992). In the 1990s, the Stanford Faculty Development Program developed and disseminated a framework for the improvement of clinical teaching (Skeff et al. 1992) composed of seven specific teaching competencies: (1) establishing a positive learning climate; (2) control of the teaching session; (3) communicating goals; (4) promoting understanding and retention; (5) evaluation; (6) feedback; and (7) promoting self-directed learning. In 2006, Skeff and a group of colleagues held a 2-day conference on Teaching as a Competency with the goal of developing and implementing a skills-development framework (Srinivasan et al. 2011). The group described a set of four core values or principles for teaching in medical education: (1) learner engagement; (2) learner-centeredness; (3) adaptability; and (4) self-reflection; they also proposed six core medical educator competencies for all medical educators (see Table 2.1).

There is a great deal of overlap between the various competency frameworks proposed thus far (and outlined in Table 2.1), including those identified for primary and secondary education in the United States by the National Board for Professional Teaching Standards (2002). The terms used in the various reports may be slightly different, or a new concept may be introduced, such as professionalism and role modeling (Srinivasan et al. 2011) or medical informatics (Harris et al. 2007); however, the overall set of competencies for teaching in the health professions is quite consistent and relatively well defined. Moreover, competency models such as the AoME domains for teaching can be used as a framework for developing a comprehensive faculty development program for health professions teachers.

Table 2.1 Relationship between various teaching competency frameworks

	AoME domains[b]	Netherlands competencies[c]	Academic competencies[d]	Competencies for medical educators[e]	Dental competencies[f]	Carnegie task force[g]
Design & planning of learning activities[a]	X	X	X	X	X	
Teaching & supporting learners[a]	X	X	X	X	X	X
Assessment & feedback to learners	X	X	X	X	X	X
Educational research	X		X		X	
Management/Administration	X	X	X	X		X
Leadership	X		X			
Evidence-based/Practice-based teaching	X					X
Systems-based learning				X		
Medical informatics			X	X		
Care management			X			
Evaluation		X				
Content knowledge				X		X
Professionalism & role modeling				X		
Multiculturalism			X			
Members of learning communities						X
Teach in a variety of settings					X	

[a] Includes learner-centeredness and communication skills

[b] AoME Domains: (1) design and planning of learning activities; (2) teaching and supporting learners; (3) assessment and feedback to learners; (4) educational research and evidence-based practice; and (5) educational management and leadership

[c] Domains in the Netherlands framework (Molenaar et al. 2009): (1) development; (2) organization; (3) execution; (4) coaching; (5) assessment; and (6) evaluation

[d] Competencies for specific Family Medicine roles (Harris et al. 2007): (1) leadership; (2) administration; (3) teaching; (4) curriculum development; (5) research; (6) medical informatics; (7) care management; and (8) multiculturalism

[e] Core teaching competencies (Srinivasan et al. 2011): (1) medical/content knowledge; (2) learner centeredness; (3) interpersonal and communication skills; (4) professionalism and role modeling; (5) practice-based reflection and improvement; and (6) systems-based learning

[f] Competencies in Dentistry (Hand 2006): (1) foundational competencies; (2) plan and evaluate teaching/learning experiences; (3) teach in a variety of settings (large group, small group, one-on-one, preclinical, clinical, laboratory, distance/continuing); (4) assess student performance; (5) plan and evaluate curriculum; and (6) competencies for the scholarship of discovery (foundational, formulate research question, design studies, write a proposal, conduct and manage research projects, collect and manage data, manage data analysis, evaluate and discuss findings, and publish)

[g] Competencies for primary and secondary educators (National Board for Professional Teaching Standards 2002): (1) teachers are committed to students and their learning; (2) teachers know the subjects they teach and how to teach those subjects to students; (3) teachers are responsible for managing and monitoring student learning; (4) teachers think systematically about their practice and learn from experience; and (5) teachers are members of learning communities

2.4   Faculty Development to Meet Teaching Competencies – Selected Examples

2.4.1   Choosing a Competency Framework

It is not the goal of this chapter to define a competency framework for health professions teachers, but instead to assist those persons planning teaching improvement programs in identifying a set of competencies for the teachers that will be involved in the resulting program. Milner et al. (2011) suggest three methods for defining faculty competencies: (1) use of the characteristics described by Bland and Schmitz (1986) for successful faculty members; (2) use of an established competency framework; or (3) expert consensus developed during workshops and conferences. For the remainder of this chapter, we will use the AoME Professional Standards to demonstrate the range of objectives that might be addressed in a comprehensive faculty development program designed to prepare faculty members to be competent teachers: (1) designing and planning learning activities; (2) teaching and supporting learners; and (3) assessing and providing feedback to learners. Although longitudinal teaching scholar or fellowship programs usually cover all of the five AoME competencies, we will leave the discussion of this specific type of faculty development program to the authors of Chap. 10. Faculty development approaches to developing the remaining two AoME competencies – educational leadership and scholarship – will be discussed in Chaps. 3 and 4.

2.4.2   Competency Domain 1: Design and Planning of Learning Activities

AoME Domain 1 is focused on the following standards for 'educational design and learning development processes' (Academy of Medical Educators 2012, p. 15): (1) using learning principles in the development of curricula; (2) developing and using needs assessment; (3) defining learning objectives; (4) selecting learning methods/activities linked to objectives; and (5) evaluating learning outcomes (see Appendix A for the specific standards). These elements are very similar to those described by Kern et al. (1998) in *Curriculum Development for Medical Education: A Six-Step Approach*:

> Step 1 – Problem identification and general needs assessment; Step 2 – Targeted needs assessment; Step 3 – Goals and objectives; Step 4 – Educational strategies; Step 5 – Implementation; Step 6 – Evaluation (Kern et al. 1998, p. 5).

The two faculty development programs described below follow the Kern et al. (1998) model for curriculum development and therefore are useful examples of faculty development programs to achieve AoMe Domain 1.

Snyder (2001) describes a component of a 1-year Family Medicine faculty development fellowship consisting of a series of workshops on curriculum development for 3 h per month for 10 months. The teaching format for the workshops included readings, short lectures, group discussions, and the development of a curricular project. Evaluation included participant satisfaction, peer-ratings of the quality of written curricular projects, and evidence of actual implementation of the curriculum. Each written curriculum project was rated with respect to the six steps in the Kern et al. (1998) model described above. Eight projects were produced: seven included a targeted needs assessment; all had goals and learning objectives; six had teaching strategies matched to those objectives, but only five had an evaluation plan. Most importantly, six of the eight curricula were implemented.

Windish et al. (2007) describe 16 years of experience in offering a faculty development program on curriculum design at Johns Hopkins University School of Medicine using the Kern et al. (1998) model:

> The goals of the program are for participants to: (1) develop the knowledge, attitudes, and skills to design, implement, evaluate, and disseminate a curriculum in medical education; and (2) design, pilot, implement, evaluate, write-up, and present a curriculum (Windish et al. 2007, p. 656).

The 10-month program consisted of a weekly half-day session with interactive workshops, readings, a mentored curriculum development project, and in-progress reporting sessions. Over a period of 16 years, 145 faculty members completed the program. For cohorts two through nine, each participant identified a peer who could serve as a control in terms of demographic characteristics, training, and professional status. Participants and controls were asked to complete pre- and post-test surveys on their demographic characteristics, academic activities, curriculum development experience, self-assessment of curriculum development skills, implementation of curricula, evaluation of curricula, and enjoyment in curricular activities. Participants also responded to open-ended questions regarding their satisfaction with the faculty development program. At baseline, non-participants rated their curriculum/program development skills and curriculum/program implementation skills significantly higher than the participants. However, the program participants rated their enjoyment of curriculum/program development higher than their peer comparison group. At post-test, the results were reversed with program participants rating their skills in all areas higher than the control group. When pre- to post-test differences were tested, the participants increased from pre- to post-test in all areas except curriculum/program evaluation skills and enjoyment. The peer comparison group also changed from pre- to post-test, but in the opposite direction, with all values decreasing from pre- to post-test. Across all cohorts of participants, 84 % partially or fully implemented a curriculum. Approximately 20 % published an article about their curriculum in a peer-reviewed journal. The vast majority of participants (86 %) worked on their projects in either pairs or teams and reported that the collaboration was an important part of the experience. Of those who worked alone, three quarters wished they had worked collaboratively. Program participants and peer control group members from cohorts two through nine were also followed longitudinally for 6–13 years after the initial post-test (Gozu et al. 2008). At long-term follow-up, participants were significantly more likely to report proficiency in developing curricular programs, implementing/administering curricular programs, and evaluating curricular programs. Participants were also more likely than controls to report implementing one or more curricula in the last 5 years; they also reported conducting a needs assessment more frequently. Only one area was not significantly different between the participants and the peer control group, 'using different educational strategies based on the objectives of the curriculum and the needs of the learners' (p. 689). These results indicate that not only were there immediate self-reported differences between participants and non-participants, but that those differences were maintained over many years.

These two programs are interesting in that they both use the Kern et al. (1998) model for curriculum development within a single institution; however, the first program evaluated the actual curricula developed to determine if the preferred process was followed by participants, and the second program relied on self-report, albeit over an extended period of time. Mitcham and Gillette (1999) report on a national faculty development program offered by the American Occupational Therapy Association to recruit, train, and retain newly qualified occupational therapy (OT) faculty members with a focus on curriculum design and evaluation. The program started as an intensive week-long in-person 3-credit course offered at the Medical University of South Carolina (MUSC) for new OT faculty from any institution. After completion of the course, participants returned to their home institutions and developed and implemented a curriculum or new instructional materials for a course, which were submitted for grading as part of their MUSC course. This allowed participants in the program to implement what they had learned and receive feedback via a grade for their efforts. Although this course was well received, feedback from participants led to the evolution of the week-long course to a 3-day workshop in which curriculum development remained a key focus that was offered as part of an existing OT conference. Over a 5-year period, ten workshops were offered with 354 participants. A retrospective pre-to-post survey on their perceived mastery of 17 teaching elements revealed self-reported improvement in curriculum development areas: 'construction of a syllabus,' 'construction of teaching plans,' and 'creativity in presentation of content' (Mitcham et al. 2002, p. 337). In addition, participants were asked to share if there were any changes in student evaluations of their teaching. Of those who reported having teaching evaluations, '48 % reported improvements in their evaluations after attending one or more of the ten workshops (Ten percent of respondents had not yet been evaluated…)' (p. 338). An open-ended question asked respondents to indicate the three most important principles that they had learned and used in their own teaching. The most common responses were improved objectives, better exams, and improved congruence between objectives and test items. They also indicated that these principles were commented on by their students in their course/instructor evaluations.

Very few faculty development programs devoted to curriculum development can be found in the health professions education literature. Participants in each of the three examples above met the core objective of the faculty development program – to develop and implement a curriculum. These programs provide evidence that faculty development can be used successfully to improve the curriculum development skills if a significant amount of time and support is available for the faculty development program.

2.4.3   Competency Domain 2: Teaching and Supporting Learners

Core elements of AoME Domain 2 include: (1) teaching/learning methods; (2) the learning environment; (3) feedback on teaching; (4) active learning; and (5) reflection (see Appendix A). Faculty development programs to meet these competencies are the most common type of faculty development described in the literature.

A prime example in this domain is the Stanford Faculty Development Program, which has focused on the teaching of a variety of special topics based on understanding and responding effectively to the ways in which content, learners, teachers, and context interact to promote learning. The Stanford Program was first implemented in 1985 (Skeff et al. 1992), and through its graduates, it has been implemented in medical schools across North America and in other countries, notably China (Wong and Fang 2012) and Russia (Wong and Agisheva 2007). The month-long Stanford Faculty Development Program has trained more than 300 clinical and basic science faculty members from 141 institutions since its initial implementation in 1986 (Stanford Faculty Development Center for Teachers 2012). Faculty members from other institutions travel to the Stanford School of Medicine for a month of training, and then return to their home institutions to implement the teaching improvement program with their own colleagues. The Stanford Program consists of seven 2 h seminars, readings, discussion, video-taped practice teaching of one of the seminars with feedback, and additional practice teaching sessions to prepare to teach the program at their home institution. This train-the-trainer dissemination concept builds on the idea that 'change agents with characteristics of their target audience have strong credibility for disseminating new ideas to their colleagues.' (Skeff et al. 1992, p. 1156).

The most important goal of the Stanford Faculty Development Program is to prepare participants to effectively implement the program at their home institution and to evaluate its impact by using a retrospective pre-post assessment format in which institutional participants report on changes in their clinical teaching behaviors (Skeff et al. 1992). However, when the program was implemented in China, there were challenges; 'although this project was an adaption from a well-studied and successful model, it remains a great challenge to successfully overcome differences in culture, language, and educational systems' (Wong and Fang 2012, p. 357).

Even so, there was a significant increase in scores on the retrospective pre-post assessment on the overall portion and on the Specific Teaching Skills portion of the survey instrument. Comments from participants most frequently described improvement of the learning climate, promoting understanding and retention, feedback, and promoting self-directed learning (Wong and Fang 2012). In another study of the Stanford Program, Berbano et al. (2006) evaluated the implementation of the Stanford program with eight faculty members using a direct measure of teaching behaviors with an Objective Structured Teaching Evaluation (OSTE). Each participant completed three OSTE stations before and 1 month after completing the program, discussing a case with a third-year medical student, an intern, and an internal medicine resident. From pre- to post-test, participants changed the types of questions asked and the type of feedback given. The total number of questions decreased significantly at post-test. During the case discussion, factual questions decreased (80–59 %) and the number of higher-level questions requiring analysis/synthesis increased (10 to 34 %, respectively). This study adds to the evidence that the Stanford Program is effective given the direct evaluation of teaching skills versus the use of self-report that is found in most studies.

While workshops and presentations are the most common methods used to help faculty members and residents to improve teaching skills, programs using guided reflection, coupled with practice and feedback, suggest that a broader array of approaches can be effective (Alteen et al. 2009; Branch et al. 2009; Cole et al. 2004; Kumagai et al. 2007; Rabow et al. 2007; Steinert et al. 2010; Tang et al. 2009). A multi-institutional study of a longitudinal faculty development program to improve clinical teaching using reflection deserves special note. Five medical schools in the United States collaboratively developed and implemented a program to foster the teaching of humanistic values and behaviors during the process of patient care (Branch et al. 2009). This 18-month program used self-reflective discussion and narrative writing as core teaching methods. The authors studied outcomes of the program using a quasi-experimental post-test only control group design. Students and residents of program participants and faculty members willing to serve as controls were surveyed regarding their teachers' effectiveness in teaching the human dimension of care. Participants were scored significantly higher on all ten items on the Humanistic Teaching Practices Effectiveness Questionnaire than were controls. Some sample items included: inspires me to grow personally and professionally (88 % vs. 76 %); actively uses teaching opportunities to illustrate humanistic care (86 % vs. 73 %); serves as an outstanding role model (89 % vs. 77 %); explicitly teaches communication and relationship-building skills (83 % vs. 72 %); and inspires me to adopt caring attitudes toward patients (90 % vs. 80 %). The strength of this study is that a standard faculty development curriculum was implemented at multiple medical schools and was evaluated by comparing participants' and controls' teaching behaviors as reported by their trainees. Although selection bias could contribute to these results, at one of the participating medical schools, an historical pre-test compared evaluations by residents of participants and controls and found no significant differences at baseline.

Kumagai et al. (2007) and Tang et al. (2009) describe a novel approach to teaching improvement using interactive theater to stimulate reflection and to provide a venue for practical experience with new teaching behaviors. Forum Theater is a type of interactive theater 'in which the traditional barrier between the actors and the audience is broken down, and the audience becomes directly involved in determining the course of the play' (Kumagai et al. 2007, p. 336).

At the University of Michigan, first- through third-year students work on longitudinal cases in small groups. These cases may contain controversial and contentious issues that should be discussed sensitively and not avoided. In fact, the facilitators are 'expected to assure a safe and respectful environment for everyone in the group, and to raise questions, identify contradictions, and stimulate discussion that encourages individual and shared reflection of these issues and their consequences' (Kumagai et al. 2007, p. 336).

In order to prepare the small group facilitators for this task, a 3.5 h faculty development session using Forum Theater was introduced in 2004. The University Center for Research on Learning and Teaching (CRLT) has members (i.e. the Players) who are trained in acting and how to reflect upon their own and others' biases, especially with respect to gender, ethnicity, sexual orientation, and socio-economic status. For the Forum Theater faculty development program, the CRLT Players enacted a scenario based on the discussion observed in an actual small group in the course. After the scenario was performed, the faculty development participants (15 at each of two sessions) could ask questions of the Players, all of whom responded within their scenario role. The participants then engaged in a discussion of possible resolutions to the problems demonstrated in the scenario. Then the CRLT Players re-enacted the scenario using the suggestions from the faculty development participants. Participants were surveyed about the experience upon the conclusion of the workshop and also 9–15 months later. A week after the survey, participants were invited to a focus group. The results indicated that the Forum Theater experience led the facilitators to reflect upon their own teaching and have more awareness of the issues affecting women and minorities; it also provided new strategies for dealing with difficult conversations within the small groups. The survey item with the highest rating was 'led me to reflect on how my actions in the classroom affect students' (Kumagai et al. 2007, p. 338). At the focus group, one facilitator shared that the workshop had made him/her 'more sensitive to the cultural aspects of our discussions' (Kumagai et al. 2007, p. 338). The authors felt that the Forum Theater workshop had been quite successful in leading facilitators to reflect on their teaching in a new way that would ultimately improve the discourse within their small groups, especially around sensitive cultural issues.

These examples are meant to illustrate a range of approaches and contexts in which faculty members can be helped to develop improved teaching skills. Of particular interest in two of these examples is the power of collaboration among institutions in the design, implementation, and evaluation of teaching improvement programs.

2.4.4   Domain 3: Assessment and Feedback to Learners

The last AoME area to be addressed in this chapter, Domain 3, focuses on assessment and feedback to learners. Faculty development programs in this domain generally focus on (1) test development; (2) general training in the use of a variety of assessment methods; and (3) feedback. The range of assessment tools used in health professions education includes various forms of knowledge examination types, tools for evaluating competencies during clinical care, and performance evaluation exercises in simulated clinical settings (Wass and Archer 2011). However, this area of teaching improvement has been less well described in the literature, which may reflect that it is less often being addressed in faculty development programs.

There are few studies of faculty development programs in the health professions that focus on improvement of test development and standard setting. Jozefowicz et al. (2002) showed that untrained test item writers are not as good at writing exam items as those who are trained using a standard method, such as the one outlined in the National Board of Medical Examiners (NBME) text on item-writing, *Constructing Written Test Questions for the Basic and Clinical Sciences* (Case and Swanson 1998). Naeem et al. (2012) implemented a 1-week full-time faculty development program to teach faculty members to write multiple-choice questions, short-answer questions, and to develop checklists for an Objective Structured Clinical Examination (OSCE). To evaluate the effects of the program, the authors asked participants to submit an example of their 'best' item for each of the item categories prior to the start of the program. Participants then rewrote their test items after each phase of the intervention. The test items were scored at pre-test, at mid-point, and after the second intervention. There was a significant increase in scores from pre-test to mid-point assessment and from mid-point to post-test with strong effect sizes. These results, along with the study by the NBME, provide evidence that the quality of test items can be improved through faculty development.

The Medical College of Wisconsin's (MCW) longitudinal fellowship program evolved over 10 years into a modular system – Excellence in Clinical Education and Leadership (ExCEL). In this system, faculty members can complete one module on a specific topic or string together a set of modules to complete a longitudinal program of learning (Simpson et al. 2006) This modular system allows faculty members to create their own individualized learning plan that meets their own needs and the needs of their departments. The MCW modular faculty development system includes an 'assessment of learner performance' module. This assessment module includes practical and fun exercises, such as the 'Wisconsin State Fair Chocolate Judging' in which faculty members learn about measurement theory by developing criteria to describe the best chocolate. The work culminates in the judging of a variety of chocolates, some well-known and others submitted for competition at the Wisconsin State Fair. Faculty members learn about bias and measurement error using their taste buds. In another assignment, faculty members work in small groups to development an OSCE station. This exercise includes all aspects of an OSCE, from the development of the case objectives, the writing of the standardized patient script, the development of the checklist, and even producing the door signs for the station. During the exercise, faculty members are reminded to consider the issues of reliability and measurement error. The assessment module also requires faculty members to develop their own assessment tool based on a real educational need. They then pilot test the assessment instrument and determine the measurement characteristics. Each of these assessment exercises employ active learning methods, are practical for the learner, and employ elements of fun while learning. Evidence of the success of the ExCEL program is its ongoing enrollment levels. These exceeded the planners' expectations with 23 primary care faculty members participating per module with an 85 % completion rate. Retrospective self-report of change from pre-to-post completion of the modules indicates that the program objectives were met. In addition, between 2002 and 2005, the 30 participants 'averaged five accepted peer-reviewed presentations at regional national meetings and published more than 20 articles and 50 abstracts. Ten of their durable products were accepted to the AAMC's MedEdPORTAL between May and November 2005' (Simpson et al. 2006, p. 950).

Although giving effective feedback is often the skill that faculty members list as one in which they would like to become more skilled, there are few reported studies that focus on training in the art of feedback, especially ones that provide evaluation data beyond participant satisfaction. Walsh et al. (2009) evaluated the outcome of a 2 h workshop on giving feedback using case discussions, role playing, and reflection on how to change teaching practices. A pre-test survey of participants consisted of items on what constituted effective feedback and possible barriers to effective feedback. An immediate post-test survey asked participants to indicate anticipated changes in their teaching practices. Three to four months after the workshop, participants were asked to complete a follow-up survey indicating if they had made the planned changes to their teaching behavior or any unplanned changes. Only 20 % at pre-test felt that effective feedback should be timely or constructive. At immediate post-test, 76 % reported that they planned to make 'a definite change in their teaching practices' (Walsh et al. 2009, p. 48) and 41 % indicated a specific change. The 4-month follow-up survey indicated that approximately 75 % of respondents had interacted with a learner since the workshop and all reported that they had made at least one of their planned changes to the way they gave feedback. Some (37 %) even reported unplanned changes to their teaching. Other studies of programs to train faculty members in feedback skills exist, but a number have resulted in negative results (McAndrew et al. 2012; Stone et al. 2003). Each of these programs to develop skills in providing feedback were short workshops. Development and evaluation of more extensive faculty development programs in this area will likely be needed as medical education moves quickly into competency-based and developmental (i.e. achievement of milestones along the educational continuum) educational models (Dath and Iobst 2010; Holmboe et al. 2011; Ross et al. 2011).

2.5 Designing Teaching Improvement Activities

Evaluation studies of specific teaching improvement interventions provide limited guidance on the most powerful design for teaching improvement activities. Most programs have largely relied on participants' ratings of quality or usefulness. Others have relied on self-reports of changes in knowledge, attitudes and beliefs about learning and teaching and sometimes actual change in teaching practices. Few evaluation studies have included control groups or focused on changes in students' ratings of the teaching behaviors or actual learning outcomes (Steinert et al. 2006). Those few studies associated with actual changes in teaching behaviors or learner outcomes suggest that certain teaching improvement formats are more effective than others (Chism and Szabo 1997; Steinert et al. 2006; Wilkerson and Irby 1998).

In a systematic review of studies in faculty development, Steinert et al. (2006) concluded:

> Key features of effective faculty development contributing to effectiveness included the use of experiential learning, provision of feedback, effective peer and colleague relationships, well-designed interventions following principles of teaching and learning, and the use of a diversity of educational methods within single interventions (p. 497).

New approaches to teaching improvement activities will likely capitalize on the growing use of social media and other methods of brief electronic communication, such as those already being used in clinical teaching to 'push' information to learners (Boulos et al. 2006), but there is little in the literature currently that describes or evaluates the use of these tools for teaching improvement purposes, although Web-based modules on teaching skills have been available for many years (e.g. Practical Doc, http://www.practicaldoc.ca/teaching/practical-prof/). In one new approach using e-mail, Matzie et al. (2009) used a spaced education approach for teaching residents to give feedback in a general surgery program. The 55 participating residents were stratified by year of training and whether they had attended a 1 h didactic program on giving feedback; they were randomized to either receive or not receive a weekly email for 9 months containing one succinct tip on giving feedback (e.g. keep feedback focused and avoid trying to accomplish too much). Students rotating on the surgery clerkship were asked to evaluate the feedback frequency and quality provided by residents with whom they had worked over the previous 2 weeks. Residents in the spaced practice intervention were rated as providing significantly more feedback and feedback that was more useful than those in the control arm. Spaced education uses repetition and time to reinforce knowledge and skills learned, as opposed to massed or one-time learning. Use of e-mail reminders, or in the future possibly the use of Twitter to serve as an adjunct to faculty development, may become more common. As more millennial students become faculty members, we may need to examine how we deliver faculty development to a generation that is accustomed to receiving bits of information through texting and Twitter and using social media for communication.

Whatever the methods employed in teaching improvement programs, it is important to focus on the critical goal – change. O'Sullivan and Irby (2011) have suggested that we need a more complex model of faculty development in order to better understand the features that lead to desired changes in teachers, learners, organizations, and patients. The authors suggest the need to include a focus on the faculty development community of participants and the workplace community rather than focusing only on the individual participants. They suggest four components essential to the planning and evaluation of faculty development – the participants, the program content, the skills and attitudes of the facilitators, and the organizational contexts in which participants actually teach in order to extend our understanding of essential faculty development features. In the book, *Influencer: The Power to Change Anything*, Patterson et al. (2008) suggest that the likelihood of change is increased when individual and organizational 'six sources of influence' are included: making the undesirable desirable; capitalizing on peer pressure and developing organizational rewards and accountability measures; building the individual's personal commitment to change; reinforcing new abilities through the engagement of others; and structuring the environment so that the targeted behaviors are rewarded. This interplay of personal, social, and structural sources of influence are drawn from social psychology and organizational change. The development of competencies for teachers at the school, institution, and national level is changing how we prepare and reward competent teachers. There is a long history of faculty development for teaching improvement. How we as faculty developers design, implement, and disseminate our successful programs should help us move the field forward to meet the needs and challenges put forth to us by our stakeholders – the trainees, patients, faculty members, and accreditation bodies – who will demand of us the tools and training to make our faculty the most competent teachers possible.

2.6 Implications for Teaching Improvement Activities in Faculty Development

As teaching as a scholarly activity and educational scholarship (Boyer 1990) become more valued faculty activities in health professions education and assume a more influential place in the promotion and tenure process, it is likely that more institutions, and perhaps more governments, will follow the lead of the Netherlands. We believe that a competency framework, such as the one developed by the AoME, is a useful guide for faculty developers in creating programs to train faculty members to meet teaching standards. In this chapter, we have described a number of successful faculty development programs that trained faculty to develop curricula, to teach, and to assess and provide feedback to learners. In some areas, such as curriculum development and assessment, there is a paucity of published studies that go beyond student satisfaction as an outcome. A challenge for us is to document and rigorously study the work that we are doing. A number of the studies described went beyond self-report of behavioral change following participation in a faculty development program. Examples of these are evaluating a curriculum for quality (Snyder 2001), assessing teaching behaviors via an objective structured teaching evaluation (Berbano et al. 2006), or evaluating test items (Jozefowicz et al. 2002; Naeem et al. 2012).

Resources get scarcer all the time. Budgets are smaller and time seems to be ever shrinking. If we as faculty developers are to justify our continued existence within our professional schools, we will likely need to meet greater scrutiny to demonstrate that our programs are worthwhile to our faculty members and institutions in general. Can we do that by designing comprehensive faculty development programs that train our faculty members to meet specific measureable competencies, just as students and other trainees must do? Should we also consider a developmental model (Dreyfus and Dreyfus 1986; Green et al. 2009) that will demonstrate that we can train our faculty members to achieve varying levels of competency and maintain their competency over time? O'Sullivan and Irby (2011) suggest that participants identify a knowledge gap and then develop their own methods to demonstrate that they have filled that gap. The use of a competency framework should inform faculty members about the values and expectations of the institution, allowing them to evaluate their own needs to meet identified standards as teachers. Using the competency framework within a comprehensive faculty development program could inform not only the individual faculty member but also the larger community of faculty members, affecting the context in which they teach and work. This is consistent with O'Sullivan and Irby (2011) who suggest that this is the ultimate goal of faculty development. They contend that the system is complex and requires us to consider the various communities of practice that are affected by our programs and where our programs are situated. Is a successful faculty development program one that only affects the participant or is the program successful when it affects the larger community and context of the institution? One may also ask if making expectations for our teachers more explicit, such as using a competency framework, is the first step in influencing the community of practice. If faculty members know what is expected of them to demonstrate that they are effective teachers, must we provide the tools for them to improve their teaching in a way different from what we do today? At the Medical College of Wisconsin (Simpson et al. 2006), the longitudinal faculty development program was changed to a modular system to better meet the needs of participants. Is a more individualized system the future of faculty development? If O'Sullivan and Irby's approach (2011) is correct, this may be the case if we can also create community within these smaller units of instruction. Only time and the use of rigorous outcome measures will inform us if this new approach to improving teaching is successful.

2.7 Conclusion

In the 1950s, faculty development to improve teaching was one of the first types of faculty development to emerge in higher education. Today, it is still the most common form of faculty development in the health professions. In this chapter, we reviewed a number of competency frameworks to improve teaching for health professions teachers. We found that most of these frameworks had considerable overlap with each one including: (a) skills in curriculum design; (b) teaching and supporting learners; and (c) assessment and feedback. Several best practice examples from the faculty development literature demonstrate how these three competencies might be learned and illustrate what is known about the effectiveness of a variety of teaching improvement activities. The literature is limited in the quality of evidence available about what works for teachers, their students, and the systems in which both education and patient care occur. As faculty developers, we will need to continue to innovate in defining and teaching the competencies necessary for our health professions teachers as they progress from novice to master teachers.

2.8   Key Messages

- Faculty development to improve teaching is the most common type of faculty development activity reported in the health professions literature.
- Many competency frameworks for improving the teaching of health professions teachers exist; most of these include: (a) skills in curriculum design; (b) teaching and supporting learners; and (c) assessment and feedback.
- The competency framework developed by the Academy of Medical Educators in Great Britain is a useful guide for faculty developers who wish to create programs to train faculty members to meet teaching standards.
- Many successful faculty development programs have trained faculty members to develop curricula, to teach, and to assess and provide feedback to learners. Many have also gone beyond self-report of behavioral change following participation in a faculty development program and have included more rigorous evaluation methods.
- In the future, faculty developers should consider developing comprehensive faculty development programs that train our faculty members to meet specific measureable competencies.

Appendix A

First three Domains of the 2012 Professional Standards of the Academy of Medical Educators (Re-printed with permission from the Academy of Medical Educators (2012) *Professional Standards.*)

Domain 1: Design and Planning of Learning Activities

This domain outlines the expected standards for medical educators involved in educational design and learning development processes. Applicants must demonstrate and referees must corroborate these capabilities.

Element	Standard level 1
Learning and teaching principles	*1.1.1* Shows how the principles of learning and teaching are incorporated into educational developments
	1.1.2 Is aware of different ways of learning and teaching
Learning needs	*1.1.3* Shows how the needs of learners are considered
Learning outcomes	*1.1.4* Is aware of the need to define what is to be learned
Learning and teaching methods and resources	*1.1.5* Is aware of a range of learning methods, experiences and resources and how they may be used effectively
Evaluation of educational interventions	*1.1.6* Responds appropriately to feedback and evaluation of educational interventions

Standard level 2	Standard level 3
1.2.1 Applies learning and teaching principles in the design of a unit, module or subject area	1.3.1 Applies learning and teaching principles in the design of a curriculum for a whole course or degree program
1.2.2 Matches course design to support different ways of learning and teaching	
1.2.3 Gathers and interprets basic information on the needs of learners	1.3.2 Conducts complex learning needs analyses including those of learners, groups, professions or healthcare systems
1.2.4 Constructs appropriate learning outcomes that can be measured or judged	1.3.3 Defines learning outcomes within theoretical frameworks
1.2.5 Matches learning methods, experiences and resources to intended outcomes	1.3.4 Is adaptive and effective in securing resources and dealing with constraints
1.2.6 Develops learning resources for planned courses	
1.2.7 Evaluates and improves educational interventions	1.3.5 Conducts, interprets, acts on and disseminates evaluations of learning programs

Domain 2: Teaching and Supporting Learners

This domain outlines the expected standards for medical educators in relation to teaching and facilitating learning. Applicants must demonstrate and referees must corroborate these capabilities.

Element	Standard level 1
Delivering teaching	2.1.1 Appropriately uses a range of learning and teaching methods and technologies
Maintaining an effective learning environment	2.1.2 Is aware of the importance of establishing a safe and effective learning environment
Learning and teaching methods and resources	2.1.3 Is aware of a range of learning methods that may be used in learning and teaching activities
Feedback on learning	2.1.4 Understands the importance of seeking, receiving and responding to feedback about learning and teaching
Participation	2.1.5 Describes ways of involving learners in actual practice e.g. experiential learning opportunities
Reflection	2.1.6 Is aware of the importance of reflection on practice

Standard level 2	Standard level 3
2.2.1 Appropriately uses a broad range of learning and teaching methods and technologies	2.3.1 Is adaptive and innovative in respect to learning and teaching
	2.3.2 Supports others to innovate
2.2.2 Establishes an effective learning environment	2.3.3 Monitors and manages complex learning environments

(continued)

(continued)

Standard level 2	Standard level 3
2.2.3 Provides educational, personal and professional support in relevant contexts	2.3.4 Proactively seeks to improve the learning environment
2.2.4 Applies learning and teaching methods that are relevant to programme content	2.3.5 Adapts learning and teaching methods to unexpected circumstances
2.2.5 Uses learning resources appropriately	2.3.6 Develops innovative learning resources
2.2.6 Develops self-awareness in learners	2.3.7 Develops self-awareness in learners and teachers
2.2.7 Listens actively and provides effective feedback to learners using a range of methods	2.3.8 Interprets, synthesizes and deals with conflicting information arising from feedback from learners and educators
	2.3.9 Effectively demonstrates to learners the rationale for changing or not changing teaching and learning activities in response to feedback
2.2.8 Engages learners in reflective practice	2.3.10 Actively seeks to incorporate learners into a community of practice
2.2.9 Uses systems of teaching and training that incorporate reflective practice in self and others	2.3.11 Demonstrates a commitment to reflective practice in self, learners and colleagues

Domain 3: Assessment and Feedback to Learners

This domain outlines the expected standards for medical educators in making and reporting judgments that capture, guide and make decisions about the learning achievement of learners. Applicants must demonstrate and referees must corroborate these capabilities.

Element	Standard level 1
The purpose of the assessment	3.1.1 Is aware of the general purpose of assessment
The content of the assessment	3.1.2 Is aware that assessment should align with the course learning outcomes
The development of assessment	3.1.3 Is aware that good assessment practices are integral to course development
Selecting appropriate assessment methods	3.1.4 Is aware that assessment methods are chosen on the basis of the purpose, content and level of the assessment
	3.1.5 Uses a basic range of methods to assess learners
Maintaining the quality of assessment	3.1.6 Is aware that assessment practices require continuous monitoring and improvement

Standard level 2	Standard level 3
3.2.1 Relates the purposes of assessments to the context of the course or programme	*3.3.1* Designs complex assessment strategies and blueprints
3.2.2 Demonstrates that the contribution of any assessment addresses the learning outcomes and the assessment blueprint	*3.3.2* Maintains and manages assessment blueprints for one or more courses or levels
3.2.3 Contributes to the construction of assessment items	*3.3.3* Leads design and development of assessments utilising accepted good practice such as in the determination of reliability, validity, acceptability, cost effectiveness and educational impact
3.2.4 Selects assessment methods that match the purpose, content and level of the learner	*3.3.4* Assesses learners using a wide range of methods
3.2.5 Uses a broad range of methods to assess learners	
3.2.6 Interprets accurately assessment reports in relation to educational quality management	*3.3.5* Contributes under guidance to standard setting processes
	3.3.6 Applies standard setting procedures most relevant to particular methods and format
	3.3.7 Interprets technical data about effectiveness of assessment practices
	3.3.8 Prepares assessment reports for learners, examination boards and external stakeholders

References

Academy of Medical Educators. (2008). *Annual report and financial statements: 30 September 2008.* Available from: http://www.medicaleducators.org/aome/assets/File/Annual%20 Report%202008%20final.pdf

Academy of Medical Educators. (2012). *Professional standards.* London, UK: Academy of Medical Educators. Available from: http://www.medicaleducators.org/index.cfm/linkservid/180C46A6-B0E9-B09B-02599E43F9C2FDA9/showMeta/0/

Academy of Medical Educators. (n.d.). *Educational Supervisors Project.* Available from: http://www.medicaleducators.org/index.cfm/profession/edsupervisors

Alteen, A. M., Didham P., & Stratton C. (2009). Reflecting, refueling, and reframing: A 10-year retrospective model for faculty development and its implications for nursing scholarship. *Journal of Continuing Education in Nursing, 40*(6), 267–272.

Association of American Medical Colleges. (1977). *Second preliminary report of the faculty development survey: Special report.* Washington, DC: Distributed by ERIC Clearinghouse.

Berbano, E. P., Browning, R., Pangaro, L., & Jackson, J. L. (2006). The impact of the Stanford Faculty Development Program on ambulatory teaching behavior. *Journal of General Internal Medicine, 21*(5), 430–434.

Bergquist, W. H. & Phillips, S. R. (1975). *A handbook for faculty development.* Washington, DC: Council for the Advancement of Small Colleges.

Bland, C. J. & Schmitz, C. C. (1986). Characteristics of the successful researcher and implications for faculty development. *Journal of Medical Education, 61*(1), 22–31.

Boulos, M. N. K., Maramba, I., & Wheeler, S. (2006). Wikis, blogs and podcasts: A new generation of web-based tools for virtual collaborative clinical practice and education. *BMC Medical Education, 6*, 41.

Boyer, E. L. (1990). *Scholarship reconsidered: Priorities of the professoriate.* Princeton, NJ: Carnegie Foundation for the Advancement of Teaching.

Branch, W. T. Jr., Frankel, R., Gracey, C. F., Haidet, P. M., Weissmann, P. F., Cantey, P., et al. (2009). A good clinician and a caring person: Longitudinal faculty development and the enhancement of the human dimensions of care. *Academic Medicine, 84*(1), 117–125.

Case, S. M. & Swanson, D. B. (1998). *Constructing written test questions for the basic and clinical sciences.* Philadelphia, PA: National Board of Medical Examiners.

Centra, J. A. (1976). *Faculty development practices in U. S. colleges and universities.* Princeton, NJ: Educational Testing Service.

Chism, N. V. N. & Szabo, B. (1997). How faculty development programs evaluate their services. *Journal of Staff, Program and Organizational Development, 15*(2), 55–62.

Cole, K. A., Barker, L. R., Kolodner, K., Williamson, P., Wright, S. M., & Kern, D. E. (2004). Faculty development in teaching skills: An intensive longitudinal model. *Academic Medicine, 79*(5), 469–480.

Dath, D. & Iobst, W. (2010). The importance of faculty development in the transition to competency-based medical education. *Medical Teacher, 32*(8), 683–686.

Dreyfus, H. L. & Dreyfus, S. E. (1986). *Mind over machine: The power of human intuition and expertise in the era of the computer.* New York, NY: Free Press.

Gaff, J. G. (1975). *Toward faculty renewal.* San Francisco, CA: Jossey-Bass.

Green, M. L., Aagaard, E. M., Caverzagie, K. J., Chick, D. A., Holmboe, E., Kane, G., et al. (2009). Charting the road to competence: Developmental milestones for internal medicine residency training. *Journal of Graduate Medical Education, 1*(1), 5–20.

Gozu, A., Windish, D. M., Knight, A. M., Thomas, P. A., Kolodner, K., Bass, E. B., et al. (2008). Long-term follow-up of a 10-month programme in curriculum development for medical educators: A cohort study. *Medical Education, 42*(7), 684–692.

Hand, J. S. (2006). Identification of competencies for effective dental faculty. *Journal of Dental Education, 70*(9), 937–947.

Harden, R. M. & Crosby, J. (2000). AMEE guide no. 20: The good teacher is more than a lecturer – The twelve roles of the teacher. *Medical Teacher, 22*(4), 334–347.

Harris, D. L., Krause, K. C., Parish, D. C., & Smith, M. U. (2007). Academic competencies for medical faculty. *Family Medicine, 39*(5), 343–350.

Holmboe, E. S., Ward, D. S., Reznick, R. K., Katsufrakis, P. J., Leslie, K. M., Patel, V. L., et al. (2011). Faculty development in assessment: The missing link in competency-based medical education. *Academic Medicine, 86*(4), 460–467.

Hueppchen, N., Dalrymple, J. L., Hammoud, M. M., Abbott, J. F., Casey, P. M., Chuang, A. W., et al. (2011). To the point: Medical education reviews - Ongoing call for faculty development. *American Journal of Obstetrics and Gynecology, 205*(3), 171–176.

Irby, D. M. (1978). Clinical teacher effectiveness in medicine. *Journal of Medical Education, 53*(10), 808–815.

Irby, D. M. (1994). What clinical teachers in medicine need to know. *Academic Medicine, 69*(5), 333–342.

Jason, H. (1962). A study of medical teaching practices. *Journal of Medical Education, 37*(12), 1258–1284.

Jason, H. & Westberg, J. (1982). *Teachers and teaching in U. S. medical schools.* Norwalk, CT: Appleton-Century-Crofts.

Jozefowicz, R. F., Koeppen, B. M., Case, S., Galbraith, R., Swanson, D., & Glew, R. H. (2002). The quality of in-house medical school examinations. *Academic Medicine, 77*(2), 156–161.

Kern, D. E., Thomas, P. A., Howard, D. M., & Bass, E. B. (Eds.). (1998). *Curriculum development for medical education: A six-step approach.* Baltimore, MD: Johns Hopkins University Press.

Kumagai, A. K., White, C. B., Ross, P. T., Purkiss, J. A., O'Neal, C. M., & Steiger, J. A. (2007). Use of interactive theater for faculty development in multicultural medical education. *Medical Teacher, 29*(4), 335–340.

Matzie, K. A., Kerfoot, B. P., Hafler, J. P., & Breen, E. M. (2009). Spaced education improves the feedback that surgical residents give to medical students: A randomized trial. *American Journal of Surgery, 197*(2), 252–257.

McAndrew, M., Eidtson, W. H., Pierre, G. C., & Gillespie, C. C. (2012). Creating an objective structured teaching examination to evaluate a dental faculty development program. *Journal of Dental Education, 76*(4), 461–471.

Metz, J. C. M., Zwierstra, R. P., Fluit, C. R. M. G. & Scherpbier, A. J. J. A. (1996). Didactische en onderwijskundige scholing van docenten geneeskunde. [Didactic and educational development of medical teachers.] *Nederlands Tijdschrift voor Geneeskunde, 140*(16), 894–896.

Miller, G. E. (1980). *Educating medical teachers*. Cambridge, MA: Harvard University Press.

Milner, R. J., Gusic, M. E., & Thorndyke, L. E. (2011). Perspective: Toward a competency framework for faculty. *Academic Medicine, 86*(10), 1204–1210.

Mitcham, M. D. & Gillette, N. P. (1999). Developing the instructional skills of new faculty members in occupational therapy. *American Journal of Occupational Therapy, 53*(1), 20–24.

Mitcham, M. D., Lancaster, C. J., & Stone, B. M. (2002). Evaluating the effectiveness of occupational therapy faculty development workshops. *American Journal of Occupational Therapy, 56*(3), 335–339.

Molenaar, W. M., Zanting, A., van Beukelen, P., de Grave, W., Baane, J. A., Bustraan, J. A., et al. (2009). A framework of teaching competencies across the medical education continuum. *Medical Teacher, 31*(5), 390–396.

Naeem, N., van der Vleuten, C., & Alfaris, E. A. (2012). Faculty development on item writing substantially improves item quality. *Advances in Health Sciences Education, 17*(3), 369–376.

National Board for Professional Teaching Standards. (2002). *What teachers should know and be able to do*. Retrieved January 22nd, 2013, from http://www.nbpts.org/sites/default/files/documents/certificates/what_teachers_should_know.pdf

O'Sullivan, P. S. & Irby, D. M. (2011). Reframing research on faculty development. *Academic Medicine, 86*(4), 421–428.

Patterson, K., Grenny, J., Maxfield, D., McMillan, R., & Switzler, A. (2008). *Influencer: The power to change anything*. New York, NY: McGraw Hill.

Peyton, J. W. R. (Ed.). (1998). *Teaching and learning in medical practice*. Rickmansworth, UK: Manticore Europe.

Price, D. A. & Mitchell, C. A. (1993). A model for clinical teaching and learning. *Medical Education, 27*(1), 62–68.

Rabow, M. W., Wrubel, J., & Remen, R. N. (2007). Authentic community as an educational strategy for advancing professionalism: A national evaluation of the Healer's Art course. *Journal of General Internal Medicine, 22*(10), 1422–1428.

Ross, S., Poth, C. N., Donoff, M., Humphries, P., Steiner, I., Schipper, S., et al. (2011). Competency-based achievement system: Using formative feedback to teach and assess family medicine residents' skills. *Canadian Family Physician, 57*(9), e323–e330.

Schön, D. A. (1987). *Educating the reflective practitioner*. San Francisco, CA: Jossey-Bass.

Shulman, L. S. (1986). Those who understand: Knowledge growth in teaching. *Educational Researcher, 15*(2), 4–14.

Simpson, D., Marcdante, K., Morzinski, J., Meurer, L., McLaughlin, C., Lamb, G. et al. (2006). Fifteen years of aligning faculty development with primary care clinician-educator roles and academic advancement at the Medical College of Wisconsin. *Academic Medicine, 81*(11), 945–953.

Skeff, K. M., Stratos, G. A., Berman, J., & Bergen, M. R. (1992). Improving clinical teaching: Evaluation of a national dissemination program. *Archives of Internal Medicine, 152*(6), 1156–1161.

Snyder, S. (2001). A program to teach curriculum development to junior faculty. *Family Medicine, 33*(5), 382–387.

Sorcinelli, M. D., Austin, A. E., Eddy, P. L., & Beach, A. L. (2006). *Creating the future of faculty development: Learning from the past, understanding the present.* Bolton, MA: Anker Publishing.

Srinivasan, M., Li, S. T., Meyers, F. J., Pratt, D. D., Collins, J. B., Braddock, C., et al. (2011). 'Teaching as a competency': Competencies for medical educators. *Academic Medicine, 86*(10), 1211–1220.

Stanford Faculty Development Center for Medical Teachers. (2012). *Stanford Faculty Development Center - Background.* Available from: http://sfdc.stanford.edu/background.html

Steinert, Y., Boudreau, J. D., Boillat, M., Slapcoff, B., Dawson, D., Briggs, A., et al. (2010). The Osler Fellowship: An apprenticeship for medical educators. *Academic Medicine, 85*(7), 1242–1249.

Steinert, Y., Mann, K., Centeno, A., Dolmans, D., Spencer, J., Gelula, M., et al. (2006). A systematic review of faculty development initiatives designed to improve teaching effectiveness in medical education: BEME Guide No. 8. *Medical Teacher, 28*(6), 497–526.

Stone, S., Mazor, K., Devaney-O'Neil, S., Starr, S., Ferguson, W., Wellman, S., et al. (2003). Development and implementation of an objective structured teaching exercise (OSTE) to evaluate improvement in feedback skills following a faculty development workshop. *Teaching and Learning in Medicine, 15*(1), 7–13.

Tang, T. S., Skye, E. P., & Steiger, J. A. (2009). Increasing patient acceptance of medical student participation: Using interactive theatre for faculty development. *Teaching and Learning in Medicine, 21*(3), 195–200.

van Keulen, H. (2006). *Staff development and basic teaching qualification systems in the Netherlands, with a focus on Utrecht University.* International Consortium for Educational Development 2006 International Conference: Sheffield, UK. Retrieved August 2nd, 2012, from http://igitur-archive.library.uu.nl/ivlos/2006-1221-201509/keulen%20-%20towards%20a%20national%20system.pdf

Walsh, A. E., Armson, H., Wakefield, J. G., Leadbetter, W., & Roder, S. (2009). Using a novel small-group approach to enhance feedback skills for community-based teachers. *Teaching and Learning in Medicine, 21*(1), 45–51.

Wass, V. & Archer, J. Assessing learners. (2011). In T. Dornan, K. Mann, A. Scherpbier, & J. Spencer (Eds.), *Medical education: Theory and practice,* (pp. 229–255). Edinburgh, Scotland: Churchill Livingstone Elsevier.

Wilkerson, L. & Anderson, W. A. (2004). Hilliard Jason, MD, EdD: A medical student turned medical educator. *Advances in Health Sciences Education, 9*(4), 325–335.

Wilkerson, L. & Irby, D. M. (1998). Strategies for improving teaching practices: A comprehensive approach to faculty development. *Academic Medicine, 73*(4), 387–396.

Windish, D. M., Gozu, A., Bass, E. B., Thomas, P. A., Sisson, S. D., Howard, D. M., et al. (2007). A ten-month program in curriculum development for medical educators: 16 years of experience. *Journal of General Internal Medicine, 22*(5), 655–661.

Wong, J. G. & Agisheva, K. (2007). Developing teaching skills for medical educators in Russia: A cross-cultural faculty development project. *Medical Education, 41*(3), 318–324.

Wong, J. G. & Fang, Y. (2012). Improving clinical teaching in China: Initial report of a multihospital pilot faculty development effort. *Teaching and Learning in Medicine, 24*(4), 355–360.

Chapter 3
Faculty Development for Leadership and Management

Tim Swanwick and Judy McKimm

3.1 Introduction

When we think of leadership in health professions education, it is tempting to be drawn to images of medical school deans, principals of colleges and heads of academic departments. Institutional leadership. Ivory tower. Arcane. But the vast majority of those involved in educational leadership (particularly at postgraduate levels) work primarily in hospitals and community settings, are practicing clinicians, and deliver care to patients while carrying the responsibility for systems of education and training that must prepare the professionals of the future. And all of this occurs within a rapidly changing healthcare context that is increasingly challenging and uncertain.

The foregrounding of leadership as an essential 'non-technical skill' (Fletcher et al. 2002) for health professionals is emphasized in standards frameworks and core curricula around the world (e.g. Royal College of Physicians and Surgeons of Canada 2010; General Medical Council 2009). Effective leadership is widely considered a prerequisite for the delivery of high quality healthcare (Institute of

T. Swanwick, MA, MBBS, FRCGP, MA, FAcadMEd (✉)
Postgraduate Medical Education, Health Education North Central and East London, London, UK
e-mail: tim.swanwick@ncel.hee.nhs.uk

J. McKimm, MBA
College of Medicine, Swansea University, Swansea, West Glamorgan, UK
e-mail: j.mckimm@swansea.ac.uk

Y. Steinert (ed.), *Faculty Development in the Health Professions: A Focus on Research and Practice*, Innovation and Change in Professional Education 11, DOI 10.1007/978-94-007-7612-8_3, © Springer Science+Business Media Dordrecht 2014

Medicine 2011; King's Fund 2011) and a range of publications cite leadership as a fundamental underpinning of professional practice (e.g. van Mook et al. 2012). Nowhere is this more true than for those health professionals who have the challenge of working in the dual contexts of the academic institution (which awards professional qualifications) and the clinical environment in which much of the learning takes place.

As a result, faculty development plays a vitally important role in ensuring that those who lead and manage the education and training of health professionals have the knowledge, skills and attitudes appropriate to their role and organization. In this chapter, we use the term 'educational leadership' – as opposed to the 'clinical leadership' of teams, departments, units and specific clinical situations – to include the leadership and management of organizations, departments, resources, research studies, projects, curricula, assessment and innovations. Common to both the educational and clinical contexts, leadership can be found at 'all levels', distributed or dispersed, throughout the organization. And both clinical and educational leadership involve autonomous professionals with their own professional identities, with the consequence that leadership often requires the mobilization of both positional and professional power. We explore these issues later in the chapter.

For some professions, such as medicine, learners will be engaged in training programs for anything up to 15 years. Ensuring that curricula and competency frameworks genuinely help prepare learners for independent professional practice is a huge challenge given the slow pace of change in academic organizations. Alongside these pedagogic issues, educators (particularly in academic institutions) are increasingly required to perform more administrative and management functions, respond to demands from regulators and funding bodies around quality assurance, carry out research activities, and teach more students within increasing economic constraints. Delivering a high quality learning experience on this 'crowded stage' challenges educators across all health professions more than keeping up to date with subject discipline and educational knowledge and skills (McKimm and Swanwick 2011).

Such challenges also raise some specific issues for faculty members as many come through a vocational clinical route into education or research and, in doing so, have to make career transitions from clinician to teacher, and then from teacher/researcher to manager and leader. Other educators from academic, biomedical or social science environments are required to make similar transitions. And whilst (in high income countries at least) the professionalization of teachers in higher education and clinical settings is becoming embedded, with a plethora of courses and programs available for health professionals to help develop their understanding and skills as teachers (see Chap. 2), faculty development targeted specifically at leadership and management is relatively new. This chapter sets out the rationale for introducing such provision and describes some of the ways in which healthcare and academic organizations and individuals might 'learn leadership'.

3.2 Models, Concepts and Theories of Leadership

Concepts of leadership have developed over the last 60 years as leaders and leadership emerge in response to preoccupations of the time and socio-cultural change. In trying to describe 'what works' (and what doesn't), a range of theoretical models have been generated. It is important to note, however, that the emergence of a new model does not mean that older models are discarded; rather, they are reconceptualized. A Google™ search on 'leadership' brings up over 120,000,000 sites, and so we can only just touch on some of the main theories and concepts about leadership in this section.

Leadership models and theories can be categorized in a number of ways. Although there is clearly some overlap between theories, for the purposes of this chapter, which discusses the faculty development of health professions educators, we will group them as follows:

1. Those which focus on the personal qualities or personality of the leader as an individual.
2. Those which relate to the interaction of the leader with other people.
3. Those which seek to explain leadership behaviors in relation to the environment or system.

Considering the theories from these perspectives enables faculty development activities to be tailored to achieve the desired outcomes of the individual, the team or the organization. Table 3.1 lists some of the commonly described theories, concepts and models that can be found in the vast literature on leadership. The numbers in brackets (i.e. 1, 2 or 3) relate to how the theories relate to the three categories described above.

Kouzes and Posner (1995) suggest that leadership is an observable, learnable set of practices. Leadership is not something mystical and ethereal that cannot be

Table 3.1 Some commonly described leadership theories, concepts and models[a]

Leadership theories, concepts and models	
Adaptive leadership (3)	Engaging leadership (2)
Affective leadership (1, 2)	Followership (2)
Authentic leadership (1, 2)	Leader-member-exchange (LMX) theory (2)
Charismatic leadership (narcissistic) (1)	Ontological leadership (1)
Complex adaptive leadership (3)	Relational leadership (2)
Collaborative leadership (2, 3)	Servant leadership (1, 2, 3)
Contingency theories (2, 3)	Situational leadership (2, 3)
Dialogic leadership (2)	Trait ('great man') theory (1)
Distributed, dispersed, shared leadership (2, 3)	Transactional leadership (2, 3)
Eco-leadership (3)	Transformational leadership (1, 2, 3)
Emotional intelligence (EI) (1, 2)	Value led, moral or wise leadership (1, 2)

[a]For those interested in exploring leadership theories and concepts in more depth, Northouse (2012) provides a useful starting point

understood by ordinary people. Given the opportunity for feedback and practice, those with the desire and persistence to lead – to make a difference – can substantially improve their abilities to do so (p. 386). Taking the idea that leaders and leadership can be developed, how can faculty developers use these theories or models to help explain why certain leadership approaches might work best in the context of healthcare education and training? Let us consider each in turn.

3.2.1 Theories Focusing on Leaders' Personal Qualities or Personality

Trait theories have a long history in that 'great' leaders were often seen as endowed with certain characteristics, which sometimes related to their position (e.g. religious leaders or monarchs). Such characteristics or qualities include being consistent, trustworthy, inspiring and authentic, and displaying appropriate emotion, values and moral courage (Avolio and Gardner 2005; Kouzes and Posner 2002). Despite the doubt cast on such 'great man' theories, personality traits appear to be an important pre-condition of effective leadership with positive, if weak, correlations found between the personalities of those in leadership positions and the 'Big Five' factors of extraversion, openness to new experience and conscientiousness and a negative correlation with neuroticism or anxiety (Judge et al. 2002). Such individualistic approaches have been criticized for venerating the 'hero leader' (King's Fund 2011). However, concepts such as servant leadership (Greenleaf 2002), in which the leader 'serves first', ontological leadership (Erhard et al. 2010; Souba 2010), which is about 'being' a leader rather than 'doing leadership,' or the 'incomplete', fallible leader (Ancona et al. 2007), who is authentic in their behaviors, all seem very relevant to leadership in the health professions, where professional behaviors and role modeling are vitally important. The idea of leaders being in tune with their emotions as they engage in 'people work' (affective leadership) also resonates well with educators' primary role of developing the next generation of health professionals (Held and McKimm 2012). Nonaka and Takeuchi (2011) suggest that leaders need to develop practical wisdom or 'phronesis', which Hilton and Slotnick (2005) suggest is a core component of medical professionalism. These wise leaders are able to:

> … assess what is good; quickly grasp the essence of situations; create contexts for learning; communicate effectively; exercise political power to bring people together; and encourage the development of practical wisdom in others through apprenticeship and mentoring (Nonaka and Takeuchi 2011, p. 61).

Based on these perspectives, faculty development activities would aim to primarily develop the individual's leadership behaviors, competencies and potential over the long-term. Strategies and activities that have been found to be helpful in developing individuals' self-insight and understanding of their impact on others include personal development planning, analysis of strengths and areas for development, mentoring and coaching, workplace based feedback (e.g. multisource feedback) and the use of psychometric tests such as the Myers-Briggs Type Indicator (Myers et al. 1998) or Hogan Personality Inventory (http://www.hoganassessments. com/hogan-personality-inventory).

3.2.2 Theories Relating to the Interaction of Leaders with Others

Most leadership theories understandably offer explanations of how leaders can best work with others to engage and influence them and facilitate change. Early models, such as transactional leadership (Burns 1978) and leader-member-exchange theory (Seibert et al. 2003), looked at how leaders worked with others reciprocally to improve organizational performance by offering rewards, imposing sanctions and enabling participation in the leaders' 'in-group' (Heifetz and Linsky 2004). Models such as Goleman's work on Emotional Intelligence (EI) and leadership styles (2000) can be helpful in offering a framework for leaders to consider different contexts and situations and adopt an appropriate style or approach to motivate others and regulate disruptive emotions. Goleman (2000) suggests that the emotionally intelligent leader requires competencies in self-awareness, self-regulation/management, social awareness, empathy and relationship management.

The idea that leaders can adopt different approaches, behaviors or styles from some sort of 'menu' suggests that (a) leadership can be learned and developed through training and feedback, and (b) that leadership behaviors are contingent on situations or those involved (i.e. contingency theories, situational leadership). This perspective also moves us away from the idea of leadership being primarily rooted in personality. Team development activities (very pertinent to the health professions where much of the work is carried out in teams) and developing understanding of erred ways of working in teams can be helpful. Faculty development activities that focus on working with whole (often multidisciplinary) teams to develop and hone leadership and team working skills can also be very powerful. Such activities might include simulated scenarios of clinical or managerial difficult situations which may involve manikins or actors simulating others or case study scenarios around service redesign using role play.

Unlike some management activities which might be carried out in isolation (such as writing a report or strategy document), leadership is relational and dia- logical and therefore primarily involves working with people (Isaacs 1999; Lieff and Albert 2010; Souba 2011; Uhl-Bien 2006). We explore the distinctions between leadership and management later in the chapter. Leaders need 'followers' and there is a growing literature considering the concept of 'followership'. Grint and Holt's (2011) typology of followership is based on authority, certainty and uncertainty in considering the complexity and types of problems ('wicked' or 'tame') that orga- nizations face. Other writers (e.g. Kellerman 2007; Kelley 1988) consider the nature of power relations between leaders and followers, highly relevant to healthcare and health professions education in which there are longstanding power and status differentials between professional groups, hierarchically structured organizations, and students, patients and teachers.

Faculty development activities building on these perspectives would focus on developing the leader's competence in relation to others, through team-based activities or multi-source feedback supported by the acquisition of a knowledge base to provide frameworks which the leader can use in work situations.

3.2.3 Theories Explaining Leadership in Relation to the Environment or System

These theories are probably the most recent in terms of the business and health environments, considering the organization (or subsets thereof) as complex and dynamic social systems, and the leader as 'adaptive' (Doll and Trueit 2010; Fullan 2005; Mennin 2010). A leader's role here is to understand the internal system (formal and informal structures and processes) and its relationship with the external environment, From this perspective, change is effected through alignment of people and processes and pushing the system towards emergent change. Bolman and Gallos (2011) suggest that the use of metaphor or 'frames' is helpful in assisting academic leaders to conceptualize the organization from the different perspectives of those working and learning within it.

A primary leadership role is that of 'change agent' and leaders need to work with followers to effect lasting and transformational change (Fullan 2007; Kellerman 2008). The concept of 'transformational leadership' (Bass and Avolio 1994) has been highly influential in public services, in which leaders work with others to motivate and inspire them to higher order thinking and value–based change. Although transformational leadership enshrines elements of all three categories, it has been criticized for focusing too much on the individual 'charismatic' (potentially narcissistic and dangerous) leader rather than focusing on system-wide interventions and the building of 'social capital' (Bolden et al. 2009). Many organizations have been led into failure by a combination of the charismatic, powerful leader operating without effective governance and monitoring systems. The concepts of shared, distributed, dispersed and collaborative leadership (King's Fund 2011) are now starting to come to the fore, replacing concepts primarily vested in individuals. Not only does this approach sit more comfortably with health professionals' values and ways of working, but it also enables organizations to spread risk and build organizational resilience. More recently, echoing a focus on sustainability as a key feature of all systems, the concept of eco-leadership has been described as an emerging discourse within these post-heroic paradigms (Western 2011). Eco-leadership emphasizes connectivity, inter-dependence and an ethical, socially responsible stance – similar in some ways to servant leadership.

Seen through this lens, faculty development therefore needs to focus on system-wide interventions, developing organizational capacity to adapt to the changing environment, building sustainable leadership at all levels and empowering health professionals to collaborate interprofessionally and transprofessionally to effect meaningful and lasting change. Leadership development is most effective when linked with organizational development and although it may prove costly, taking a holistic organizational approach to leadership development (e.g. employing external consultants to work with all departments and individuals) can help deliver long-standing and deep-rooted cultural change.

In the above, we have discussed leadership as if it exists as a discrete entity. In reality however, health professionals are appointed to *managerial* positions or given managerial responsibilities from which they are *expected* to lead, so they must be able to understand management, and possess managerial skills as well as those of leadership. Described further below, the implications of this for faculty developers is that they must fully understand leadership and management theory as applied to the healthcare professions education context, so that the most relevant theoretical approaches can be taken. The ever-changing dynamic between rapidly evolving leadership theory and health services in constant flux means that faculty developers who deliver leadership development need to be fully aware of both the academic and health service contexts, so that theory can be closely aligned and applied appropriately.

3.3 Management, Administration and Leadership

In the past (and currently in more traditional settings) academics were seen as primarily responsible for the academic content and structure of programs, for ensuring appropriate program delivery, for designing assessments, and for evaluating educational effectiveness and quality. Academics also carried out research as well as teaching, and conducted some administrative tasks such as chairing committees, managing budgets or collating examination results. University administrators were seen as providing support for academic endeavors and programs and ensuring that appropriate management systems and processes were in place. Today, educational leaders are increasingly required to demonstrate effective managerial skills, blurring the boundary between the academic and the administrative. This in itself can cause tension and a need to negotiate responsibilities for all those involved in planning, delivering and evaluating educational programs; however, the reality is that the educational leader (at whatever level) needs to have many more skills than before, ranging from business management and entrepreneurship to program administration and evaluation.

Mirroring the merging of academic and administrative functions, the lines between leadership and management described in the literature are also less clearly drawn than they once were. Until relatively recently, leadership was seen

Table 3.2 Traditional distinctions between leadership and management

Management	Leadership
Produces order and consistency through	*Produces change and movement through*
Planning and budgeting	Setting direction
Problem solving	Problem defining
Organizing and staffing	Building commitment
Controlling and monitoring	Motivating and sustaining

Adapted from Northouse (2012)

as a sub-set of management and much of the business literature focused on management rather than leadership. More recently, leadership has become the ascendant term, promoted in almost all walks of life as a panacea for most world problems.

Typologies that distinguish between leadership and management abound and a typical description is provided in Table 3.2. But these are entwined, complementary and mutually dependent activities and a number of writers (Bolman and Deal 1997; Covey et al. 1994; Gosling and Mintzberg 2003; Kotter 1990a, b) highlight that separating leadership from management at best simply does not reflect the real world and is, at worst, dangerous. Leaders who cannot manage effectively risk alienation and disconnection from those who work with them and from their organization's goals and priorities. This can potentially cause destruction and damage through, for instance, financial mismanagement or ignorance of legal or human resource processes. Conversely, management without wise and visionary leadership can result in dispirited organizations, unable to respond to change. What organizations, teams and groups need is a combination of effective leadership and good management: leadership that aligns, empowers and inspires people and creates vision, change and movement, and management that ensures stability, consistency and order.

In Sect. 3.2 we discussed differing models and concepts of leadership. Depending on the theoretical framework selected, each naturally infers their own (broadly similar) sets of leadership competencies. Indicative curriculum content in relation to leadership development is also provided later on in the chapter, but at this point it seems appropriate to surface the many (sometimes seen as less glamorous) skills that educators need to develop that clearly fall under the umbrella of 'management'. Table 3.3 describes some common management activities, summarizes why these are important in the context of health professions education and suggests some work-based development activities that might help educators acquire and develop these skills. Most organizations will have courses available to senior educators, although these are typically offered once a person has attained a management position and not offered as a routine part of development or succession planning. We discuss below how taking a 'whole organization' approach to embedding leadership development at all levels can help better prepare people for management positions and strengthen the organization.

Table 3.3 Management activities for educators in the health professions

Management activities	Why is this important?	Development activities
Understanding, controlling and managing budgets	Vital to stay within budgets, to do this you need to know what the budget allocation is and be able to actively manage it through setting priorities and sensible procurement	Find out who is responsible for what budget and how the planning and budgeting cycle works
	You can make educational changes once you know the budget, to fund new initiatives or change priorities in response to internal or external changes	Ask to be involved in budget setting and management for your area of work
	Education and training budgets are often amongst the first to be cut – stay ahead of the game	Get involved in (or offer to chair) finance committees and other resource allocation groups
	Budgets that support clinical teaching and training at all levels are often very complex	Find out about how budgets for clinical placements and training are allocated, nationally, regionally and locally
Human resource (people) management	Organizations invest most of their time and money in people	Learn about the formal processes in place in your organization
	Being able to delegate and work with people is vital to get tasks done (and done well)	Get feedback on the way you work with others, through multisource feedback or more informally
	Understanding formal processes (recruitment, appraisal, performance management, etc.) will help you support and develop your team	Practice delegating, don't take on everything yourself
		Offer to get more involved with recruitment (e.g. writing job descriptions, interview panels) and appraisal
Physical resources and facilities	Classrooms, equipment, laboratories, clinical placements/appropriate case mix, simulation, communication and IT facilities are all vital to deliver high quality experiences but are expensive	Find out how facilities are planned for, allocated and managed: is there a teaching resources/facilities plan?
	As teaching/learning experiences and students and other stakeholder's expectations change, learning resources need to adapt	Visit other establishments, and find out what the requirements of future education are going to be
	Faculty development is required to keep pace with technological or educational changes	Discuss internally whether your facilities are appropriate for current and future learning and what new facilities might be needed

(continued)

Table 3.3 (continued)

Management activities	Why is this important?	Development activities
Business planning (e.g. strategic, departmental and operational plans)	These set out organizational and lower level goals, priorities and a strategy so that everyone is working in the same direction Aims and goals help determine the strategy (what needs to be done to achieve the goals) Without a plan, you can't set priorities or allocate budgets and other resources, recruit and retain people and develop new initiatives Reviewing plans enables evaluation of activities and planning of next steps	Look at your organization's strategic plan (which should be in the public domain) and also departmental plans Set out a plan for your team, program or initiative in line with organizational plans Find out about some basic management tools (e.g. SWOT analysis)
Curriculum/program management	A beautifully designed program that won't work in practice will fail and falter Need to work out to the finest detail how a curriculum will be operationalized with clear systems and processes Managing requires everyone to know their responsibilities and resources to be allocated appropriately Effective program management reassures internal and external stakeholders and provides a basis for review and change	Find out about how curricula/programs are managed in your organization Are roles and responsibilities clearly stated, how do academic and administrative staff work together, how do committees function? Get involved in curriculum planning, management and review, take on a key responsibility
Project management	All short term activities can benefit from a project management approach Project managing helps identify and manage risks, options, key stakeholders, budget, time and other resources required Many healthcare organizations have formal project planning processes in place	Find out about basic project management techniques (e.g. GANTT charts, critical path analysis) project planning and put them into practice with a project or initiative Get involved in projects and look at the project plan (often required for funding bodies)
Understanding the internal environment	Understanding the formal structures, processes, roles and responsibilities of your organization is essential for good management and to effect change Understanding the 'shadow side' (the informal rules, rituals, power struggles and ways of working) can also help you influence change and make things happen	Find out about your organization: managerial hierarchy/organizational tree; committee structures and terms of reference; departmental structure; etc. Consider the informal side – who wields influence, do you know the key players, how would you get things done, what are the rules and rituals in your organization?

Understanding the external environment	Because health professions education is carried out in multiple contexts, understanding the external environment, systems, stakeholders and processes is essential	Find out about the key external organizations that your program/organization interacts with and their own internal structures and processes Use tools such as PESTLE (political, economic, socio-demographic, technological, legal, environmental) to assess the key factors in the external environment and how these might impact on your organization/program
Understanding and developing management systems (including IT) and processes	Educational management is increasingly IT based Effective management systems improve quality and data handling and support a range of activities The technical system should not drive the educational process – but it often does	Learn to use (or use better) the management and educational IT systems that support your program delivery and evaluation See what other organizations have in place – is there anything you might use Make sure you understand the basics of data protection legislation
Educational quality, evaluation	Quality assurance, management and enhancement mechanisms and reports are required by internal higher stakeholders (e.g., universities) as well as external bodies (funders, regulators, professional bodies) Thorough and robust QA mechanisms enable issues to be identified and addressed early and for longer-term program review and reform	Find out what the QA requirements are for your program/curriculum and from whom Look at reports from stakeholders (internally and in the public domain) What internal processes are in place Get involved with preparing reports and internal and external evaluation reviews
Time management (self and others)	Effective time management makes best use of everyone's time and gets more done It is the basis of many other management activities (e.g. projects, chairing meetings etc.)	Agree priorities (for yourself and others) and review regularly Make a plan, write lists (and stick to them) Build in time for interruptions and dealing with administration and emails (all part of work, not an add on)
Chairing or being involved in committees	Committees are the formal ways in which organizational decisions are made Understanding how committees work can help you get your ideas discussed and make effective changes	Get involved, offer to participate or chair committees, project groups and working parties Learn how to set an agenda (it will differ in different contexts), chair effectively (by observing others) and produce good minutes/records (reading minutes for sense making and clarity)

3.4 General Approaches to Leadership Development

So when it comes to leadership, what is the best way to approach the development of this range of complex social processes?

Across the board, there is a dearth of high quality evidence to support a growing range of leadership development practices. Indeed, this was one of the findings of a recent BEME review which looked at the evidence for interventions used in the leadership development of faculty members in the health professions (Steinert et al. 2012), as outlined in Table 3.4. The key, then, may be to go back to the *object* of the activity. Leadership, management and organizational development can be seen as being part of the same process, that of 'increasing the capacity of organizations and the people within them to better achieve their purpose' (Bolden 2010, p. 117). This takes us beyond historical, but continuingly pervasive conceptions of leadership development that focuses on training individuals to take on increasingly responsible and complex roles and involves a shift in emphasis from the *development of*

Table 3.4 Faculty development initiatives designed to promote leadership in medical education: Key findings of a BEME systematic review

Review of the evidence identified:
41 studies of 35 different interventions
Lack of methodological rigor and sophistication of research design
Most evaluation data were collected post-intervention and consisted of participants' responses to questionnaires and interviews

Participants reported:
High satisfaction with faculty development programs, finding them useful, and of personal and professional benefit
Positive changes in attitudes toward their own organizations as well as their leadership capabilities
An increased awareness of, and commitment to, their institution's vision and challenges
A greater self-awareness of personal strengths and limitations, increased motivation, and confidence in their leadership roles
A greater sense of community and appreciation of the benefits of networking
Increased knowledge of leadership concepts, principles, and strategies
Gains in specific leadership skills
Increased awareness of leadership roles in academic settings
Changes in leadership behavior
Limited changes in organizational practice

Features contributing to positive outcomes included the use of:
Multiple instructional methods within single interventions
Experiential learning and reflective practice
Individual and group projects
Peer support and the development of communities of practice
Mentorship
Institutional support

Adapted from Steinert et al. (2012)

individual leaders to that of *leadership development*. Leadership development is an investment in social capital which builds the organization's leadership capacity at all levels as well as the human capital of individual competence and capability.

Within this shifting paradigm, a number of secondary themes in the wider leadership development literature can be identified, summarized as an evolution in thinking about:

- **The educational approach**: moving from the provision of training to a focus on ongoing leadership development embedded in systems and organizational processes (e.g. appraisal).
- **Where learning is situated**: relocating from the classroom to the workplace.
- **How career development is considered**: reprioritizing from organizational requirements to a consideration of individual needs.

These trends point us in the direction of some particular strategies for program design and the selection of appropriate faculty development interventions.

3.4.1 From Training to Development

At the centre of the argument about the effectiveness of leadership development lie some fundamental questions about whether or not leadership can be learned. As we discussed earlier, trait theories of leadership suggest that there are innate qualities that mark our leaders, whereas behaviorist and competency-based movements maintain that leadership behaviors can be acquired. The truth probably lies somewhere in between. More recently, along with the development of how we think about leadership, has come about a paradigm shift in leadership development from instructor-centered teaching to learner-centered personal transformation. Antonacopoulou summarizes:

> The transformation paradigm, with intellectual roots in constructivism, social constructiv-ism and interactionism, emphasizes co-creation, interpretation, discovery, experimentation and a critical perspective. Rather than learning leadership as it is known by others, learners make sense of their own experiences, discover and nurture leadership in themselves and in each other, not in isolation but in community (Antonacopoulou 2004, p. 82).

The rationale for such an approach, argues Antonacopoulou (2004), is that if leadership's prime purpose is to make sense to others of a constantly changing world, then the crucial question in leadership development becomes not *what* to learn but *how* to learn (i.e. how to remain receptive and adaptable to new situations, new con-texts and new configurations of human and organizational relationships). Conversely, as Hodgson (1999) highlights, 'People who have learned leadership as a series of rules will have an inherent inflexibility which will eventually be their downfall... telling people how to lead is roughly equivalent to painting by numbers' (p. 129).

A useful taxonomy that exposes some of these underlying assumptions of lead-ership development is proposed by Holman (2000). Each of Holman's four 'models of management education' highlights differing philosophical beliefs about learning

Academic liberalism	Experiential vocationalism
Aims to pursue objectivity in order to produce the management 'scientist'. Delivery occurs through lectures, case studies, seminars.	Aims to equip managers with the skills they need for 'the job'. Competence-based approaches, including short courses, assignments and e-learning, predominate.
Experiential liberalism	**Experiential/critical**
Aims to create the reflective practitioner capable of applying theory thoughtfully to practice. Delivery is grounded in action-learning and self-development	Aims to foster a more reflexive approach and a higher order of criticality resulting in a practitioner able to challenge established forms of action. What is the delivery?

Fig. 3.1 Models of management education (From Holman 2000)

and the nature of management (see Fig. 3.1). As advice to program designers, Holman counsels that an over-reliance on either theory ('academic liberalism'), or action ('experiential vocationalism') is unlikely to achieve the desired results, favoring instead interventions that are built around critical reflection and action learning.

3.4.2 From the Classroom to the Workplace

Mintzberg argues that 'using the classroom to help develop people already practicing management is a fine idea, but pretending to create managers out of people who have never managed, is a sham' (Mintzberg 2004, p. 5). Mintzberg's jibe at the proliferation of classroom-based MBAs concords with a growing consensus that leadership development should be both drawn from, and embedded in, work-based activities. McCall et al., at the Center for Creative Leadership, summarized this neatly as far back as 1988 (cited in Lombardo and Eichinger 2000), proposing that in effective leadership development programs, 70 % should be work or project-based; 20 % should occur through personal development as a result of, for example, working and interacting with others, multisource feedback and coaching; and 10 % can be provided through formal training programs such as attendance at courses.

The following principles for best practice in leadership development, summarized in a review by Gosling and Mintzberg (2004), further emphasize the primacy of work-based learning:

- Leadership development only makes sense for people who have current leadership responsibilities.
- While the staff of development programs should be clear about what they want to teach, participants should be able to weave their own experience into the process.
- Leadership development should leverage work and life experience as fully as possible.

- The key to learning is thoughtful reflection. This means allowing time for it.
- Leadership development should be embedded and result in organizational development.
- Leadership development becomes a process of interactive learning.
- Every aspect of the education should aim to facilitate learning and development.

What these principles also, paradoxically, suggest, is that to reap the benefit of management and leadership development requires the design of 'appropriate approaches for specific situations rather than the adoption of a universal model of best practice' (Burgoyne et al. 2004, p. 49). So, a program that aims to develop research leadership skills may involve new principal investigators (i.e. they have leadership responsibilities); use case examples from good and failing research projects; include skills such as budget and project management and team building; and utilize relevant leadership theory (e.g. collaborative leadership for multi-centre projects). Alternatively, a program geared to develop health professions leaders in developing countries deliver public health strategies would focus on health management case studies, include strategic health systems management skills, and explore the impact of organizational structures, processes and culture on delivering effective healthcare. A wide range of leadership theories would also be included, as these leaders need a broad repertoire from which to draw.

3.4.3 Balancing Organizational Requirements with Individual Needs

Finally, in any leadership development program the career aspirations of individuals need to be considered. Indeed the goal of any successful program of continuing professional development is the alignment of organizational goals with individual needs. This balance is illustrated by a range of approaches identified in business leadership development by Clarke et al. (2004). In considering the 'who' and 'what' of leadership development, the authors develop four distinguishable approaches to how such programs may be presented within an organization. The resulting four approaches, which we can see at play in programs across the higher education and health sectors, are summarized in Fig. 3.2.

However, in contrast to the corporate universe of business and enterprise, in the increasingly complex world of health professions education, portfolio-working (i.e. having a number of different roles, jobs or employers) is the norm, and faculty members more often than not, maintain a clinical commitment as 'the day job'. Add to that, the impact of an increasingly feminized healthcare workforce with its attendant family and lifestyle decisions and 'organisations can no longer assume that those with identifiable potential will aspire to the management positions they would like them to occupy' (Sturges 2004, p. 263). For example, there is currently a severe shortage of clinical (medical) academics in the UK with some disciplines and specialties particularly affected. This affects not only research and educational

Who? What?	Leadership development targeted at individuals	Leadership development offered across the organisation
Individualized Content	High performing individuals are nurtured through tailored pro-grammes	Open opportunities provided for development but left to self-direction of the individual
Consistent Content	Planned activities for specific groups are driven by the needs of the organisation	Organisation-wide provision is cascaded down and available to all

Fig. 3.2 Approaches to leadership development (From Clarke et al. 2004)

activities in those areas, but also means that there are fewer role models in leadership positions with longer-term implications for strategic development and recruitment. Careers have become the 'property' of the individual, rather than the organization. And this is an important distinction, as organizational control over *who* they develop for positions of leadership and management diminishes, the control over *how* and *when* this occurs, is also severely weakened. Organizations also become less likely to invest in the leadership development of individuals who may move on or who work part-time and thus may offer more ad hoc, short, just-in-time courses rather than long term programs. Leadership development of course serves other purposes (both for the organization and the individual) than the purely developmental, and the benefits to both, of relationship-building, retention and renewal of a sense of shared purpose, should not be underestimated.

3.5   Specific Leadership Development Interventions

The design principles discussed above appear to move us from a pre-determined 'course' to a personalized 'program' rooted in real-world experience. But what does that look like in practice? No two leadership development programs will be the same, but a number of potential interventions are available for consideration, and a selection of these are briefly described.

3.5.1   Courses, Seminars and Workshops

With these principles of leadership development in mind, what can we hope to gain from leadership courses? There are a number of immediately tangible benefits. Courses and formal learning opportunities provide a cohort of participants with a sense of community and unity of purpose; they also offer participants a new shared language to think about and discuss salient issues. They provide time out for reflection and, through the support and challenge of others, encourage new ways of thinking about familiar situations. Although a one-off short course is unlikely to do much other than refresh or update skills, or perhaps enthuse a group of participants new to leadership and management concepts, programmatic approaches to short course development can punctuate work-place activities, coaching and feedback with vital fora for discussion and reflection. Beyond the immediate benefits, formal programs will often result in the establishment of a sustained, working network, either informal, supported by social media, or as part of a structured alumnus program.

3.5.2 Action Learning

'Action learning is a continuous process of learning and reflection, supported by colleagues, with the intention of getting things done' (McGill and Beaty 2001, p. 11). Individuals engaged in action learning work on real life problems with a small group of peers, where a combination of reflection, a commitment to act, and the support and challenge of peers creates a powerful environment for change and development. One variation on action learning is the technique of 'step back', where the problem is presented by a participant who then 'steps back' to listen and observe whilst the group works on the problem.

3.5.3 Coaching and Mentoring

Coaching and mentoring, and related activities (e.g. supervision, counseling, preceptorship) are often carried out to support leadership development. (See also Chap. 8.) For our purpose, we shall consider coaching and mentoring to lie on the same continuum of developmental conversations, with coaching tending to focus on the short term achievement of specific objectives and mentoring on the longer term advancement or development of an individual within an organization or community of practice. Many organizations provide formal mentoring schemes for faculty who are new to the organization or have been promoted to a leadership or management position (e.g. http://www.london.nhs.uk/leading-for-health/programmes/leadership-coaching). Such developmental conversations can be used synergistically with 360° appraisal, psychological tests or in aiding the transfer of classroom learning to the workplace.

3.5.4 Multi-source Feedback

Also known as 360° appraisal, the widespread adoption of multi-source feedback in human resource development is well documented (Alimo-Metcalfe and

Alban-Metcalfe 2006). Multisource feedback is now, of course, a familiar feature of the health professions education landscape, although care needs to be taken in how such tools are applied in practice. In the context of leadership development, Chappelow (2004) offers some helpful guidelines on how to use these tools to best benefit learners, namely that:

- 360° appraisal should not be used as a stand-alone event; rather, it should be integrated within a developmental program of challenge and support.
- Commitment from participants to engage with developmental goals arising from the appraisal and support from line managers are critical ingredients for success.
- The process works best when it starts at the top (i.e. the use of such tools is seen as a culturally acceptable norm).
- Poor administration of a 360° appraisal process within an organization can have disastrous consequences.
- Timing is crucial (e.g. to avoid redundancies).

3.5.5   Simulation

Simulation is a particularly effective vehicle for the rehearsal of leadership behaviors in the team context. Simulations may include a focus on practicing one-to-one communication skills, such as how to give constructive feedback to a colleague or deal with a difficult work-based situation, through to full immersion simulations involving whole teams or organizations. The problem, as with clinical simulation, is how the skills and approaches then 'transfer' to the workplace setting. Again, simulation is a tool best integrated within a program of development rooted in work-based activities. Ensuring that participants in simulation activities receive appropriate and constructive feedback, both in the moment and through structured debriefs, is essential as this is part of developing more insight and understanding into the impact of one's behaviors on others and how this can be improved.

3.5.6   Psychometric Tools That Help Facilitate Self-Insight

Zaleznik's somewhat chilling statement that 'leadership is a psychodrama in which a brilliant, lonely person must gain control of himself or herself as a precondition for controlling others' (Zaleznik 1977, p. 75) may be questionable 40 years on, but the emphasis on developing self-knowledge and insight in leadership development is as strong as ever. Programs of leadership selection and development employ a barrage of psychometric tests ranging from parlor games to high reliability psychological assessments. When used thoughtfully, they can provide a quick route to finding out information about people that may not be readily available through observation. They can also provide a neutral language and framework for discussing a participant's strengths and weaknesses. But psychometrics come with a number of health warnings; many instruments (including several in widespread use) have poor scientific underpinnings, the results of such tests rely on a degree of self-knowledge, and it is often the combination of resultant factors, rather than an individual 'trait', 'attribute' or 'preference', that is significant. As with multi-source feedback, psychometric tests should be included in any program but are best used as a starting point for discussion rather than being seen as offering some absolute truth.

3.5.7 Work-Based Initiatives

Shadowing, project work, consultancy, internships, and fellowships are all useful work-based vehicles for getting into the machinery of organizations. Coupled with coaching or action learning, the learning that results through participation can be real and powerful. See Chap. 7 for more information about work-based learning.

3.5.8 E-learning

Despite the convenience for students, attrition rates for e-learning are often high even in the more successful knowledge-based specialties (Martinez 2003). Romiszowski's review of e-learning (2004) is critical that the 'l' is often subjugated by the 'e'; that is, programmers tend to focus on the technology rather than the learning, although the rise of social media (Facebook, Twitter) coupled with mobile technologies have provided a new generation with a powerful vehicle for networking and support. Global communities of practice can now come together with ease, with near instant access to network members across the world. E- and m-learning (mobile learning using smart phones and other mobile technologies) can be very useful for keeping in touch and networking, as well as for gaining easy and round-the-clock access to 'theory', articles and web resources; however, because leadership development focuses on development of the individual, face-to-face learning is essential.

3.6 A Framework for Faculty Development

Whilst the short courses, workshops and development activities described above can be delivered on an ad hoc basis, if we take on board the idea of developing organizational capacity and social capital, a programmatic approach to faculty development in leadership needs to be taken. We therefore propose five principles for designing leadership development programs which should:

- *Be practical*: through the incorporation of the development of key skills such as coaching, change management and negotiation.

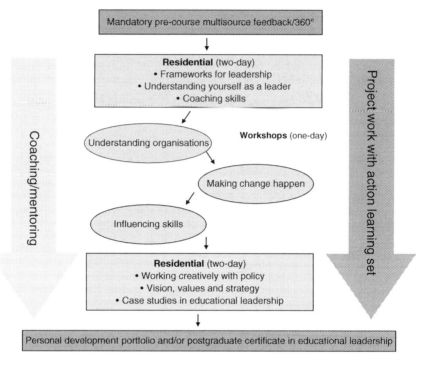

Fig. 3.3 Sample structure for a leadership development program (as outlined in Sect. 3.6)

- *Be work-oriented*: by including project work as a key component supported by action learning sets.
- *Be supportive of individual development*: through 360° feedback, coaching and mentoring.
- *Link theory to practice*: through the provision of selected leadership and management literature relevant to the educational context.
- *Build networks*: through action learning, coaching and social networking.

A sample structure for a leadership development program building on these principles is shown in Fig. 3.3. This generalized example, taken from a number of development programs in which the authors have been involved, incorporates a programmatic approach to leadership development, embodying the principles outlined above, coupled with a learner-centered approach to weaving theory with practical work-based projects, gathering feedback and processing this in a safe environment.

As far as more detailed 'curriculum content' is concerned, there are a growing number of leadership frameworks in the literature, from a wide range of different fields. Many institutions and professional bodies will have their own and, with minor variations, a similar list of competencies and topics tends to be covered in each. As with any program development, it is essential to clearly define the needs of the learners and the aims and outcomes required, and to select which of the vast array of theories, models and concepts will best underpin the activities and intended learning. Clearly, depending on the trainers' philosophical approaches, background and experience, and the needs of individuals and organizations, different approaches and emphases will be taken. Figure 3.4 illustrates two typical frameworks for health professionals, to which all the provisos contained in this chapter can be adapted and used to guide leadership development for faculty members in health professions education.

3.7 Conclusion

In a report from an 'Independent Commission' published in *The Lancet* in 2010, 20 professional and academic leaders from around the world expound their shared vision of the future of health professions education in an interdependent world (Frenk et al. 2010). The ten recommendations for reform are both challenging and illustrative of the increasingly complex system in which we operate. These recommendations can be seen as the 'to do' list for faculty members in the forthcoming century, one in which, as the Commission highlights, 'Professional educators are key players since change will not be possible without their leadership and ownership' (Frenk et al. 2010, p. 1954). If we were to search for a guiding purpose to underpin the faculty development of education leaders in the health professions, then the list in Table 3.5 would be an excellent starting point.

It is clear that developing the leadership and management skills, approaches and understanding of faculty members is central to effecting such transformational change and we have discussed some of the ways in which this might be achieved. The 'transformational' educator described above, who is required to work and lead health education organizations, curricula and teams in an increasingly complex global environment, will not only need to have subject discipline expertise and understanding of educational principles and practice but will also need to develop and demonstrate a range of leadership and management competencies. The establishment of system-wide leadership development therefore needs to be actively and proactively managed and embedded in curriculum design and delivery, faculty and educational development programs, performance management approaches and recruitment and retention policies. This in turn requires leaders at all levels to believe in and communicate a coherent vision and direction so that strategies and policies that enable educational change that ultimately improves health services can be implemented effectively. Developing and supporting faculty in this endeavor through 'learning leadership' is central to achieving this task.

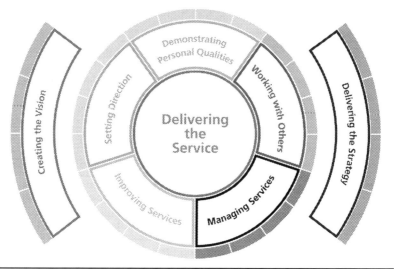

a NHS Leadership Framework (UK)

Demonstrating
Personal Qualities

Setting Direction

Creating the Vision

Working with Others

Delivering
the
Service

Delivering the Strategy

Improving Services

Managing Services

b NCHL Health Leadership Competency Model (US)

The NCHL model provides
breakthrough research and
a comprehensive database
for defining the competencies
required for outstanding
healthcare leadership
for the future.

TRANSFORMATION
Achievement Orientation
Analytical Thinking
Community Orientation
Financial Skills
Information Seeking
Innovative Thinking
Strategic Orientation

EXECUTION
Accountability
Change Leadership
Collaboration
Communication Skills
Impact and Influence
Information Technology
  Management
Initiative
Organizarional Awareness
Performance Measurement
Process Management/
  Organizational Design
Project Management

HEALTH LEADERSHIP

PEOPLE
Human Resources
  Management
Interpersonal
  Understanding
Professionalism
Relationship Building
Self Confidence
Self Development
Talent Development
Team Leadership

© Copyright 2004 National Center for Healthcare Leadership, All rights reserved.

Fig. 3.4 Leadership development competency frameworks. (**a**) *Leadership Framework (UK)* (NHS Leadership Academy 2011) © 2011 NHS Leadership Academy. All rights reserved (Permission granted to use the diagram by NHS Leadership Academy. Full details at www.leadershipacademy. nhs.uk). (**b**) *Health Leadership Competency Model (US)* (National Center for Healthcare Leadership 2010) (Permission granted to use the diagram by NCHL, full details at http://nchl.org)

Table 3.5 Proposed reforms for health professions education

Proposed reforms
1. Adoption of responsive, competency-based curricula that include competencies for dealing with global health issues and complex health and social systems.
2. Promotion of interprofessional and transprofessional education that enhances collaboration and team work and includes transferable competencies such as communication skills and analytical abilities.
3. Exploitation of the capacity and possibilities of IT in management and data handling systems to enable transformative education that equips learners for mastering large flows of information.
4. Harnessing global resources for local adaptation and implementation, including curricula, materials, and faculty and student exchange.
5. Strengthening educational capacity, capability and resources and investing in faculty development.
6. Developing and promoting a common set of professional attitudes, values and behaviors for all health professionals to prepare them for their role as change agents, accountable resource managers and promoters of evidence-based policies.
7. Establishing joint mechanisms to engage key stakeholders in policy and strategy development and in planning and managing resources, including the health workforce.
8. Expanding health education out of academic centers into system wide processes that engage primary care and communities.
9. Establishing global and regional consortia, networks and alliances to overcome the limitations of individual organizations or countries and share resources equitably.
10. Nurturing a culture of critical inquiry which mobilizes scientific knowledge, ethical debate and public reasoning to generate enlightened social transformation.

Adapted from Frenk et al. (2010)

3.8   Key Messages

- Leaders in the education of the health professions typically carry a dual responsibility of ensuring high quality education and safe and effective healthcare.
- Effective organizations require leadership at all levels and leaders need to learn to lead.
- Both leadership and management are vital for organizational performance.
- Leadership development requires specific solutions for different situations.
- Faculty development programs should be practical and work-focused, support individual development, link theory to practice and build networks.
- Longitudinal programs of development are required – in addition to short courses.

References

Alimo-Metcalfe, B. & Alban-Metcalfe, J. (2006). More (good) leaders for the public sector. *International Journal of Public Sector Management, 19*(4), 293–315.

Ancona, D., Malone, T. W., Orlikowski, W. J., & Senge, P. M. (2007). In praise of the incomplete leader. *Harvard Business Review, 85*(2), 92–100.

Antonacopoulou, E. P. (2004). Methods of 'learning leadership': Taught and experiential. In J. Storey (Ed.), *Leadership in organizations: Current issues and key trends*, (pp. 81–102). Abingdon, UK: Routledge.

Avolio, B. J. & Gardner, W. L. (2005). Authentic leadership development: Getting to the root of positive forms of leadership. *The Leadership Quarterly, 16*(3), 315–338.

Bass, B. M. & Avolio, B. J. (Eds.). (1994). *Improving organisational effectiveness through transformational leadership*. London, UK: Sage.

Bolden, R. (2010). Leadership, management and organisational development. In. J. Gold, R. Thorpe & A. Mumford (Eds.), *Gower handbook of leadership and management development*, 5th Ed., (pp. 117–132). Farnham, UK: Gower.

Bolden, R., Petrov, G., & Gosling, J. (2009). Distributed leadership in higher education: Rhetoric and reality. *Educational Management, Administration and Leadership, 37*(2), 257–277.

Bolman, L. G. & Deal, T. E. (1997). *Reframing organizations: Artistry, choice and leadership*. San Francisco, CA: Jossey-Bass.

Bolman, L. G. & Gallos, J. V. (2011). *Reframing academic leadership*. San Francisco, CA: Jossey-Bass.

Burgoyne, J., Hirsh, W., & Williams, S. (2004). The development of management and leadership capability and its contribution to performance: The evidence, the prospects and the research need. London, UK: Department for Education and Skills. Available from: https://www.education.gov.uk/publications/eOrderingDownload/RR560.pdf

Burns, J. M. (1978). *Leadership*. New York, NY: Harper & Row.

Chappelow, C. T. (2004). 360 degree feedback. In C. McCauley & E. Van Velsor (Eds.), *The Center for Creative Leadership: Handbook of leadership development*, (pp. 58–84). San Francisco, CA: Jossey-Bass.

Clarke, M., Butcher, D., & Bailey, C. (2004). Strategically aligned leadership development. In J. Storey (Ed.), *Leadership in organizations: Current issues and key trends*, (pp. 271–292). Abingdon, UK: Routledge.

Covey, S., Merrill, A. R., & Merrill, R. R. (1994). *First things first*. New York, NY: Simon and Schuster.

Doll Jr., W. E. & Trueit, D. (2010). Complexity and the health care professions. *Journal of Evaluation in Clinical Practice, 16*(4), 841–848.

Erhard, W. H., Jensen, M. C., & Granger K. L. (2010). *Creating leaders: An ontological model*. Harvard Business School: Harvard Working Paper Series. Retrieved February 15th, 2013, from http://hbswk.hbs.edu/item/6570.html.

Fletcher, G. C. L., McGeorge, P., Flin, R. H., Glavin, R. J., & Maran, N. J. (2002). The role of non-technical skills in anaesthesia: A review of current literature. *British Journal of Anaesthesia, 88*(3), 418–429.

Frenk, J., Chen, L., Bhutta, Z. A., Cohen, J., Crisp, N., Evans, T., et al. (2010). Health professionals for a new century: Transforming education to strengthen health systems in an interdependent world. *The Lancet, 376*(9756), 1923–1958.

Fullan, M. (2005). *Leadership and sustainability: Systems thinkers in action*. Thousand Oaks, CA: Corwin Press.

Fullan, M. (2007). *The new meaning of educational change (4th Ed.)*, Abingdon, UK: Teachers College Press.

General Medical Council. (2009). *Tomorrow's doctors: Outcomes and standards for undergraduate medical education*. Retrieved August 7th, 2012, from http://www.gmc-uk.org/education/undergraduate/tomorrows_doctors.asp

Goleman, D. (2000). Leadership that gets results. *Harvard Business Review, 78*(2), 78–90.

Gosling, J. & Mintzberg, H. (2003). The five minds of the manager. *Harvard Business Review, 81*(11), 54–63.

Gosling, J. & Mintzberg, H. (2004). The education of practicing managers. *MIT Sloan Management Review, 45*(4), 19–22.

Greenleaf, R. K. (2002). *Servant leadership: A journey into the nature of legitimate power and greatness (25th anniversary edition)*. Mahwah, NJ: Paulist Press.

Grint, K. & Holt, C. (2011). *Followership in the NHS*. Commission on Leadership and Management in the NHS. London, UK: The King's Fund. Available from: http://www.kingsfund.org.uk/sites/files/kf/followership-in-nhs-commississon-on-leadership-Management-keith-grint-claire-holt-kings-fund-may-2011.pdf

Heifetz, R. A. & Linsky, M. (2004). When leadership spells danger. *Educational Leadership, 61*(7), 33–37.

Held, S. & McKimm, J. (2012). Emotional intelligence, emotional labour and affective leadership. In M. Preedy, N. Bennett, & C. Wise (Eds.), *Educational leadership: Context, strategy and collaboration*, (pp. 52–64). Milton Keynes, UK: Open University Press.

Hilton, S. R. & Slotnick, H. B. (2005) Proto-professionalism: How professionalisation occurs across the continuum of medical education. *Medical Education, 39*(1), 58–65.

Hodgson, P. (1999). Leadership, teaching and learning. In Royal Society of Arts (Ed.), *On work and leadership*. Aldershot, UK: Gower.

Holman, D. (2000). Contemporary models of management education in the UK. *Management Learning, 31*(2), 197–217.

Institute of Medicine of the National Academies. (2011). *The future of nursing: Leading change, advancing health*. Washington, DC: The National Academies Press.

Isaacs, W. N. (1999). Dialogic leadership. *The Systems Thinker. 10*(1), 1–5.

Judge, T. A., Bono, J. E., Ilies, R., & Gerhardt, M. W. (2002). Personality and leadership: A qualitative and quantitative review. *Journal of Applied Psychology, 87*(4), 765–780.

Kellerman, B. (2007). What every leader needs to know about followers. *Harvard Business Review, 85*(12), 84–91.

Kellerman, B. (2008). *Followership: How followers are creating change and changing leaders*. Boston, MA: Harvard Business School Press.

Kelley, R. E. (1988). In praise of followers. *Harvard Business Review, 66*(6), 142–148.

King's Fund Commission on Leadership and Management in the NHS. (2011). *The future of leadership and management in the NHS: No more heroes*. London, UK: The King's Fund. Available from: http://www.kingsfund.org.uk/sites/files/kf/future-of-leadership-and-management-nhs-may-2011-kings-fund.pdf

Kouzes, J. M. & Posner, B. Z. (1995). *The leadership challenge: How to keep getting extraordinary things done in organizations*. San Francisco, CA: Jossey-Bass.

Kouzes, J. M. & Posner, B. Z. (2002). *The leadership challenge*. San Francisco, CA: Jossey-Bass.

Kotter, J. P. (1990a). What leaders really do. *Harvard Business Review, 68*(3), 103–111.

Kotter, J. P. (1990b). Management and leadership. In J. P. Kotter (Ed.), *A force for change: How leadership differs from management*, (pp. 3–8). New York, NY: Free Press.

Lieff, S. J. & Albert, M. (2010). The mindsets of medical education leaders: How do they conceive of their work? *Academic Medicine, 85*(1), 57–62.

Lombardo, M. M. & Eichinger, R. W. (2000). *The career architect development planner, (3rd Ed.)*. Minneapolis, MN: Lominger Limited.

Martinez, M. (2003). High attrition rates in e-learning: Challenges, predictors, and solutions. *The e-Learning Developers' Journal*. Retrieved December 9th, 2012, from http://www.elearningguild.com/pdf/2/071403MGT-L.pdf

McGill, I. & Beaty, L. (2001). *Action learning: A practitioner's guide (Revised 2nd Ed.)*. London, UK: Kogan Page.

McKimm, J. & Swanwick, T. (2011). Educational leadership. In T. Swanwick & J. McKimm (Eds.), *ABC of clinical leadership*, (pp. 38–43). Oxford, UK: Blackwell Publishing.

Mennin, S. (2010). Self-organisation, integration and curriculum in the complex world of medical education. *Medical Education, 44*(1), 20–30.

Mintzberg, H. (2004). *Managers not MBAs: A hard look at the soft practice of managing and management development*. San Francisco, CA: Berrett-Koehler Publishers Inc.

Myers, I. B., McCaulley, M. H., Quenk, N. L., et al. (1998). *MBTI manual: A guide to the development and use of the Myers-Briggs Type Indicator, (3rd Ed.)*. Palo Alto, CA: Consulting Psychologists Press.

National Center for Healthcare Leadership. (2010). *Health Leadership Competency Model*. Retrieved August 16th, 2012, from www.nchl.org/Documents/NavLink/Competency_Model-summary_uid31020101024281.pdf

NHS Leadership Academy. (2011). *Leadership framework*. Coventry, UK: NHS Institute for Innovation and Improvement.

Nonaka, I. & Takeuchi, H. (2011). The wise leader. *Harvard Business Review, 89*(5), 58–67.

Northouse, P. G. (2012). *Leadership, theory and practice, (6ᵗʰ Ed.)*. Thousand Oaks, CA: Sage Publications.

Romiszowski, A. J. (2004). How's the e-learning baby? Factors leading to success or failure of an educational technology innovation. *Educational Technology, 44*(1), 5–27.

Royal College of Physicians and Surgeons of Canada. (2010). *CanMEDS Physician Competency Framework*. Retrieved August 12th, 2012, from http://www.royalcollege.ca/portal/page/portal/rc/canmeds/framework

Seibert, S. E., Sparrowe, R. T., & Liden, R. C. (2003). A group exchange structure approach to leadership in groups. In C. L. Pearce & J. A. Conger (Eds.), *Shared leadership: Reframing the hows and whys of leadership*, (pp. 173–192). Thousand Oaks, CA: Sage Publications.

Souba, C. (2010). Perspective: The language of leadership. *Academic Medicine, 85*(10), 1609–1618.

Souba, W. (2011). Perspective: A new model of leadership performance in health care. *Academic Medicine, 86*(10), 1241–1252.

Steinert, Y., Naismith, L., & Mann, K. (2012). Faculty development initiatives designed to promote leadership in medical education. A BEME systematic review: BEME Guide No. 19. *Medical Teacher, 34*(6), 483–503.

Sturges, J. (2004). The individualisation of the career and its implications for leadership and management development. In, J. Storey (Ed.), *Leadership in organisations: Current issues and key trends,* (pp. 249–268). Abingdon, UK: Routledge.

Uhl-Bien, M. (2006). Relational leadership theory: Exploring the social processes of leadership and organizing. *The Leadership Quarterly, 17*(6), 654–676.

van Mook, W. N. K. A., Gorter, S. L., Kieboom, W., Castermans, M. G. T. H., de Feijter, J., de Grave, W. S., et al. (2012). Poor professionalism identified through investigation of unsolicited healthcare complaints. *Postgraduate Medical Journal, 88*(1042), 443–450.

Western, S. (2011). An overview of the leadership discourses. In M. Preedy, N. Bennett, & C. Wise (Eds.), *Educational leadership: Context, strategy and collaboration*, (pp. 11–24). Milton Keynes, UK: The Open University.

Zaleznik, A. (1977). Managers and leaders: Are they different? *Harvard Business Review, 55*(3), 67–78.

Chapter 4
Faculty Development for Research Capacity Building

Brian Hodges

4.1 Introduction

University faculty members typically strive to balance research and teaching, and for clinical faculty members, there is the further challenge of patient care. To support the latter clinical role, faculties have developed continuing education programs and for development of teaching skills, faculty development programs. Yet despite the almost universal imperative for scholarly productivity in addition to teaching (and clinical work), programs to help faculty members develop skills in research are not widely available. For example, in a survey of 110 physiotherapy programs in the United States, Rothman and Rinehart (1990) found few organized plans to help faculty members achieve scholarly goals or to foster growth in this area. The situation is similar in nursing, where the lack of programs for scholarly development has been described (Foley et al. 2003). In medicine, there have been substantial critiques of research quality and repeated calls for more research training (Beckman et al. 2009; Chen et al. 2004; Cook et al. 2008; Gruppen et al. 2011; Whitcomb 2002). Taken together, these papers shine light on a significant challenge in advancing scholarship and research in health professions faculties. To address this gap, Steinert (2011) has recommended an expansion of the traditional domains of faculty development (the development of teachers and pedagogical skill) to include specific development for scholarship and research. This chapter takes up that challenge and examines faculty development for research capacity. There is much wisdom to be

B. Hodges, MD, Ph.D., FRCPC (✉)
Department of Psychiatry, University of Toronto, Toronto, ON, Canada

University Health Network, Toronto, ON, Canada

Wilson Centre for Research in Education, Health Professions Education Research,
University of Toronto, Toronto, ON, Canada
e-mail: brian.hodges@utoronto.ca

Y. Steinert (ed.), *Faculty Development in the Health Professions: A Focus on Research and Practice*, Innovation and Change in Professional Education 11, DOI 10.1007/978-94-007-7612-8_4, © Springer Science+Business Media Dordrecht 2014

gained from the descriptions and evaluations of existing programs, but an even greater opportunity for the creation of new and innovative faculty development programs to foster research and scholarship.

4.1.1 Sources

In preparation for this chapter, information was gathered from leaders engaged in developing research and researchers in Canada, the USA and Europe, with a focus on health professions education research. These consultations and the more systematic literature review arose from a particular context: primarily colleagues and authors who write in English and work in Euro-American countries. As such, conclusions about what is good "evidence" and which practices are "best practices" require confirmation and validation when applied in other contexts and cultures.

4.1.2 Literature Review

The literature search was undertaken in English using Ovid Medline and repeated in Ovid Healthstar using the terms health professions/medical/nursing education (and their variations), research (and its variations) and faculty development. There is a relatively large literature on faculty development for research, ranging from the specific ('how to') to the conceptual ('faculty development and the mission of the university'), spanning from about 1984 to 2012. There was a flurry of writing on the topics from 2000 to 2006. The preliminary search yielded 376 abstracts, all of which were reviewed. Relevant articles were hand searched to identify secondary sources. A subtotal of 93 articles were read in depth and used to prepare this chapter: 36 from the search on medical education and faculty development, 29 from the search on nursing or other health professions and faculty development, 26 from the search of the general faculty development literature, and 2 from the search on faculty development and research generally; a further 36 were identified through hand searching secondary references across all of these categories.

4.2 Creating, Nurturing and Evaluating Programs of Faculty Development for Research

O'Sullivan and Irby (2011) have described the limitations of what they call the 'traditional' (p. 422) model of faculty development, which is organized around a linear notion that education flows from faculty members to learners to patients. This linear model is limited, they say, because it implies that patient-related outcomes (improved care, improved health) are achieved *via* student outcomes. They also critique this model because it leaves no place for context. A similar argument is made in nursing by Drummond-Young et al. (2010) who emphasize that a comprehensive faculty development program must involve instructional development, professional development, leadership development and organizational development. O'Sullivan and Irby identify four elements: context, participants, program and facilitator(s), all of which form an integrated community of practice for faculty development that they call a 'teaching commons' (2011, p. 324). This community of practice is itself embedded in a second and larger workplace community of teaching practice. In the literature, many agree with the notion that the context in which faculty members' work is at least as important as (some say more important than) the formal pedagogical instruction they receive. For this reason, I have taken up the challenge of O'Sullivan and Irby's model (if not the full model itself) throughout this paper. O'Sullivan and Irby themselves further elaborate their model in Chap. 18. In the next section, we explore participants, context, program (curriculum) and the role of mentors.

4.2.1 The Participants

Health professions schools spend a huge amount of time designing selection criteria and screening tools to identify applicants who will succeed as students. Oddly, the concept of matching faculty to development programs has received almost no attention. Yet there is literature on the characteristics associated with research productivity. For example, Levinson and Rubenstein (2000) argue that successfully undertaking research requires 'an intellectual commitment to discovery' (p. 910). Bland and Schmitz (1986) document ten critical features associated with successful researchers. Not surprisingly, this includes an in-depth knowledge of the research area and a mastery of methodological skills. However, they point out that other features are critical: having been socialized to academic values, the ability to form a relationship with a mentor, disciplined work habits, the ability to communicate and maintain professional contacts, being highly motivated, and the ability to work autonomously. 'Besides prerequisite knowledge and skills in a research area, successful researchers have academic values and attitudes derived from specific socialization experiences' (Bland and Schmitz 1986, p. 22).

Elen et al. (2007) argue that research development requires a different focus than the pedagogical 'skills paradigm' (p. 135). In the latter, academic development focuses on 'the development of concrete teaching competencies, often through training of well-defined teaching strategies or the presentation of 'tips and tricks' (Elen et al. 2007, p. 136). Rather than learning skills, Elen et al. suggest that the most important quality of a research educator is the development of a 'sophisticated epistemological belief system' (2007, p. 134). They argue that such a belief system is a disposition and that it is important that faculty members gain insight into the belief system of the research communities they wish to join. Further, it should not be assumed that just because an individual is experienced or even successful in previous research that they can undertake *any kind* of research. It has been suggested, for example, that basic scientists may have difficulty adapting to the contexts and approaches of education research (Brawer 2008).

There is, of course, great variation in the jobs that individual researchers have, ranging from those for whom research is a very minor component of a multi-faceted academic career, through to individuals for whom research is their principle academic activity. Attention to specific roles and networks in which individuals are embedded is important to ensuring the relevance and effectiveness of a program of development for research (Bakken et al. 2006).

4.2.2   The Context

As Arnold (2004) writes, 'although the characteristics of individual researchers influence productivity, the quality of research environments is even more important for generating scientific work' (p. 966). First and foremost then, faculty development for research must attend to context. Bland and Ruffin's (1992) 30-year review of literature on research productivity emphasizes the *delicate structure* required to successfully foster research and articulates 12 characteristics of a productive research environment. In medical education, Arnold (2004) similarly provides a helpful summary of elements of successful research groups based on eight case studies in the USA, Canada and Europe, all of which demonstrate the centrality of institutional support and investment of resources. Bakken et al. (2006) emphasize the interaction of individual characteristics and context and suggest specific interventions to optimize the career development of clinician researchers. These include: reducing role conflicts, providing continuity of research training, creating a positive mentorship culture and creating positive outcome expectations.

The context may be even more challenging in institutions that are *not* research intensive. Feldman and Acord (2002), writing about nursing, note 'colleges and universities without the resources of research-intensive universities face a special challenge to support faculty research' (p. 140). Mundt (2001) also describes the importance of creating programs that nurture research and scholarship in environments that do not naturally foster such activities. Such programs include linking faculty with external mentors who come from outside institutions that have a greater research focus.

Hafler et al. (2011) highlight a 'hidden curriculum' (p. 440) that greatly affects the lives and activities of faculty members. Their paper extends Hafferty's (1998) well-known argument about the effects of the hidden curriculum on student learning and asks why we educators have ignored the powerful hidden curriculum that drives faculty behavior. They note that 'efforts to improve the instructional value, impact, and/or relevance of formal faculty development programs will be dictated in part by the broader array of cultural messages that faculty members encounter as they go about learning what being a 'good faculty member' means' (Hafler et al. 2011, p. 442). The key elements of the hidden curriculum for faculty members, they write, are: promotion and tenure processes, space and time issues, salary structure and leadership. Shedding light on context and the faculty-level hidden curriculum specifically may be helpful to untangle the sobering evidence that, despite participation in activities designed to foster research (sometimes as extensive as a Masters program), many participants do not conduct more or better research.

It is clear that faculty development programs for research that neglect these contextual factors in the creation of programs for research development risk having reduced long-term impact. In addition to negative factors, there are important organizational and structural elements that help researchers flourish in some settings. Faculty development for organizational development is considered in Chap. 6. Institutions that wish to foster research will have to attend as much to organizational development as to faculty development.

4.2.3   The Program

In this section, we consider the key elements of a faculty development program for research, beginning with needs assessment and then focusing on various curricular structures, content requirements and pedagogical methodologies that can be used, before turning to consider the qualities and roles of facilitators and mentors.

4.2.3.1   Needs Assessment

As with any educational program, curriculum content and structure should respond to the needs of participants. And both should be based on a coherent set of objectives that are meaningful and achievable. It perhaps reflects the pressure for research productivity that faculty members face that they sometimes harbor fantasies of being able to master all the skills of research in a half-day course. Thus, one of the first tasks is to align participants' expectations with *realistic* course goals; defining course goals, in turn, is based on a solid needs assessment.

The literature suggests a strong desire for faculty members' research development. For example, a 2010 survey of 860 individuals in 76 countries (Huwendiek et al. 2010) explored perceptions about priorities for medical faculty development. The study, which achieved a 36 % response rate from an initial sample of 2,200 members of the Association for Medical Education in Europe mailing list, revealed that at the very top of a long list of priority areas was research methodology. This contrasted with areas in which participants reported having sufficient expertise (in their own view) such as: principles of teaching, assessment, curriculum development and other pedagogical topics. A similar, smaller study in nursing (Foley et al. 2003) surveyed 24 programs in the United States and noted that although few had formal faculty development programs, where they did exist, the focus was on teaching skills. Yet when individuals were asked about their priorities, research mentoring, scholarly writing and skills to obtain grants were at the top of the list.

In terms of the need for faculty development in specific areas, information can be gleaned from papers that critique the quality of current research. Common themes (that could be used to create a faculty development curriculum) include the need to: understand and define the link between interventions and patient outcomes (Whitcomb 2002); better align the objectives of study with appropriate methodology (Cook et al. 2008); and employ conceptual frameworks and theory to design better research projects (Bordage 2009).

An important issue to consider in program design is *which* research theories and methodologies will be taught, given that no one course, not even a PhD, could cover the whole breadth of research theory and methodology. Yet a solid grasp of theory and skillful command of methodology is key to doing good research. Therefore, difficult as it is, faculty developers working in this area have to make choices. Just as undergraduate programs suffer from trying to cover too many different topics, faculty developers should think long and hard about programs for research development that cram in too many different (and often theoretically incompatible) approaches. Is there time to deal with the fundamentally different underlying conceptions of positivism and constructivism, for example? Will there be time to deal with both the naturalistic, observational qualitative methods and controlled, experimentalist approaches? Will it be possible to deal with both coding and interpretation of language-based data as well as statistical approaches to numerical data?

These questions go to the heart of the critiques of quality in research generally and in health professions education specifically. Bordage (2000) observed that much research is undertaken in opportunistic settings, without a theoretical base, with little funding, and by isolated researchers, who publish in a dispersed fashion. If we take these observations as a starting point for a good curriculum, at a minimum it should address: sampling and study design; literature searching; using theory/conceptual frameworks; finding funding; developing a research team; and publishing systematically.

Choices for program structure range from short workshops, through longitudinal courses, mentorship programs and research groups, to graduate degrees. In the next section, we have aligned each of these approaches with a set of feasible purposes (Table 4.1) and provide references for published models and resources. Naturally, choice of curriculum content and model should rest on the needs assessment.

4.2.3.2 Short Workshops and Modular Programs

It is evident that a one-size-fits-all short workshop will not a competent researcher make. Yet a meaningful short workshop can be used to:

- Develop an approach to reading and using research as a *consumer.*
- Whet the appetite for a greater personal engagement in research.
- Develop knowledge/skills in a focal area: for example, getting grant funding, developing a research team/collaboration, or conducting an in-depth discussion about sampling strategies or of a particular form of data analysis.

Table 4.1 A classification of faculty development programs for research

Program type	Feasible purposes	Model programs	Resources
Short workshops and modular programs	Ability to approach research as a 'consumer' Wheting the appetite for greater engagement in research Asking good research questions Development of knowledge or skills in a focal area Introduction to research theories or methods (may be in more depth if a focused course)	Medical Education Research Certificate (AAMC Group on Educational Affairs, Gruppen et al. 2011) RESME/AMEE (http://www.amee.org/index.asp?pg=45) Wilson Centre Atelier (http://cre.med.utoronto.ca/About/AtelierHome.aspx)	RESME research guide (Ringsted et al. 2011) 12 tips for getting a grant (Blanco and Lee 2012) Workshop for writing in medical education (Steinert et al. 2008) Workshop for scholarly writing in nursing (Shatzer et al. 2010)
Longitudinal fellowships and scholars programs	Executing a scholarly project with support (not necessarily discovery research)	Medical Education Scholars Program (Gruppen et al. 2003)	Developing a scholarly project in education: A primer for medical teachers (Beckman and Cook 2007) Special edition of *Academic Medicine* (volume 81, issue 11, 2006) focusing on fellowships and scholars programs
Fulltime research fellowship programs (often linked to Masters programs)	Advanced skill development in research, with mentorship, aiming for a completed research project Core elements of research: design, literature review, ethics, data collection, analysis, publication, presentation	Wilson Centre Fellowship Program (Hodges 2004; Parker et al. 2010) University of California at San Francisco, Research Fellowship Program (Irby et al. 2004)	Education fellowship programs: Common themes and overarching issues (Gruppen et al. 2006)
Masters and doctoral degrees	Comprehensive research project or thesis External examination/peer review of work Peer-reviewed publication		Index of Masters and their curricula (Cohen et al. 2005) Worldwide inventory of Masters programs (Tekian and Harris 2012)

One common targeted use of a workshop is to develop skills of academic publication and grant writing. Paul et al. (2002), for example, found that grant writing seminars were associated with greater research productivity among occupational therapists. Blanco and Lee (2012) provide a helpful guide called 'Twelve tips for writing educational research grant proposals' that can be used in a workshop. Steinert et al. (2008) describe a workshop for academic writing in medical education consisting of a half-day workshop supplemented by peer writing groups and a manual for independent work. Shatzer et al. (2010) describe a program for nurses involving a workshop and mentorship program to develop scholarly writing. Their program focused on the fear of failure and writing anxiety, and they use a curriculum designed to bolster self-efficacy in writing.

Some use workshops to help educators effectively 'collaborate with more experienced researchers' and become 'better consumers of medical education scholarship' (Gruppen et al. 2011, p. 123). Given the pressure experienced by faculty members to be productive researchers themselves, workshop objectives of this kind must be clear to participants so as to avoid disappointing them.

However, the value and impact of a workshop may be extended with longitudinal components. For example, Coates et al. (2010) describe how the foundational knowledge introduced through a research certificate program (the Medical Education Research Certificate - MERC program) was extended to support the development of a real world research project by 'identifying persons with similar interests and establishing a consortium within which to conduct more robust research studies…' (p. 835). Indeed, evidence from continuing education research demonstrating that *one-shot* education sessions are of less value and produce fewer enduring results than longitudinal approaches (Davis et al. 1999) suggests that it is advisable to try to include a longitudinal component wherever possible.

International conferences such as the annual meetings of the Association for Medical Education in Europe (AMEE), Association of American Medical Colleges (AAMC) and the Canadian Conference on Medical Education (CCME), all provide short workshops on research. Some lead to a certificate, such as the Research Essentials in Medical Education (RESME) course that is associated with AMEE and the longer, modular Medical Education Research Certificate (MERC) developed by the AAMC Group on Educational Affairs (Gruppen et al. 2011). Indeed, many international meetings now include offerings in research skills development as conference organizers become aware that the huge demand for such courses is an opportunity for revenue generation. Goldszmidt et al. (2008) have noted, however, that even in a relatively wealthy country (Canada), nearly 50 % of their study participants report being discouraged from participating in such courses because of the cost.

The MERC program mentioned above was created in 2004 and provides 11 main topics, six of which are required to earn the certificate. (The curriculum is published in Gruppen et al. 2011.) The topics are: formulating research questions and designing studies; searching and evaluating the medical education literature; data management and preparing for statistical consultation; measuring educational outcomes with reliability and validity; research ethics; qualitative analysis methods in medical education; program evaluation and evaluation research; questionnaire design and survey research; qualitative data collection methods; scholarly writing and publishing; and hypothesis-driven research. Gruppen et al. (2011) underscore that the program is explicitly *not* designed to develop independent researchers, again an important message when communicating with potential participants. They also note that while the program committee experiences constant pressure to modify the program to do just that, they have held firm to their belief of the value and appropriateness of what they call the more 'modest goal' of 'providing participants with enough knowledge…to ask informed and focused questions of consultants and experts who can help plan studies and analyze results' (Gruppen et al. 2011, p. 125). The program has been successful and has grown consistently in enrolment, with over 140 individuals earning the certificate up to 2011. The authors highlight a number of challenges including the need for constant attention to the business model – sustainability being heavily influenced by tuition, facilitator stipends and number of participants per course.

The Research Essentials in Medical Education (RESME) course, created by AMEE in 2007, takes a somewhat different approach. This course is a self-contained, 4-day curriculum given during an AMEE (or other) conference. Major topics include an orientation to the field of medical education research; asking research questions; an introduction to quantitative design and analysis; and an introduction to qualitative design and analysis. The formal part of the curriculum is published in a manual that is used in the course (Ringsted et al. 2011). The balance of the course involves hands-on activities individually and in small groups to analyze and critique the actual research abstracts, posters and presentations given during the same conference. During the course, participants are expected to create the rough outline of a research proposal that can be refined in the year following the course through mentorship with one of the course facilitators. This course has also proved successful and has enrolled over 160 learners. In summary, modular, multi-day programs, though expensive and time-consuming, have met with considerable popularity.

4.2.3.3   Longitudinal Fellowships and Scholars Programs

In the last two decades, a popular model for faculty development in the health professions is the longitudinal program for education scholars, which involves a cohort of faculty members in a one to two-year curriculum (Fidler et al. 2007). Longitudinal programs are discussed in more detail in Chap. 10. Scholars programs and many fellowships, unlike the full-time programs described later, do not require faculty members to step out of their clinical or academic responsibilities on a full-time basis. A common model is a half-day session on a regular basis (weekly, bi-monthly or monthly depending on the program). While scholars programs and fellowships cover a range of topics including educational theory, pedagogical methods and assessment and leadership, most include a focus on scholarship broadly defined and some also include a component on research. (Many such programs are described in a special edition of *Academic Medicine* e.g. Hatem et al. 2006; Robins et al. 2006; Steinert and McLeod 2006; see also Wilson and Greenberg 2004).

To take but one of many examples, the Medical Education Scholars Program established at the University of Michigan in 1998 includes a research methods and design component in its curriculum as well as a required research project. Two published program evaluations document that participants were involved in more research publications, presentations and grants following the program (Gruppen et al. 2003; Frohna et al. 2006). Studies of other programs suggest increases in productivity, grant funding and promotion among participants in scholars programs (e.g. Coates et al. 2010; Steinert and McLeod 2006), though evaluations generally consist of uncontrolled study designs and self-reported outcomes.

Few articles report the actual objectives or curriculum for research embedded in a scholars programs. An exception is the University of California, San Francisco program (Muller and Irby 2006), which describes seven program objectives: develop skills in educational research sufficient to propose, conduct, analyze, and present a study; write a proposal with a well-defined research question; select appropriate research designs and measures; devise an analytical plan; identify characteristics of accepted and rejected studies; write an abstract; critique an educational research article (p. 962). Most programs require some sort of scholarly project, though generalizing across a diverse set of programs, these projects focus most often on development of curricula, assessment methods, and other innovations or application of new techniques and program evaluation, reflecting an emphasis on Boyer's (1990) categories of scholarship of application and of teaching, more than on research (Frohna et al. 2006; Muller and Irby 2006). This is logical given the comprehensive focus of scholars programs. Gruppen et al. (2011) however caution that:

> [E]mbedding an instruction strand on research skills into a broad faculty development curriculum has some definite strengths, but it also has limitations. One limitation is the risk that research skills receive diminished visibility when 'competing' with topics like teaching skills and educational methods (p. 122).

They go on to note that many institutions lack the infrastructure, resources and expertise to provide a robust curriculum in research skills.

A variation on the scholars program is to create a research support group. Beckman and colleagues (Beckman et al. 2009) created a program at Mayo Clinic that involves regular meetings of a group of scholars who are expected to participate in, present and critique a presentation on an actual project each month. The authors note that certain elements are necessary to make this model effective, including accountability (attendance and tracking of participants' scholarly activity), a spirit of mentorship, a focus on works-in-progress, and the deployment of protected time and money which is distributed to the group in a competitive fashion. They report a wide range of scholarly projects, with approximately one third consisting of research. This program uses a framework also published by Beckman and Cook (2007) for developing a scholarly project including: key steps of refining research questions, identifying designs and methods, and selecting outcomes. As with many of the programs in this category, the authors report that 'one problem is that … scholarly productivity is achieved by a minority of its members' (Beckman et al. 2009, p. 520).

4.2.3.4 Full-Time Research Fellowship Programs

More targeted still are fellowships specifically focused on research. There is a long tradition of such fellowships in clinical departments created to producing clinician-scientists with a graduate degree. This model was relatively unknown in health professions education until the last decade. One of the first published examples of a medical education research fellowship was by Irby et al. (2004) who described a program at the University of California. Meant to follow on from an education scholars program or general education Masters degree, the fellowship included funding support for protected time. The program was deliberately small, focusing on individuals thought to be good candidates for extramural funding and leadership.

On a larger scale, the Wilson Centre for Research in Education at the University of Toronto offers a fellowship program of 2–5 years for more than 30 individuals at a given time, placing a focus on research skills development and on one-to-one supervision and mentorship (Hodges 2004). Fellows must take a research-oriented graduate degree in Toronto or internationally. The emphasis of the Wilson Centre Fellowship Program is capacity building to develop researchers who can 'engage in their own program of high-quality research, to collaborate with a diverse set of research colleagues [who will be] the next generation of researchers in this field' (Parker et al. 2010, p. 1097). A formal description and review of this program has been published and emphasizes the importance of both formal elements (clear procedures, structured objectives, formal community activities) and informal elements (diversity of fellows and supervisors, flexibility of expectations, fostering of healthy independence) (Parker et al. 2010). In summary, while longitudinal programs are useful for fostering a comprehensive set of educational and leadership skills, to develop research skills specifically a targeted curriculum may be needed.

4.2.3.5 Masters Degrees

Researchers in many fields pursue graduate studies as a way of deepening their research skills. While it is beyond the scope of this chapter to review the whole field of graduate education for research, it is well within our scope to review the important and sometimes debated question of graduate degrees for individuals who are already members of faculty. Levinson and Rubenstein (2000) argue that formal graduate education for researchers is essential. They argue that while helping clinicians to develop rudimentary skills in scholarship will allow them to engage in projects that will, in turn, help them to be promoted academically, such introductory training is not sufficient to function successfully as an independent researcher. They suggest that for junior faculty members to develop research careers, they need: 'protected time, uninterrupted by clinical or teaching responsibilities, mentorship from senior research faculty, space and a financial commitment' (Levinson and Rubenstein 2000, p. 908) and a graduate degree. They place emphasis on having a 'clear road map' (Levinson and Rubenstein 2000, p. 908) for their career that will lead to success.

This is a challenging undertaking for already busy faculty members who must add the demands of a graduate program to their clinical, teaching and administrative commitments. Yet this approach has been rising in popularity (Cohen et al. 2005). Indeed, in the field of medical education, there has been a rapid growth of Masters programs (Tekian and Harris 2012). Interestingly, few actually include research. As with the scholars programs described above, many Masters programs (particularly Masters of Education) focus on a wide array of topics and some contain no research training at all. Goldszmidt et al. (2008) brought this important observation to the fore. Their paper, entitled 'It's not just a question of "degree"', reported that, of a purposive sample of 108 medical faculty members at one Canadian medical school who had an interest in medical education, 40 % had taken formal full-time fellowship or Masters. While many were involved in scholarly projects, few had attained funding or had published their work, and no significant difference was found between those with and without formal education training. In fact, a quarter of the participants indicated that a major weakness of the degree program they had taken was its inability to prepare them for conducting research. Those who felt that the degree had a positive impact on their scholarship reported completing a thesis and having greater exposure to education literature.

Goldszmidt et al. (2008) note that more important than obtaining a degree was research support, enhancing colleague interactions and ongoing development activities. Major barriers included lack of protected time, lack of access to a context and support staff that sustains research, and a lack of knowledge of research methodology. Strongly underscoring the role of context, the authors concluded that:

> Many medical faculty perceive that they are not adequately equipped to pursue education scholarship, especially education research. An advanced education program on its own, such as the Master degree may not provide all of necessary training if the plan is to pursue education scholarship. On-going institutional support and faculty development is required (Goldszmidt et al. 2008, p. 34).

Taken together, these results suggest that formal graduate training (or a full-time research fellowship program) may be an important part of preparation for a research career; however, on its own, it is not sufficient. The Goldszmidt et al. (2008) study is a clear caution about assuming that Masters or fellowship training contains adequate training to undertake research; it also highlights once again that a supportive culture and access to resources are crucial factors.

4.2.3.6 Doctoral Degrees

In most university departments and faculties, other than faculties of medicine, a doctoral degree is required for appointment. Thus, PhDs and their graduate students largely populate research centers in universities. An exception to this has been physician-scientists, many of whom do not undergo PhD training.

Levinson and Rubenstein (2000) were among the first to suggest that in order to conduct independent research, clinical researchers might benefit from PhD training. They also recommended that clinician scientists so trained devote at least 75 % of their time to research in order to be productive. While they noted at the time of their paper in 2000 that the number of MD-PhDs who had made major contributions to the field (of education) was very small, they foresaw the importance of having a critical mass of such clinician researchers. Indeed, today there is growing interest in PhD programs in many areas. Most PhD programs, by their nature, require an intensive research-based thesis. This is true, for example, of PhD programs in health professions education at the University of Maastricht in the Netherlands, the University of Chicago in the United States, and at the University of Toronto and McMaster University in Canada, to name just a few. The number of clinicians holding a PhD is rising steadily and some are finding roles as clinician scientists in education research centers (Hodges 2004). However, MD-PhD training is expensive and time-consuming and appropriate for a very few. While the role of PhD researchers is likely to continue to expand, this approach is not likely to be feasible or useful for the majority of clinical faculty members who wish to engage in some form of scholarship. Thus, considering a track toward a doctoral program for those who wish to go this route is important, all the while recognizing that doctoral education will not be the most important or practical form of research faculty development for most.

4.2.4 Facilitators and Mentors

Having reviewed needs assessment, curriculum content and structure, we turn to the last consideration – the individuals who will play the role of facilitators and mentors in programs of faculty development for research. As we have seen, the research environment is crucial, as is the availability of sufficient time and financial support. In addition, the role of a research mentor also plays a crucial part. Many papers, and the nursing literature in particular, focus on the central role of mentorship (Morrison-Beedy et al. 2001). Chapters 5 and 8 focus on mentorship in more depth.

In examining factors that lead to research productivity in occupational therapy, Paul et al. (2002) noted the pivotal role of having a research mentor who helps to develop short and long-term goals. A similar point is made in nursing by Morrison-Beedy et al. (2001) who write that key factors for effective research mentoring include: setting clear goals for projects; defining expectations for protégés; establishing and maintaining good team communications; and sharing values related to research and nursing. Mundt (2001), also writing about nursing, outlines a set of key activities for research mentors that allowed the University of Louisville to rapidly develop a culture of research growth and productivity. These include: development of a 5-year research career trajectory, plans to develop or strengthen the research program, development and critical review of proposals for extramural funding and of manuscripts, and the provision of advice to strengthen research development. The role of mentorship, then, appears to be particularly important in research development.

Another key issue is the role of facilitators who provide more generic research support to researchers versus mentors who develop individual researcher skills. Some universities hire staff to provide statistical, design and IRB consultation while others hire research scientists who provide mentorship across the range of research developmental levels. Where should scarce resources be invested? It has been noted that busy clinicians, under pressure to do research, may fall into a dependence on some kinds of support which, though helpful, may in the long run work against capacity building. An extreme example was recounted by a PhD scientist who, shortly after being hired was asked to carry a pager so that physicians could call for micro-consultations on their research between cases in the operating room. Colleagues at larger centers for research around the world struggle with finding the right balance between what Albert et al. (2007) call 'service' and 'science' (p. 103). In general, for capacity building, mentorship probably has a greater long-term impact than technical service provision.

An illustrative example from the literature, now nearly 30 years old, was the creation of an office for support of education research at Michigan State College of Human Medicine (Downing et al. 1983). The office was staffed to provide services such as clarifying research questions, designing studies, statistical analysis, and the preparation of manuscripts and oral presentations. The office was inundated with requests and in the first year alone, 62 new projects were initiated. Tellingly, 38 % of the participants reported that they would not have undertaken the project without the help of the research office and only 41 % reported that they would be willing to pay for similar services. After running the office for 2 years, the authors stated that 'guiding them through a positive, initial research experience is educationally valuable but unlikely to generate external funding' (Downing et al. 1983, p. 904) This begs the question of the degree to which this kind of research support fosters sustainability versus dependence. Said the authors, 'providing research opportunities for a large number of inexperienced researchers, many of whom will not advance their research skills any further, presents many obstacles' (Downing et al. 1983, p. 902). While such resources are important, and indeed can propel the research productivity of an institution, the degree to which they create sustainability and increased capacity through development of faculty members skilled in research is less clear. A balance between skills development and mentorship programs on one hand, and direct research support service and facilitation provision on the other, must therefore be struck.

Lave and Wenger's (1991) notion of *legitimate peripheral participation* is helpful in conceptualizing how a novice researcher engages with a new research community. In their concept, novices move from a peripheral to a more central role in a community of practice. The research mentors helps individuals gradually move from a peripheral, observer role to one of more active participants. Some (but not all) will then move to the central role of researcher, leading his or her own research program. Finally, O'Sullivan and Irby (2011) emphasize the importance of bringing together faculty members from different disciplines to learn from one another and support development. This would seem to be an essential part of achieving Boyer's

(1990) second level of scholarship of integration. However, it is more than that. Bringing together individuals with different disciplinary, epistemological and methodological perspectives is an important part of developing a culture of broad thinking, and may be accelerated by co-locating research in dedicated research centers, units or departments.

4.3 Conclusion

Faculty development for research capacity building is a complex undertaking and is, in many ways, distinct from other forms of faculty development. However, a relatively well-developed literature, including several published models accompanied by program evaluations, is available to guide those wishing to embark on this challenge. If there is one overarching theme that emerges clearly from the literature reviewed in this chapter, it is that faculty developers must focus not only on course content, the participants, the mentors and the facilitators but above all else, the context to which participants will return.

Our field will benefit from scholars and researchers trained to a variety of levels. An appreciation for, and literacy in, research is good for everyone; the ability to participate in research is useful for a smaller, but significant number of faculty members; and the skill to conduct an independent research program is a necessity for a few. The format of programs presented here could be seen as a progression, perhaps even as a developmental scheme: progressing from awareness, to personal engagement, to leadership in research. Such a model, accompanied by an appropriately supportive work environment might better allow faculty members to progress to each successive level according to their needs, interest and abilities. Such a model also emphasizes the *development* in faculty development.

4.4 Key Messages

- Faculty development for research capacity building can draw from, but is not identical to, faculty development in other domains.
- Consideration of the context in which participants work is crucial; the context to which they return and the support they receive may be more of a determinant in their research productivity than their educational development.
- Development should be considered sequential and progressive with focused introductory programs giving way to longer multi-component courses and workshops which in turn may lead, for some, to fellowships or graduate programs.

Acknowledgements The author would like to acknowledge Elisa Hollenberg for support in the literature search and formatting of the manuscript and references. Thanks also to Yvonne Steinert, David Irby and Pat O'Sullivan for very helpful comments and suggestions.

References

Albert, M., Hodges, B., & Regehr, G. (2007). Research in Medical Education: Balancing service and science. *Advances in Health Sciences Education, 12*(1), 103–115.

Arnold, L. (2004). Preface: Case studies of medical education research groups. *Academic Medicine, 79*(10), 966–968.

Bakken, L. L., Byars-Winston, A., & Wang, M. F. (2006). Reflections: Viewing clinical research career development through the lens of social cognitive career theory. *Advances in Health Sciences Education, 11*(1), 91–110.

Beckman, T. J. & Cook, D. A. (2007). Developing scholarly projects in education: A primer for medical teachers. *Medical Teacher, 29*(2–3), 210–218.

Beckman, T. J., Lee, M. C., & Ficalora, R. D. (2009). Experience with a medical education research group at the Mayo Clinic. *Medical Teacher, 31*(6), 518–521.

Blanco, M. A. & Lee, M. Y. (2012). Twelve tips for writing educational research grant proposals. *Medical Teacher, 34*(6), 450–453.

Bland, C. J. & Ruffin, M. T. IV (1992). Characteristics of a productive research environment: Literature review. *Academic Medicine 67*(6), 385–397.

Bland, C. J. & Schmitz, C. C. (1986). Characteristics of the successful researcher and implications for faculty development. *Journal of Medical Education, 61*(1), 22–31.

Bordage, G. (2000). La recherche en pédagogie médicale en Amérique du Nord: Tour d'horizon et perspectives. *Pédagogie Médicale, 1*(1), 9–12.

Bordage, G. (2009). Conceptual frameworks to illuminate and magnify. *Medical Education, 43*(4), 312–319.

Boyer, E. L. (1990). *Scholarship reconsidered: Priorities of the professoriate.* Princeton, NJ: Carnegie Foundation for the Advancement of Teaching.

Brawer, J. R. (2008). The reincarnation of a biomedical researcher: From bench science to medical education. *Medical Teacher, 30*(1), 86–87.

Chen, F. M., Bauchner, H., & Burstin, H. (2004). A call for outcomes research in medical education. *Academic Medicine, 79*(10), 955–960.

Coates, W. C., Love, J. N., Santen, S. A., Hobgood, C. D., Mavis, B. E., Maggio, L. A., et al. (2010). Faculty development in medical education research: A cooperative model. *Academic Medicine, 85*(5), 829–836.

Cohen, R., Murnaghan, L., Collins, J., & Pratt, D. (2005). An update on master's degrees in medical education. *Medical Teacher, 27*(8), 686–692.

Cook, D. A., Bordage, G., & Schmidt, H. G. (2008). Description, justification and clarification: A framework for classifying the purposes of research in medical education. *Medical Education, 42*(2), 128–133.

Davis, D., O'Brien, M., Freemantle, N., Wolf, F. M., Mazmanian, P., & Taylor-Vaisey, A. (1999). Impact of formal continuing medical education: Do conferences, workshops, rounds and other traditional continuing education activities change physician behavior or health care outcomes? *JAMA, 282*(9), 867–874.

Downing, S. M., Richards, R. K., Maatsch, J. L., & Peirce, J. C. (1983). Development of a community-based office of research consultation. *Journal of Medical Education, 58*(11), 902–904.

Drummond-Young, M., Brown, B., Noesgaard, C., Lunyk-Child, O., Matthew-Maich, N., Mines, C., et al. (2010). A comprehensive faculty development model for nursing education. *Journal of Professional Nursing, 26*(3), 152–161.

Elen J., Lindblom-Ylänne, S. & Clement, M. (2007). Faculty development in research-intensive universities: The role of academics' conceptions on the relationship between research and teaching. *International Journal for Academic Development, 12*(2), 123–139.

Feldman, H. R. & Acord, L. (2002). Strategies for building faculty research programs in institutions that are not research intensive. *Journal of Professional Nursing, 18*(3), 140–146.

Fidler, D. C., Khakoo, R., & Miller, L. A. (2007). Teaching scholars programs: Faculty development for educators in the health professions. *Academic Psychiatry, 31*(6), 472–478.

Foley, B. J., Redman, R. W., Horn, E. V., Davis, G. T., Neal, E. M., & Van Riper, M. L. (2003). Determining nursing faculty development needs. *Nursing Outlook, 51*(5), 227–232.

Frohna, A. Z., Hamstra, S. J., Mullan, P. B., & Gruppen, L. D. (2006). Teaching medical education principles and methods to faculty using an active learning approach: The University of Michigan Medical Education Scholars Program. *Academic Medicine, 81*(11), 975–978.

Goldszmidt, M. A., Zibrowski, E. M., & Weston, W. W. (2008). Education scholarship: It's not just a question of 'degree'. *Medical Teacher, 30*(1), 34–39.

Gruppen, L. D., Frohna, A. Z., Anderson, R. M., & Lowe, K. D. (2003). Faculty development for educational leadership and scholarship. *Academic Medicine 78*(2), 137–141.

Gruppen, L. D., Simpson, D., Searle, N. S., Robins, L., Irby, D. M., & Mullan, P. B. (2006). Educational fellowship programs: Common themes and overarching issues. *Academic Medicine, 81*(11), 990–994.

Gruppen, L. D., Yoder, E., Frye, A., Perkowski, L. C. & Mavis, B. (2011). Supporting medical education research quality: The Association of American Medical Colleges' Medical Education Research Certificate Program. *Academic Medicine, 86*(1), 122–126.

Hafferty, F. W. (1998). Beyond curriculum reform: Confronting medicine's hidden curriculum. *Academic Medicine, 73*(4), 403–407.

Hafler, J. P., Ownby, A. R., Thompson, B. M., Fasser, C. E., Grigsby, K., Haidet, P., et al. (2011). Decoding the learning environment of medical education: A hidden curriculum perspective for faculty development. *Academic Medicine, 86*(4), 440–444.

Hatem, C. J., Lown, B. A., & Newman, L. R. (2006). The academic health center coming of age: Helping faculty become better teachers and agents of educational change. *Academic Medicine, 81*(11), 941–944.

Hodges, B. (2004). Advancing health care education and practice through research: The University of Toronto, Donald R. Wilson Centre for Research in Education. *Academic Medicine, 79*(10), 1003–1006.

Huwendiek, S., Mennin, S., Dern, P., Friedman Ben-David, M., Van Der Vleuten, C., Tönshoff, B., et al. (2010). Expertise, needs and challenges of medical educators: Results of an international web survey. *Medical Teacher, 32*(11), 912–918.

Irby, D. M., Hodgson, C. S., & Muller, J. H. (2004). Promoting research in medical education at the University of California, San Francisco, School of Medicine. *Academic Medicine, 79*(10), 981–984.

Lave, J. & Wenger, E. (1991). *Situated learning: Legitimate peripheral participation.* Cambridge, UK: Cambridge University Press.

Levinson, W. & Rubenstein, A. (2000). Integrating clinician-educators into academic medical centers: Challenges and potential solutions. *Academic Medicine, 75*(9), 906–912.

Morrison-Beedy, D., Aronowitz, T., Dyne, J., & Mkandawire, L. (2001). Mentoring students and junior faculty in faculty research: A win-win scenario. *Journal of Professional Nursing, 17*(6), 291–296.

Muller, J. H. & Irby, D. M. (2006). Developing educational leaders: The teaching scholars program at the University of California, San Francisco, School of Medicine. *Academic Medicine, 81*(11), 959–964.

Mundt, M. H. (2001). An external mentor program: Stimulus for faculty research development. *Journal of Professional Nursing, 17*(1), 40–45.

O'Sullivan, P. S. & Irby, D. M. (2011). Reframing research on faculty development. *Academic Medicine, 86*(4), 421–428.

Parker, K., Shaver, J., & Hodges, B. (2010). Intersections of creativity in the evaluation of The Wilson Centre fellowship programme. *Medical Education, 44*(11), 1095–1104.

Paul, S., Stein, F., Ottenbacher, K. J., & Liu, Y. (2002). The role of mentoring on research productivity among occupational therapy faculty. *Occupational Therapy International, 9*(1), 24–40.

Ringsted, C., Hodges, B., & Scherpbier, A. (2011). 'The research compass': An introduction to research in medical education: AMEE Guide no. 56. *Medical Teacher, 33*(9), 695–709.

Robins, L., Ambrozy, D., & Pinsky, L. E. (2006). Promoting academic excellence through leadership development at the University of Washington: The Teaching Scholars Program. *Academic Medicine, 81*(11), 979–983.

Rothman, J. & Rinehart, M. E. (1990). A profile of faculty development in physical therapy education programs. *Physical Therapy, 70*(5), 310–313.

Shatzer, M., Wolf, G. A., Hravnak, M., Haugh, A., Kikutu, J., & Hoffmann, R. L. (2010). A curriculum designed to decrease barriers related to scholarly writing by staff nurses. *Journal of Nursing Administration, 40*(9), 392–398.

Steinert, Y. (2011). Commentary: Faculty development: The road less traveled. *Academic Medicine, 86*(4), 409–411.

Steinert, Y. & McLeod, P. J. (2006). From novice to informed educator: The Teaching Scholars Program for Educators in the Health Sciences. *Academic Medicine, 81*(11), 969–974.

Steinert, Y., McLeod, P. J., Liben S., & Snell, L. (2008). Writing for publication in medical education: The benefits of a faculty development workshop and peer writing group. *Medical Teacher, 30*(8), e280–e285.

Tekian, A. & Harris, I. (2012). Preparing health professions education leaders worldwide: A description of masters-level programs. *Medical Teacher, 34*(1), 52–58.

Whitcomb, M. E. (2002). Research in medical education: What do we know about the link between what doctors are taught and what they do? *Academic Medicine, 77*(11), 1067–1068.

Wilson, M. & Greenberg, L. (2004). Overview of the educational scholarship track. *Ambulatory Pediatrics, 4*(1 Suppl.), 88–91.

Chapter 5
Faculty Development for Academic and Career Development

Karen Leslie

5.1 Introduction

There is a clear need for, and benefit to, the provision of faculty development for career development. Faculty development for individual faculty members, their mentors, and leaders in the institutions in which they work, is required to ensure that there is clarity about what is valued, how this informs specific goals, and how these goals are supported, achieved, and acknowledged. This chapter will outline the role of faculty development in the academic and career development of faculty across the career span. The literature in this area is relatively sparse; however, there are a number of areas for which faculty development has been described and many more areas for which additional program and resource development is warranted. Moreover, although the primary focus of this chapter is on academic career development, many of the recommendations and implications are relevant to health professionals regardless of their involvement in supporting the academic mission.

The academic environment is increasingly complex and rapidly changing in response to many influences. There is evidence to suggest that work stress and career dissatisfaction are frequently the result of inadequate preparation of faculty for their roles, lack of collegial relations, inadequate feedback and recognition, unrealistic expectations, insufficient resources, and a lack of balance between work and personal life (Bland et al. 2009).

Faculty development for career development is the *explicit* provision of guidance, learning opportunities and resources that enable individuals to reflect on their careers and those of others, to identify goals and required resources, to implement

K. Leslie, MD, M.Ed., FRCPC (✉)
Department of Paediatrics and Centre for Faculty Development, Li Ka Shing International Health Education Centre, University of Toronto, Toronto, ON, Canada
e-mail: lesliek@smh.ca

Y. Steinert (ed.), *Faculty Development in the Health Professions: A Focus on Research and Practice*, Innovation and Change in Professional Education 11, DOI 10.1007/978-94-007-7612-8_5, © Springer Science+Business Media Dordrecht 2014

appropriate plans and activities, and to assess the processes and outcomes of this work. The goal is for faculty to experience success and fulfillment within their contexts and cultures of practice.

Faculty development for career development should consist of formal programs including workshops and seminars, individual and group based consultation and learning (including approaches such as coaching and mentoring), as well as the provision of information about materials and resources that can be accessed by individuals to guide and advance their own career development. Steinert (2011) has proposed a model for considering the various ways in which faculty can participate in faculty development that includes individual and group, formal and informal faculty development, with mentoring as a core or central activity. It is clear that there is no one best way to provide faculty development across the career span and therefore various methods should be considered to meet the needs of faculty members and the contexts in which they work.

This chapter will begin with a discussion about several overarching concepts for career development that inform an approach to faculty development in this area. In each subsequent section of the chapter, faculty development for career development will be framed by, and incorporate where possible, the following items: (1) the alignment of values between individuals and their organizations; (2) the processes, structures and resources within institutions that relate to academic roles and respon-sibilities; (3) faculty development needs of individual faculty members; (4) faculty development needs of their institutional or organizational leaders; (5) the existing literature; and (6) recommendations for faculty development innovation.

Case examples will be used to illustrate faculty development for career devel-opment across the career span. Embedded in the ideas and content of this chapter is the understanding that our work is *part* of our lives and that our personal and professional identities and roles are interdependent.

5.2 Overarching Concepts of Career Development

There are several overarching concepts that inform faculty development for career development. These include how 'success' is applied to career progression, the alignment of personal values with those of the organizational context, and the con-cept of academic vitality. Each of these will be discussed with reference to relevant literature, followed by ideas about how faculty development could address the identified issues and needs.

5.2.1 Definitions of Success

Prior to a discussion about faculty development for career development and success, there is the need to consider what we mean by 'success' and how this is construed.

Success can be defined as 'the accomplishment of an aim or purpose' and to be successful 'as accomplishing a desired aim or result' (Oxford English Dictionary Online n.d.). The fundamental question, however, is 'Who decides what is desirable?' with the predictable answer being, 'It depends'. There are a number of perspectives that may contribute to our conceptualization of success, and for a health professional working in an academic context, this might include the perspectives of patients, students, colleagues, institutions, families and selves. Some of these perspectives may be congruent and others may not. Faculty development for career development should engage faculty in reflection on these various perspectives and how to reconcile them. How we think about success is informed by what is valued in both the *processes* and *outcomes* of an academic career. Success is a dynamic concept, one that evolves for an individual faculty member over time and within the professional communities and cultures in which that individual practices.

Satisfaction is the other term that tends to be used when referring to faculty career experiences. The term 'satisfaction', often used in the context of faculty career experiences, also requires some consideration. For this chapter, the term *fulfillment* has been used, rather than satisfaction, as it implies a higher level faculty career experience (Brown and Gunderman 2006).

5.2.2 Alignment of Values

Congruence between personal values and those of the culture in which we practice has been identified as being a fundamental aspect of career fulfillment. Individuals need to feel that they are contributing in meaningful ways to their professional community and that, in turn, the contexts in which they practice also attribute value to these contributions. Lieff (2009) proposes that meaningful work occurs at the intersection of passions/interests, strengths and values, in the context of one's practice environment. The academic health sciences organizational context is a complex one, with multiple areas and types of practice for each individual faculty member.

When clinical faculty members describe what they value in their careers, they speak about the rewards of providing clinical care and state that caring for patients is energizing. Faculty also identify how meaningful it is to be part of the teaching mission of the university and for many, this is the reason they chose to work in academia (Pololi et al. 2009b). For some faculty, a crucial career decision may involve whether to give up clinical work in order to pursue other academic opportunities.

The other element of an academic career is involvement in scholarly activity and the discovery of new knowledge. This takes many forms; however, being part of a culture that embodies a spirit of inquiry, discovery and innovation is important to faculty.

Competing tensions exist within the academic culture. Some faculty members report that in their academic culture, research is valued above clinical and teaching work (Buckley et al. 2000; Wright et al. 2012). Those who are on a tenure track, or at an institution where promotion is largely dependent on research productivity, are often less involved in teaching and other activities to the degree that they desire. In another study, those who had recently been promoted to associate professor status shared that they were now able to focus on work they enjoyed and had greater alignment with what they wanted to do versus what they felt they had to do (Field et al. 2011).

The above mentioned areas of practice make up what is commonly referred to as the 'tri-partite' mission in the academic health professions context, and at face value it appears that faculty members and the institutions in which they practice value this mission in similar ways.

There is evidence to suggest that this is not always the case, and faculty report both overt and covert messaging that creates a tension between what is stated as being of value in one's workplace and what is actually valued (Pololi et al. 2009b). Some of this is inherent in the arrangement that is the academic health care organization, where the healthcare system and the system of higher education overlap yet aren't completely congruent with each other in their priorities. Patient care is clearly the *priority* mission of healthcare, with teaching, learning and the discovery of new knowledge and understanding being the *focus* of the university.

Faculty development can assist health professionals to reflect on their values and assess their strengths and interests in the midst of these complex professional environments in order to make choices about their careers. This might be accomplished in group-based faculty development formats; however, some faculty may prefer to reflect and plan on an individual basis, either with printed or web-based materials to guide this work, or through one-to-one conversations with a mentor or colleague. Additional detail about the role of mentoring can be found in Chap. 8.

5.2.3   Faculty Vitality

There is a growing acknowledgement that institutions need to both recognize and address the importance of providing time and resources to fostering workplace environments that allow faculty to thrive and make strong contributions to the organization. Numerous authors have identified that maintaining faculty vitality is key to both the success of the faculty and to the organization as a whole (Bland et al. 2002; Bunton et al. 2012; Lowenstein et al. 2007; Pololi et al. 2009a).

Faculty vitality is a term that has sometimes been used interchangeably with faculty development as it relates to career satisfaction and productivity. Bunton et al. (2012) conducted a survey on faculty workplace satisfaction of full-time faculty members in US medical schools and identified that organization, transparency and governance within departments and the medical school were predictive of global satisfaction of faculty. Additional factors that predicted workplace satisfaction included clarity and focus of the mission, as well as workplace relationships and culture, suggesting that institutions and their leaders play key roles in establishing and promoting environments that engage faculty. Examining the factors that influence the retention of faculty members in academia is a way of understanding academic careers and faculty engagement in the academic culture. Expressing a negative perception of the academic medical culture and intent to leave an institution and/or academic practice has been associated with perceptions of low institutional support and incongruence of values (Pololi et al. 2012). Newer generations of faculty members may have different conceptions of what an academic career means, and these expectations may or may not align with those of previous generations, many of whom are in leadership positions overseeing the recruitment and retention of faculty (Bickel and Brown 2005).

The critical need for faculty development in this area of faculty wellness and vitality is evident, and many institutions are providing this through centralized programs and resources. To date, there is little literature on the evaluation of these programs, and thus, the identification of best practices in this important area is a current gap in our understanding.

These concepts of alignment of values, definitions of success, and faculty vitality should inform our thinking about career development and be embedded in the development, delivery, and assessment of outcomes of faculty development in this area.

5.3 Faculty Development for Career Development Across the Continuum

There is considerable variability in how a career evolves and this is influenced to a large degree by the individual and by the systems in which they work. There does not appear to be consensus on when someone is considered early, mid or late career. Careers take different directions, and some faculty members take on roles that have academic affiliations after having been in professional practice for some time. Traditionally, academic careers have been viewed from a university promotions perspective; however, this somewhat rigid application of career progression no longer works for a large proportion of individuals. Each institution needs to be aware of the various roles that individuals play within their own academic contexts, and identify and address their faculty development needs relative to their career development interests. Referring to these as career 'points' as opposed to career 'stages' may better address the fluid nature of how careers develop.

The following section will describe what has been identified in the literature relating to the career development needs of faculty, specific to different points in a career. Each will include a discussion of how faculty development can address the identified needs and a summary of what has been described in the literature.

Much of what is reported in the health professions education literature is limited to faculty development for career development targeted to faculty in the early stages of their careers. This is largely in the form of *just-in-case* information provided as a single session, orientation event or manual provided at the beginning of one's first days and months as a faculty member. Rather, we need to be thinking about adding in more *just-in-time* learning, delivered at the point at which it is required and often more useful and relevant. For example, while it is important for faculty members to be aware of criteria for promotion at their institution, it is unlikely that they need much detail about this in their first weeks in a new position. Faculty development should be available longitudinally, in a variety of formats, with opportunities to reflect on, and discuss application to, practice for the individual faculty member (Steinert et al. 2006). Included in these activities are programs that promote faculty members' skills in the articulation and development of career goals, identification of learning needs, and documentation of academic achievement that align with personal and institutional values. In addition to workshops and longitudinal programs, inclusion of faculty development strategies such as guided self-assessment and reflection, mentoring, coaching, and leadership development (for which there are separate chapters in this book) are needed. There should be materials and offerings readily available to faculty for when they need the information and/or skills to help them address a particular career goal or decision. In addition, those in roles that support faculty members' careers (e.g. directors, chiefs, chairs, and mentors) need to be aware of these programs and resources and be able to refer faculty to what might be most appropriate and relevant for them. This assumes that these leaders and mentors are aware of, and value, these faculty development resources.

5.3.1 Early Career Faculty

Health professionals, early in their careers, are often simultaneously developing their identities as experts in their professional field and developing an area of academic expertise or focus. For those who may have completed graduate work or some type of specialty training prior to becoming a faculty member, there may be an existing academic identity. This identity can be further developed in relation to the networks of colleagues they may seek out or be welcomed into, although not everyone manages to acquire these networks. This alignment of identity and purpose is important for faculty to be able to identify career goals and plans.

The availability of faculty development for career development can be variable between different academic roles. For example, in the research culture, there are distinct career development programs usually linked to early career grants and funding programs. These programs can include seminars and workshops, formal research mentorship and guidance, and activities that promote networking (Brown et al. 2008; Bruce et al. 2011; Byars-Winston et al. 2011). Many begin during graduate training in order to facilitate the development of established networks of colleagues and a platform for future success. Faculty members who are part of these types of programs are more successful with respect to outcomes such as publication and subsequent funding success; however, as participation in these programs often involves a competitive application process, selection bias may influence these reported outcomes (Pion and Cordray 2008). Parker et al. (2011) describe a program that included on-line learning modules in addition to the above-mentioned components. They also utilized a novel evaluation that took a developmental approach and explored identity development in addition to more traditional end point research productivity. Their research was framed by Ibarra's work that postulates that individuals *try on* different professional identities in early career stages (Ibarra 1999).

Some institutions have clear *homes* for teacher and educators, with teaching academies (Irby et al. 2004) and centers for medical education and faculty development. These entities promote both formal and informal opportunities for faculty to access additional support for career development and to identify relevant faculty development opportunities that will prepare them for their academic roles as teachers, scholars and leaders in the education realm. While these centers are resources for faculty at all points in their career, access to formal faculty development opportunities, becoming a member of a community of like-minded individuals, and having an opportunity to link with potential mentors can be an enormous advantage for those early in their career, seeking to establish their identity as teachers and educators.

In summary, faculty early in their careers can benefit from faculty development that enables them to identify their own values and career objectives, connect with a community of colleagues with similar career foci, and develop an understanding of their ongoing career development needs. This can be achieved through a variety of faculty development formats and can be supported by having one or more mentors.

Senior leaders and mentors to these early career faculty may require their own faculty development in order to understand their roles in assisting faculty with the identification of career goals that align with the institution and broker connections with faculty development resources and programs that align with these career goals.

5.3.2   Mid-Career Faculty

As mentioned earlier in this section, it is somewhat challenging to identify what can be considered to be mid-career as this necessitates clarity about whether your career will have a definitive end! Golper and Feldman (2008) suggest that mid-career faculty may experience 'loss of direction' as they may become more in demand by others to be mentors and may have taken on more administrative roles on institutional committees. To identify the career development needs of associate professors that had been recently promoted, Field et al. (2011) interviewed 39 faculty members from six departments. Faculty expressed that they felt a greater alignment between institutional expectations and their own intrinsic motivation (not entirely surprising as the promotion process is centered on what is valued by the institution). These faculty members identified the need for assistance with skill development relating to leadership responsibilities they were assuming, an area which has also been identified from surveys of faculty career development needs (Miedzinski et al. 2001; Sanfey et al. 2012). Chapter 3 provides further detail about this area of faculty development.

In summary, while faculty who are mid-career may have many of the same career development needs as those earlier in their academic career, they have additional faculty development needs with respect to the knowledge and skills required to enact formal leadership positions and to fulfill their roles as mentors.

5.3.3 Late-Career Faculty

Health professionals in the latter parts of their careers may be completing leadership positions or contemplating taking on new leadership roles within their local or national practice communities. Tannen (2008) writes about the afterlife for retiring deans and other senior administrators, and suggests that continuing in clinical, teaching and administrative roles as well as considering retirement should all be considered as career choices. Individuals at this stage in their careers have much to offer as mentors to those in earlier career stages; however, as a group, late career faculty have their own mentoring needs that are often not met, as mentoring initiatives and resources tend to be focused on more junior faculty.

There is a dearth of recent literature on late career planning and retirement issues for health professionals, in particular for those working in an academic context. Wasylenki (1978) discusses the concept of coping with change in the context of academic physician retirement and reviews the literature in this area. He suggests that knowledge of crisis theory, and how it examines loss, might be a useful lens to bring to academic physician retirement. For example, loss of identity, income, occupation and opportunities for socializing all need to be considered when thinking about faculty needs and what areas faculty development might address.

Merline et al. (2010) surveyed members of the American Academy of Pediatrics (AAP) and identified that part-time work and reduced work hours in anticipation of retirement are options that are used and desired by older pediatricians. The study authors suggest that supporting options for gradual reduction in work hours or other forms of *phasing out* of the workforce could be beneficial in extending career length. It has been suggested that department chairs can play an important role in the careers of their faculty members by raising these issues with department members when they are in their 50's (Hall 2005).

The literature on faculty development for late career and retirement planning for academic health professionals is non-existent; in fact, this is an area with much opportunity for scholarship. There are many ways that faculty development might be offered to address some of the identified needs. Workshops on retirement planning should be offered on a regular basis, addressing areas such as practice options, financial planning and resources, and health and wellness. In parallel with these sessions for faculty, faculty leaders may require faculty development in order to develop strategies to address academic human resource planning in the areas for which they are responsible and to consider ways in which the experience and expertise of the more senior members of their organizations can be valued and utilized.

Peer mentoring, either 1:1 or group based (and outlined in Chap. 8), might be a particularly valuable faculty development strategy for later career faculty, and could facilitate exchange of knowledge and shared learning about career development strategies to address common challenges relating to negotiation of late career and retirement plans.

To summarize, late career faculty members have unique needs relating to how their interests and needs can be addressed within the academic context. Faculty development for those earlier in their careers should include proactive planning for the future, including retirement. For those at later career points, faculty development is needed to assist with transition planning, whether this transition involves realignment of their academic roles and responsibilities, or retirement from academic practice.

5.4 Processes and Structures That Support Career Development

There are many opportunities within existing institutions and organizations for faculty members to receive faculty development for their career development. Many of these opportunities link with existing processes, which map onto an academic career trajectory, as outlined in Fig. 5.1.

The following section will review some of these processes, including recruitment, orientation, systems of assessment (e.g. performance reviews, promotion and tenure), ongoing professional learning, and retirement planning. Faculty development initiatives that have been developed will be cited, and opportunities will be identified where existing practices could incorporate faculty development.

5.4.1 Recruitment

> JF is a 33-year-old who has recently completed her specialty training and is now considering faculty positions at several institutions across the country. She has completed several interviews and is now deciding between two offers of employment; one being in an academic department, and the other in a community-based practice. She is primarily interested in clinical work; however, she wishes to be involved in teaching, and thinks she may aspire to an educational administrative role in the future. She is also hoping to have one or two children in the next five years and is worried about how this might affect her ability to progress academically.

The above example illustrates a number of issues that relate to the recruitment process for new faculty, the need for faculty development for career development for the individual, and recognition of the role that institutions and their leaders play in ensuring that expectations are aligned for these new potential recruits. What information does JF have about the two institutions from which she has received job

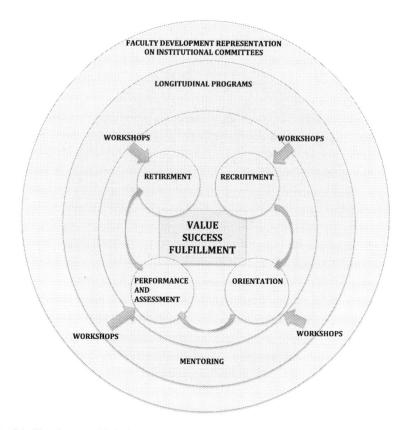

Fig. 5.1 The above model depicts the career development cycle, situated within a framework for faculty development that promotes career success and fulfillment. Specific workshops (or on-line materials and programs) can provide faculty development when it is needed, with longitudinal programs and mentorship providing opportunities for reflection and ongoing assessment of needs and learning. At the institutional or organizational level, faculty developers can contribute to the development and implementation of policies and procedures that align with, and promote, career development

Workshops: 'just-in-time' delivery (e.g. CV preparation, interviewing skills)

Longitudinal programs and formats such as certificate programs and mentoring

Faculty development at the institutional level through advocacy and contribution to development of policies and procedures (e.g. recruitment, promotion, advancement)

offers? How closely do their values align with hers? Is there a good fit with her skill set and interests? What supports are available to her as a new faculty member? While the institutions and their leaders must acknowledge the role they play in ensuring alignment of expectations, there is clearly the need for career development support for JF herself.

How might these aspects of the recruitment process be addressed by faculty development? Applicants submit a curriculum vitae that will be reviewed by prospective employers during the recruitment process. This is an opportunity for faculty development around crafting a well-organized and comprehensive curriculum vitae. For example, knowing what to delete, keep and add to a curriculum vitae that may have served you at a much earlier stage in your career, but may or may not be suitable for application for an academic position, may be invaluable. At the same time, most new positions include some description about the position and the expectations of the new faculty member. Postgraduate and graduate programs can provide faculty development to individuals to promote reflection about the alignment of their skills and interests with those of the institution through formal seminars and through mentoring. Some professional organizations also provide workshops at annual meetings to assist senior trainees with this process.

Interviews provide an opportunity for the individual and the recruiters to further explore aspects of the role, including expectations of both parties. Negotiation of what a faculty position entails is varied, and new faculty members, especially those transitioning from training, are often not in a position to have much power in this process, or perceive that they don't. Utilizing existing mentors or identifying someone to be a 'coach', and using strategies such as role playing interviews or negotiations, can be a useful faculty development strategy as these skills lend themselves to active learning approaches. These techniques could also be embedded into a workshop or seminar on interviewing and negotiation.

Leaders and administrators need to configure their recruitment strategies and approaches in such a way as to engage those recruits that they wish to bring into faculty positions. There needs to be a search for a good *fit* between the individual's and the institution's values, goals, and needs (Staveley-O'Carroll et al. 2005; Viggiano and Strobel 2009). There is a dearth of literature assessing the delivery and impact of programs or strategies that address this particular time in a faculty member's career. Similar to the scholarly work being done about admissions processes to health professions training programs, there needs to be greater study about the most effective approaches to recruitment into academic practice. This information could then be provided as faculty development to those individuals involved in supporting new recruits and responsible for developing and engaging in recruitment processes.

5.4.2 Orientation to Roles and Culture

Socialization into a profession and a culture has been identified as a fundamental aspect of career development as these informal *ways of being* are often not communicated through formal methods of instruction (Bland et al. 1990). There are a number of ways this can occur and more often than not, this occurs serendipitously, rather than intentionally. A number of factors may influence the extent to which this socialization occurs, including access to others with similar roles and identities, in addition to more formal orientation programs for new faculty that may be offered by schools, departments or programs. The provision of faculty development that explicitly offers orientation and guidance for faculty new to the academic context can augment existing formal orientation programs and the implicit socialization that already exists in a given institution.

Bland et al. (1990) proposed that there are key competencies that all faculty should acquire through socialization in order to be successful in their academic careers. She called these Professional Academic Skills (PAS), and proposed that these be formally included in faculty development curricula for new faculty, based on an extensive review of studies that examined correlates of success in academic achievement (largely in research-associated settings). These PAS include three sub-areas: Academic Values, Academic Relationships and Managing an Academic Career. *Acquiring academic values* includes understanding academic values, norms and traditions, and resolving or managing value conflicts. *Academic relationships* refer to the application of knowledge and skills at multiple professional levels, and building and maintaining relationships. *Managing an academic career* includes: setting goals and priorities, understanding reward and promotion systems, understanding the operations of the workplace, identifying one's roles and daily activities, and understanding goals and operations of relevant external organizations. Delivery of a faculty development curriculum that addresses these PAS needs to be multifaceted and longitudinal. To date, there have been no published reports of institutions that have implemented such a curriculum; however, Morzinski and Fisher (2002) used them as a basis for evaluation of their faculty development program and faculty members reported enhanced academic socialization skills and formation of relationships with career-supportive colleagues as a result of their participation in the program.

Clarity around roles, responsibilities and expectations can assist faculty with decision-making around activities in which they should engage. In an attempt to mitigate some of the challenges related to the expectation that faculty meet the 'triple threat' of having to demonstrate excellence in all areas of work, a number of institutions have developed career development frameworks. These frameworks describe the proportion of time allocated for the different academic roles, depending on the primary designation (e.g. clinician, researcher). It appears that these can make an important contribution to clarity of roles and expectations, particularly if linked to a system of assessment (Harris et al. 2007; O'Brodovich et al. 2007; Simpson et al. 2007). The program described by O'Brodovich et al. (2007) was also aligned with faculty compensation. The 'tight alignment of faculty needs, institutional priorities and academic reward structures' (Simpson et al. 2007, p. 945) are highlighted in these examples. Faculty development can assist individuals and their supervisors and mentors in becoming familiar with the utility and application of these frameworks so that they can be used to guide what faculty members choose to do within their current roles, and also what they might aspire to do in the future.

In the absence of specific job descriptions and frameworks, institutional promotions tracks can be used to provide direction to faculty as to the focus of their activities. There has been an evolution from mostly research and tenure tracks, to a diversity of tracks that include non-tenured as well as clinical and teaching faculty tracks (Coleman and Richard 2011). There continues to be wide variation between institutions, with many institutions continuing to expect that all faculty members demonstrate research achievement in the traditional paradigm of the tenure track system. Faculty development can have a role at the organizational level in promoting understanding about how different scholarly activities and achievements can be included, acknowledged and valued in promotions processes. This can be accomplished in a variety of ways, including having faculty developers sit on departmental and institutional promotions committees and contribute to the development of promotions guidelines and workshops for faculty about the promotions process.

There are a number of other tools that can assist with career development planning including CVs, dossiers and portfolios. Often these are seen as *make work* activities for faculty; however, there are creative approaches that allow them to be used to promote reflection on activities and accomplishments, and identify areas for future directions and associated goal setting. Use of these tools in the context of a supportive mentoring relationship strengthens their ability to be of use in this regard. Faculty development curricula can also address how these tools can be used to facilitate career development planning.

5.4.3   Assessment of Achievement

There are a number of benchmarks in academic systems that can provide faculty with the opportunity to reflect on their career progression. While these processes and structures are often seen as summative in nature, all have the potential to be used in a formative manner to support career development.

Performance reviews that may take place annually, or in some institutions at the 3 year mark following one's initial faculty appointment and variably thereafter, can provide information to faculty and their supervisors about achievement of academic goals within identified career roles. These reviews provide an opportunity for faculty to reflect on their existing roles and related expectations, and compare these to their own personal needs and goals, and to those of their department, hospital or university. The value of these performance reviews can be enhanced by faculty engaging in reflection and discussion prior to submitting their review materials, and in further discussion after receiving feedback about performance. Faculty development activities can be coordinated with the timing of these reviews, and can provide faculty with learning about goal setting, identification of continuing education activities that might prepare them to address these goals, and the development of ways in which they can assess the outcomes of this learning and achievement of career goals.

Pololi (2006) describes a nine-step strategy for an academic career development plan that incorporates the consideration of a desired pathway, goal setting, and the involvement of a supervisor or mentor to assist with ensuring alignment with the organizational environment. The steps begin with the identification and prioritization of values, and include identification of strengths, then short and longer term career goals, along with required skills and associated learning goals. She identifies the importance of mentoring to facilitate this process.

The promotion and tenure process can scaffold career development, and as mentioned previously in this chapter, each institution has its own set of criteria for promotion through the ranks. These criteria can be utilized proactively to guide decision-making about an individual's goals and activities. In the past, promotion criteria have not considered aspects of scholarship other than the scholarship of discovery (Boyer 1997). There has been a shift to more inclusive concepts of scholarship that have been applied to teaching, education and scholarly clinical and administrative activity (Levinson and Rubenstein 2000; Simpson et al. 2007). In addition to the traditional curriculum vitae, portfolios and dossiers are being used to document and describe these activities and achievements. Portfolios can also be utilized to monitor progress and promote reflection about ongoing faculty development needs. Zobairi et al. (2008) explored the knowledge and use of academic portfolios in primary care departments and discovered that just over half of the leaders who responded utilized portfolios for their faculty. The majority of these leaders viewed portfolios as extensions of the CV and found them useful for annual reviews and promotions purposes. Enhanced learning is also required for faculty members to construct and develop an academic portfolio so that it not only describes information that is valuable for institutional purposes, but can also be used to inform career development decisions and plans.

Faculty development can play a role in assisting health professionals to capitalize on the process of developing and reflecting on portfolios. Faculty and their mentors can learn about the ways in which information about activities and accomplishments can be identified and documented to facilitate self-assessment, the provision of feedback, and identification of ongoing learning needs. Ross and Dzurec (2010) describe an innovative approach to this process, using concept mapping as a way of capturing the processes and outcomes of various scholarly activities. The appeal of this approach is that it provides a visual collective representation of one's activities and achievements.

There have been specific faculty development initiatives described that address career development for educators, academic clinicians and researchers. Each group has distinct activities and achievements that may be valued in the promotions process, depending on the institution. There is a clear need for institutional leaders and their promotions committees to become more familiar with, and accepting of, these activities and achievements, so as to value all scholarly activity. Faculty development aimed at this level can assist with this required institutional learning. Morahan and Fleetwood (2008) describe a model created to address the needs of faculty in developing nations that combines activity (clinical, service or educational) with scholarship. They suggest that this may be a way to begin to develop different ways of thinking about scholarly activity.

Faculty development programs that incorporate learning about educational scholarship include fellowship programs (Gruppen et al. 2006) and a variety of other formats including workshops, group mentoring (Thorndyke et al. 2006), and graduate programs that provide specific skill development in the area of educational research (Cohen et al. 2005). These programs can assist faculty in acquiring the skills required to engage in scholarly educational work, and also in being able to describe and report this activity in ways that are recognized and valued with institutions. This is particularly important, as activity and achievement in teaching and education does not always align with the metrics used in the promotions process.

In comparison, the metrics by which achievement is assessed for applied and basic science research are much more widely recognized and understood. However, there are other career development challenges for those faculty members engaging in this type of career activity. Competition for increasingly scarce funding, the requirement for prolonged periods of training, and lifestyle concerns have resulted in lower numbers of junior faculty pursuing careers as researchers and scientists (Shea et al. 2011). Faculty development interventions include specific workshops providing guidance around grant preparation or manuscript writing. Specific mentorship for clinician-scientists has been identified as of paramount importance; however, it is unclear as to how this can be best provided. The majority of papers that describe mentoring programs in this regard do not include information about how mentors are chosen and prepared (a huge faculty development opportunity!) or what actual processes constituted the mentoring itself (Shea et al. 2011). Faculty development that aims to provide all faculty members with learning and practice with feedback on the development of the skills associated with effective mentoring should be an essential component of all academic programs.

5.4.3.1 Ongoing Professional Learning

ML, 44 years old, is an associate professor of nursing at his institution. He has been heavily involved and successful in his program of research, and has recently been offered (and strongly encouraged by his Department chair and others) an opportunity to take on a major leadership role at his university. ML feels he would require additional training for such a role, and also wonders what this would mean for his research program and his future promotion to full professor.

What are the career development issues in the above case scenario? Does taking on a local leadership role impact ML's ability to pursue his research career and demonstrate international impact of his work? What kind of skill development might he require if he were to consider the leadership position? Where and how might he acquire this learning? What kind of local pressure is ML under to take on this new role? Does he have adequate mentorship in order to make an informed and well thought out decision about this significant career development situation?

Career development for faculty is informed by the identification of goals and associated learning needs, and by the acquisition and application of this learning (Pololi 2006). In the academic context, faculty development is the means by which this learning can be provided, and as mentioned throughout this chapter, there are many ways in which this faculty development can be provided, including workshops, online learning, formal and informal workplace based learning, and longitudinal certificate and graduate programs.

Sabbatical leaves have also been identified and described as a strategy by which faculty can be provided with the time to pursue further learning opportunities (and/or to regenerate themselves) (Bernstein et al. 1999; Brazeau and Van Tyle 2006).

Career opportunities such as the one described in the above case provide a cue for faculty members to revisit their values, skills and career goals, and to refer to these when considering new career opportunities. During this process, the need for further faculty development and professional learning is often identified.

5.4.4 Retirement

Retirement is most often considered as an event. In fact, retirement is a career development process, about which faculty and their supervisors and leaders need to be adequately informed.

Consider the following scenario:

FR is 63 years of age and has recently completed a very successful 10-year term as a Department Chair of a large academic department. Over this time, his clinical and research activities have been reduced in order to allow him the time for his leadership role, although he has continued to be involved in teaching and as a co-investigator in several research projects. He is wondering what comes next. He is passionate about his professional work but isn't sure whether he wants to go back to the long hours on the inpatient unit or writing grant applications. He isn't confident that he is as up-to-date with his clinical field as he would like. He would also like to be able to spend more time with his three grandchildren and work in his garden more.

What are the opportunities for FR? What kinds of career goals does he have? What might the new chair of his department have in mind? Does FR have interests outside of his professional role? How is his health? Does he have a strong financial plan in place if he were to contemplate retirement? Does his institution support part-time work if this is something FR might desire?

Within the academic health professional literature, there is a paucity of information to help address some of these retirement related issues and questions. As outlined earlier in this chapter, a number of authors have identified the need for both an appreciation of, and creativity in thinking about, the roles that more senior faculty members can have in a department. Genovese (2006) proposed that: 'The key to a successful slowdown/call reduction plan resides in an understanding of the needs of the practice and the benefits that senior physicians can provide' (p. 46). There is a need for health professions faculties and departments to develop innovative models for allocation of responsibilities, in order that the experience and expertise of more senior faculty members can be leveraged as a valued resource to the organization. In their book, *The Vitality of Senior Faculty Members-Snow on the Roof-Fire in the Furnace*, Bland and Bergquist (1997) discuss that while there does not appear to be a decline in competence or productivity as faculty age, there is often a shift in their priorities and values. The importance attributed to the alignment of values has been discussed earlier in this chapter, and it is evident that it plays a role in decision making for senior faculty, as it does at all career stages.

So too does one's conceptualization of one's identity, and Viggiano and Strobel (2009) allude to the fact that one's professional identity contributes to one's personal identity; faculty development could assist faculty with preparation for the shift in identity that comes with retirement. Late career faculty contemplating retirement often have difficulty identifying suitable mentors from within their own departments; therefore, specific faculty development resources such as peer mentoring groups might address some of these career development needs.

5.5 Role of the Institution in Faculty Development for Career Development

As discussed in the preceding section, there are a variety of institutional processes that can promote faculty development for career development. This includes the provision of mentoring, as well as other programs that are supported administratively within programs, departments, hospitals and universities. It is important that there is institutional support for these entities (financial and mission based support) as this provides a strong message to faculty members that they are a valued resource to the organization.

5.5.1 Provision of Mentoring

Mentoring has been identified as an essential component of faculty success. In today's fast paced, *next deadline* work environment, carving out the time and *permission* to think about and proactively consider career opportunities does not always happen (Leslie et al. 2005). The identification and cultivation of informal mentoring relationships may be less feasible for faculty in smaller departments, or in geographically isolated workplaces. Faculty development in the form of formal mentoring programs can complement existing informal mentoring, and innovative models of mentoring, including the concept of *developmental networks*, are gaining prominence in the literature as ways to enhance opportunities for mentoring and supporting career development (Dobrow et al. 2012). Fostering faculty skills in the identification and use of these mentoring supports is important, as is further study about both processes and outcomes. This will provide greater understanding of how best to implement these supports for career success and organizational vitality.

5.5.2 Faculty Development Resources

There are numerous institutional resources that can provide leadership and co-ordination or oversight of faculty development for career development for faculty members. They may be called something different at each institution; however, their function is to oversee faculty appointments, career planning, promotion, shifting roles and responsibilities, retention, satisfaction/engagement, performance and wellness. They include such entities known as an Office of Faculty Affairs, Office/Centre for Faculty Development, Office/Department of Continuing Education/Continuing Education and Professional Development, or Office/Program for Faculty Wellness. Many institutions also have a Centre or Office of Medical Education, which can play an important role in the provision of services and supports for career development. The scope of these programs may be different between institutions, and their collective functions may be provided in distinct ways; however, they represent an explicit source of faculty development resources and programs for faculty members. Information about the establishment of faculty development programs can be found in Chap. 16.

Career development needs and the faculty development required in order to promote successful career progression and fulfillment requires attention at multiple levels in the institution, from the Dean, to Department Chairs and Chiefs, to peer mentors and colleagues. Currently, most faculty development is directed at individual faculty members. In order to address the issues identified throughout this chapter, it is evident that faculty development should include leaders, and groups within an organization who have the ability to influence changes in structures and processes. See Chap. 6 for more information about faculty development and organizational change.

5.6   Conclusion

In conclusion, there are many ways in which faculty development programs and resources can augment how faculty experience, reflect on, and plan their careers in academia. This faculty development needs to be integrated into existing programs and processes within departments, programs and institutions. There needs to be ongoing dialogue between individuals who are in leadership positions, those who have roles as mentors, and faculty across the career spectrum, as to what faculty development is needed, and how best to provide this in the local context. In reviewing the literature on career development and considering the faculty development needs related to career success and fulfillment, it is apparent that faculty development for individual faculty, their mentors, leaders and institutions is required to ensure that there is clarity about what is valued, how this informs specific goals, and how these goals are supported, achieved and acknowledged. Some combination of longitudinal programs, workshops, and on-line learning and resources, supported by ongoing individual and group based mentoring, will be required to meet the diverse needs of faculty and their work settings.

A number of areas merit additional exploration and study. The first of these is the concept of *academic identity*; how this is developed within the health professional practice context, how it evolves over a career, and how it informs professional learning and practice. Clarity about our professional identity, and in particular identity within the academic culture, is key to the alignment of values that is so crucial to success and fulfillment within an academic career. Academic identity should be considered in the development, delivery and evaluation of faculty development.

A second area for further study is how the nature of the academic affiliation frames career progression. For example, how do faculty members who wish to have part-time positions (at any career stage) align with the present system of academic recruitment, assessment and promotion? Punnett (2008) writes that women and women's issues committees originally brought forth this concept into academic medicine; however, increasingly there are other instances where part-time work is either desired or required. As more schools move to distributed campuses with associated community-based experiences for trainees, there will be increased numbers of community-based health professionals taking on part-time academic roles and faculty appointments. It is not yet clear as to how these career trajectories align with more traditional conceptions and what faculty development should look like for these health professionals.

The final point that requires a significant amount of attention is the area of assessment and evaluation of faculty development for career development. There are many papers that describe the identification of need, and the development of programs, activities and frameworks to address these needs. However, few to no rigorous and longitudinal evaluations of comprehensive career development strategies have been published in the academic health professions literature. This is clearly a complex undertaking; however, there is a need to demonstrate the impact of this work so that it can be recognized and resourced to the degree that is needed to support the most valuable resource that institutions have, that is the faculty.

> An institution is not so much a producer of great faculty as it is the product of a great faculty (Kanter 2011, p. 919).

5.7 Key Messages

- Faculty members are most effective in their roles when their values, knowledge and skills are aligned with those of the organizations in which they work.
- Faculty development that supports academic and career development is particularly important at career transitions; however, it should be provided explicitly across the career continuum.
- Faculty development for career development should consist of formal programs including workshops and seminars as well as individual and group based consultation and learning (including approaches such as coaching and mentoring).
- Faculty development for career development should be embedded as an overall organizational strategy and aimed at individuals, leaders and their institutions.

References

Bernstein, E., James, T., & Bernstein J. (1999). Sabbatical programs and the status of academic emergency medicine: A survey. *Academic Emergency Medicine, 6*(9), 932–938.

Bickel, J. & Brown, A. J. (2005). Generation X: Implications for faculty recruitment and development in academic health centers. *Academic Medicine, 80*(3), 205–210.

Bland, C. J. & Bergquist, W. H. (1997). *The vitality of senior faculty members: Snow on the roof— Fire in the furnace.* ASHE-ERIC Higher Education Report Series *25*(7). Washington, DC: George Washington University Graduate School of Education and Human Development.

Bland, C. J., Schmitz, C. C., Stritter, F. T., Henry, R. C., & Aluise, J. J. (1990). *Successful faculty in academic medicine: Essential skills and how to acquire them.* New York, NY: Springer Publishing.

Bland, C. J., Seaquist, E., Pacala, J. T., Center, B., & Finstad, D. (2002). One school's strategy to assess and improve the vitality of its faculty. *Academic Medicine, 77*(5), 368–376.

Bland, C. J., Taylor, A. L., Shollen, S. L., Weber-Main, A. M., & Mulcahy, P. A. (2009). *Faculty success through mentoring: A guide for mentors, mentees, and leaders.* Lanham, MD: Rowman & Littlefield.

Boyer, E. L. (1997). *Scholarship reconsidered: Priorities of the professoriate.* San Francisco, CA: Jossey-Bass.

Brazeau, G. A. & Van Tyle, J. H. (2006). Sabbaticals: The key to sharpening our professional skills as educators, scientists, and clinicians. *American Journal of Pharmaceutical Education, 70*(5), 109.

Brown, S. & Gunderman, R. B. (2006). Viewpoint: Enhancing the professional fulfillment of physicians. *Academic Medicine, 81*(6), 577–582.

Brown, A. M., Morrow, J. D., Limbird, L.E., Byrne, D. W., Gabbe, S. G., Balser, J. R., et al. (2008). Centralized oversight of physician-scientist faculty development at Vanderbilt: Early outcomes. *Academic Medicine, 83*(10), 969–975.

Bruce, M. L., Bartels, S. J., Lyness, J. M., Sirey, J. A., Sheline, Y. I., & Smith, G. (2011). Promoting the transition to independent scientist: A national career development program. *Academic Medicine, 86*(9), 1179–1184.

Buckley, L. M., Sanders, K., Shih, M., & Hampton, C. L. (2000). Attitudes of clinical faculty about career progress, career success and recognition, and commitment to academic medicine. Results of a survey. *Archives of Internal Medicine, 160*(17), 2625–2629.

Bunton, S. A., Corrice, A. M., Pollart, S. M., Novielli, K. D., Williams, V. N., Morrison, L. A., et al. (2012). Predictors of workplace satisfaction for U.S. medical school faculty in an era of change and challenge. *Academic Medicine, 87*(5), 574–581.

Byars-Winston, A., Gutierrez, B., Topp, S., & Carnes, M. (2011). Integrating theory and practice to increase scientific workforce diversity: A framework for career development in graduate research training. *CBE Life Sciences Education, 10*(4), 357–367.

Cohen, R., Murnaghan, L., Collins, J., & Pratt, D. (2005). An update on master's degrees in medical education. *Medical Teacher, 27*(8), 686–692.

Coleman, M. M. & Richard, G. V. (2011). Faculty career tracks at U.S. medical schools. *Academic Medicine, 86*(8), 932–937.

Dobrow, S. R., Chandler, D. E., Murphy, W. M., & Kram, K. E. (2012). A review of developmental networks: Incorporating a mutuality perspective. *Journal of Management, 38*(1), 210–242.

Field, M. B., Barg, F. K., & Stallings, V. A. (2011). Life after promotion: Self-reported professional development needs and career satisfaction of associate professors. *The Journal of Pediatrics, 158*(2), 175–177.

Genovese, B. (2006). Senior physician slowdown: Problem or opportunity? *Physician Executive, 32*(2), 42–46.

Golper, T. A. & Feldman, H. I. (2008). New challenges and paradigms for mid-career faculty in academic medical centers: Key strategies for success for mid-career medical school faculty. *Clinical Journal of the American Society of Nephrology, 3*(6), 1870–1874.

Gruppen, L. D., Simpson, D., Searle, N. S., Robins, L., Irby, D. M., & Mullan, P. B. (2006). Educational fellowship programs: Common themes and overarching issues. *Academic Medicine, 81*(11), 990–994.

Hall, J. G. (2005). The challenge of developing career pathways for senior academic pediatricians. *Pediatric Research, 57*(6), 914–919.

Harris, D. L., Krause, K. C., Parish, D. C., & Smith, M. U. (2007). Academic competencies for medical faculty. *Family Medicine, 39*(5), 343–350.

Ibarra, H. (1999). Provisional selves: Experimenting with image and identity in professional adaptation. *Administrative Science Quarterly, 44*(4), 764–791.

Irby, D. M., Cooke, M., Lowenstein, D., & Richards, B. (2004). The academy movement: A structural approach to reinvigorating the educational mission. *Academic Medicine, 79*(8), 729–736.

Kanter, S. L. (2011). Faculty career progression. *Academic Medicine, 86*(8), 919.

Leslie, K., Lingard, L., & Whyte, S. (2005). Junior faculty experiences with informal mentoring. *Medical Teacher, 27*(8), 693–698.

Levinson, W. & Rubenstein, A. (2000). Integrating clinician-educators into academic medical centers: Challenges and potential solutions. *Academic Medicine, 75*(9), 906–912.

Lieff, S. J. (2009). Perspective: The missing link in academic career planning and development: Pursuit of meaningful and aligned work. *Academic Medicine, 84*(10), 1383–1388.

Lowenstein, S. R., Fernandez, G. & Crane, L. A. (2007). Medical school faculty discontent: Prevalence and predictors of intent to leave academic careers. *BMC Medical Education, 7*, 37.

Miedzinski, L. J., Armstrong, P. W., & Morrison, M. A. (2001). Career Development Program in Department of Medicine at University of Alberta. *Annals RCPSC, 34*(6), 375–379.

Merline, A. C., Cull, W. L., Mulvey, H. J., & Katcher, A. L. (2010). Patterns of work and retirement among pediatricians aged ≥50 years. *Pediatrics, 125*(1), 158–164.

Morahan, P. S. & Fleetwood, J. (2008) The double helix of activity and scholarship: Building a medical education career with limited resources. *Medical Education, 42*(1), 34–44.

Morzinski, J. A. & Fisher, J. C. (2002). A nationwide study of the influence of faculty development programs on colleague relationships. *Academic Medicine, 77*(5), 402–406.

O'Brodovich, H., Beyene, J., Tallett, S., MacGregor, D., & Rosenblum, N. D. (2007). Performance of a career development and compensation program at an academic health science center. *Pediatrics, 119*(4), e791–e797.

Oxford English Dictionary Online. (n.d.). Available from: http://oxforddictionaries.com/definition/english/success

Parker, K., Burrows, G., Nash, H., & Rosenblum, N. D. (2011). Going beyond Kirkpatrick in evaluating a clinician scientist program: It's not 'if it works' but 'how it works'. *Academic Medicine, 86*(11), 1389–1396.

Pion, G. M. & Cordray D. S. (2008). The Burroughs Wellcome Career Award in the Biomedical Sciences: Challenges to and prospects for estimating the causal effects of career development programs. *Evaluation & the Health Professions, 31*(4), 335–369.

Pololi, L. (2006). Career development for academic medicine - A nine step strategy. *BMJ, 322*(7535), 38–39.

Pololi, L., Conrad, P., Knight, S., & Carr, P. (2009a). A study of the relational aspects of the culture of academic medicine. *Academic Medicine, 84*(1), 106–114.

Pololi, L., Kern, D. E., Carr, P., Conrad, P., & Knight, S. (2009b). The culture of academic medicine: Faculty perceptions of the lack of alignment between individual and institutional values. *Journal of General Internal Medicine, 24*(12), 1289–1295.

Pololi, L., Krupat, E., Civian, J. T., Ash, A. S., & Brennan, R. T. (2012). Why are a quarter of faculty considering leaving academic medicine? A study of their perceptions of institutional culture and intentions to leave at 26 representative US medical schools. *Academic Medicine, 87*(7), 859–869.

Punnett, A. (2008) Part-time academic medicine: Understanding culture to effect change. *Higher Education Perspectives, 4*(1), 1–16.

Ross, R., & Dzurec, L. (2010). Worth 1000 words: Concept mapping the path to tenure and promotion. *Journal of Professional Nursing, 26*(6), 346–352.

Sanfey, H., Boehler, M., Darosa, D., & Dunnington, G. L. (2012). Career development needs of vice chairs for education in departments of surgery. *Journal of Surgical Education, 69*(2), 156–161.

Shea, J. A., Stern, D. T., Klotman, P. E., Clayton, C. P., O'Hara, J. L., Feldman, M. D., et al. (2011). Career development of physician scientists: A survey of leaders in academic medicine. *American Journal of Medicine, 124*(8), 779–787.

Simpson, D., Fincher, R. M., Hafler, J. P., Irby, D. M., Richards, B. F., Rosenfeld, G. C., et al. (2007). Advancing educators and education by defining the components and evidence associated with educational scholarship. *Medical Education, 41*(10), 1002–1009.

Staveley-O'Carroll, K., Pan, M., Meier, A., Han, D., McFadden, D., & Souba, W. (2005). Developing the young academic surgeon. *Journal of Surgical Research, 128*(2), 238–242.

Steinert, Y. (2011). Commentary: Faculty development: The road less traveled. *Academic Medicine, 86*(4), 409–411.

Steinert, Y., Mann, K., Centeno, A., Dolmans, D., Spencer, J., Gelula, M., et al. (2006). A systematic review of faculty development initiatives designed to improve teaching effectiveness in medical education: BEME Guide No. 8. *Medical Teacher, 28*(6), 497–526.

Tannen, R. L. (2008). The afterlife for retiring deans and other senior medical administrators. *Clinical Journal of the American Society of Nephrology, 3*(6), 1875–1877.

Thorndyke, L. E., Gusic, M. E., George, J. H., Quillen, D. A., & Milner, R. J. (2006). Empowering junior faculty: Penn State's faculty development and mentoring program. *Academic Medicine, 81*(7), 668–673.

Viggiano, T. R., & Strobel, H. W. (2009). The career management life cycle: A model for supporting and sustaining faculty vitality and wellness. In T. R. Cole, T. J. Goodrich, E. R. Gritz (Eds.), *Faculty health in academic medicine*, (pp. 73–81). Totowa, NJ: Humana Press.

Wasylenki, D. (1978). Coping with change in retirement. *Canadian Family Physician, 24*, 133–136.

Wright, S. M., Gozu, A., Burkhart, K., Bhogal, H., & Hirsch, G. A. (2012). Clinician's perceptions about how they are valued by the academic medical center. *The American Journal of Medicine, 125*(2), 210–216.

Zobairi, S. E., Nieman, L. Z., & Cheng, L. (2008). Knowledge and use of academic portfolios among primary care departments in U.S. medical schools. *Teaching and Learning in Medicine, 20*(2), 127–130.

Chapter 6
Faculty Development for Organizational Change

Brian Jolly

6.1 Introduction

There seems to be a widely held assumption that the long-term outcomes of most faculty development initiatives will include some degree of organizational change. In many cases they do; most people engaged in faculty development have observed change at the institutional level after faculty development interventions. However, not all faculty development initiatives lead to changes and, clearly, some organizational changes take place without much faculty development.

Faculty development targeted at the individual can only achieve limited change. The degree of limitation depends on where that individual sits within the organization and how they engage with the development process. Faculty development for organizational change needs to be considered from the perspectives of all stakeholders. Each stakeholder group requires different approaches, but synergies can be obtained with a well-considered approach. Faculty development for organizational change requires attention to the educational and institutional milieu, the workforce and the organization itself. Most of the time, change will be slow and also affected by external factors. In addition, not all change will be attributable to the effect of faculty development alone. Using strategies designed to counteract, or at least acknowledge, the inhibitors of change can lead to more effective outcomes for faculty development.

This chapter will explore the mechanisms and strategies that can be used by faculty developers to promote or assist in positive organizational change. It will discuss

B. Jolly, MA (Ed), Ph.D. (✉)
Medical Education, School of Medicine and Public Health, Faculty of Health,
The University of Newcastle, Callaghan, NSW, Australia

Australian Society for Simulation in Healthcare and Health Division
of Simulation Australia, Adelaide, SA, Australia
e-mail: brian.jolly@newcastle.edu.au

Y. Steinert (ed.), *Faculty Development in the Health Professions: A Focus
on Research and Practice*, Innovation and Change in Professional Education 11,
DOI 10.1007/978-94-007-7612-8_6, © Springer Science+Business Media Dordrecht 2014

some barriers to this process and make suggestions, in the form of 'strategies for success', for faculty developers, organizational leaders and those participating in development. This will include what to focus on and how to construct faculty development, so that organizational change is more likely and aligned with organizational needs and priorities.

6.2   What Would Faculty Development for Organizational Change Look Like?

The term 'faculty development' is an indistinct one for two reasons. First, because it is so varied in its manifestations (Brew and The Society for Research into Higher Education 1995). Second, because faculty development does not have a theoretical underpinning all of its own (Steinert 2010), although to have one that is clearly identifiable would be useful (Steinert et al. 2012). Indeed, such a theory might help to construct faculty development that is ubiquitously seen as fit for purpose. In this section, we will look at how both providers and users commonly perceive faculty development, and how these perceptions might impact on its value as an organizational change agent.

There are about 12–15 commonly used definitions of faculty development (or its equivalent UK term 'staff development'). Most faculty development is currently targeted towards individuals or small groups of individuals who have common learning or development goals (e.g. the need to update teaching or management skills). However, some definitions of faculty development are couched in language that strongly implies that there are organizational imperatives (Jolly 2002). This contrast between individual and institutional needs, and the role of the institution in the provision of faculty development activities, is a key factor and is reflected in the following four definitions of faculty development:

- 'A continuous process in which opportunities are provided for professional growth of the individual within the academic environment' (Allen 1990, p. 266).
- 'A tool for improving the educational vitality of our institutions through attention to competencies needed by individual teachers and to the institutional policies required to promote academic excellence' (Wilkerson and Irby 1998, p. 388).
- 'The broad range of activities that institutions use to renew or assist faculty members in their multiple roles. Faculty development activities include programs to enhance teaching and education, research and scholarly activity, academic leadership and management, and faculty affairs, including faculty recruitment, advancement, retention, and vitality. The intent of these activities is to assist faculty members in their roles as teachers, educators, leaders, administrators and researchers' (1st International Conference on Faculty Development in the Health Professions 2011).
- 'A broad concept which covers the systematic identification of the present and anticipated needs of an organization and its members, and the development of programmes and activities to satisfy these needs. It [faculty development] is concerned with all aspects of a person's work' (Elton 1987, p. 55).

The last of these seems to be the one most applicable to organizational change, (even though the third is the most recent). The utility of Elton's 1987 definition is that it focuses on a systematic process that is aimed at both the individual's and the organization's benefit and addresses 'all aspects' of professional life. The broad compass of this definition may be tenable in our current academic and healthcare organizations, but only if the way that we promote, deliver and evaluate faculty development undergoes some radical change. Elton's conceptualization of faculty development clearly implies that personal development activities are being undertaken by academic and clinical staff in educational corporations and that, as a result, some progress or growth will occur. The benefits of this growth are defined and achieved by both the faculty member and by the organization. Typically, in commercial business communities, while personal growth is undeniably important, it is normally the case that this growth is encouraged primarily because the organization requires it, and will profit or become more competitive in some way from it (an idea which is further discussed in Sect. 6.9). However, by comparison, in universities, the notions of competition and profit generation as legitimate goals of the institution, although increasing in strength (Wildavsky 2010), are highly dependent on the local cultural context, including the extent of government funding for institutions and the intensity of the struggle to attract research income and students, a context which is markedly variable across different countries. The contrast between individual learning and organizational change will be discussed further in Sects. 6.4 and 6.8.

6.3   What Does Faculty Development Currently Include?

The types of activity that comprise faculty development are diverse and have been modeled on numerous approaches including lectures (Davis et al. 1999), mixed methods (Khan et al. 2013), action groups, survival or physical exertion courses (Marinac and Gerkovich 2012), psychotherapy, and academic 'speed dating' (Laprise and Thivierge 2012; Muurlink and Matas 2011). This testifies to the almost limitless and indistinct boundaries, both in content and in methods, of what has become known as 'faculty development'. The context in which faculty development operates is also varied and has included, in general terms, personal development, as in the sabbatical or elective; professional development, such as study for a higher degree or specialist qualification; and workforce 'tuning', where a slight change or redeployment can deliver a lot more by making work more effective and/or more efficient. Sometimes faculty development seems almost indistinguishable from similar activities that could be called 'continuing professional development'. Certainly both faculty development and continuing professional development share common ground in the educational strategies and methods used. They also both currently embody and perpetuate a perspective that puts the individual at the focus of both types of activities. So where does faculty development sit in the organizational framework?

6.4   In What Context Does Faculty Development Operate and How Does It Work?

In academia, the idea of institutional benefit is pitched against the cherished value of academic freedom. This tension often becomes intense when universities are threatened by economic downturns, resulting in reductions in student enrolments in previously expanded areas, and the only way to reap institutional benefit is to reduce academic staff numbers or cut departments (e.g. see Meyers 2012, who cites over-expansion of student numbers and, somewhat forcefully, excessive interest in the pedagogy of higher education as contributors). However, it also comes to a head in the simmering tensions between research and teaching, the two major foci of aca-demic life that are supposed to be complementary, though frequently in opposition (Rust 2011). Hence, although faculty development frequently means developing personnel more fit for the (twofold) purpose of the institution, this has been a challenging concept in institutions of professional learning or medical research. This is largely because traditionally, individual personal and professional qualities (e.g. intellect and empowerment), especially in research capacity, have often been valued above institutional ones and, more importantly, above humanistic and educa-tional ones (Handy 1999). For example, Handy (1999) describes the cultures operat-ing in medical and academic institutions as 'person culture', where charisma and expertise dominate the power hierarchy. This conflict between institutional or soci-etal needs and personal autonomy has been epitomized in several Australian univer-sities, and discussed generically in the UK, over the last decade, when attempts to introduce compulsory faculty development on teaching skills for incoming staff were resisted by some senior academics because the time devoted to this was per-ceived to harbor potential detrimental effects on research capacity (Onsman 2009; UK Department for Education and Employment 1999).

How the institution and the individuals within it perceive faculty development will determine how it is used. In the definitions above, Wilkerson and Irby (1998) are saying that faculty development should concentrate on the things that teachers do that can promote quality teaching and academic excellence. But Elton (1987), a prolific and major researcher in higher education, suggests that the goal and content of faculty development should be much broader than this. Indeed, it is becoming increasingly common in most large universities for faculty development to address a wide range of issues: financial and management skills, including the management of change, conflict resolution, leadership, innovation, creativity, and cultural com-petence. However, the precise nature of the institutional, as opposed to the personal, goal (i.e. what type of benefit should ensue?) is often not made explicit. If faculty development is seen in an institution to be only for the benefit of an individual, maybe as a right, or at least as an essential concomitant of academic life, it is unlikely to be regarded as a force for change in that organization.

This means that if faculty development is to be an instrument of change in an organization, it should encompass promotion of its role within the institution as a mechanism both to enhance the skills of individuals and as a means to develop the academic capital of the institution. Consequently, to be contemporary, relevant and organizationally acceptable, faculty development will need reframing so that it has a broader perspective than a focus on the individual. For example, faculty developers should find out before they start a project how their colleagues currently view the faculty development programs in their organization. Are these being run primarily to generate external income or goodwill from outside the organization? Are they responsive to faculty members' needs? Do they work, as far as the typical recipient is concerned? Is there a faculty development 'centre' and is it lofty and insular, or responsive, collaborative and outgoing?

Thus, a first strategy in using faculty development to achieve organizational change might be as follows: **Faculty development must be defined for, and promoted to, an institution's members in a manner that clearly connects with its capacity to contribute to organizational change.** This means that an explanation of why a program is being developed should be identified in the program's rationale, promotional material and development activities. For example, promotional material for a faculty development activity in a university might say, 'This University is not seen by its students as offering sufficient, or timely, feedback to enable students to improve their work and this is having a deleterious impact on national ratings and government funding streams. So that we can do better, a systematic literature review has isolated the main features of a useful feedback strategy, a needs assessment conducted to determine training requirements, and a program devised for faculty that will promote a more sensitive, systematic and effectively delivered approach to feedback....'. Although this example, which will also serve later when we come to strategy number two, uses the university as the primary focus, there is no reason why other organizations could not exhibit similar traits.

However, there are dangers in the use of such a strategy. How will the movement towards this rationalization portray units or academics engaged in faculty development? Will they be seen as sufficiently freethinking or mainly as agents of control for the organization, as could be typified for example by courses on conflict resolution, financial management, and how to deal with unruly students?

6.5 What Is the Organizational Potential of Faculty Development Initiatives?

Healthcare organizations and universities are run by people, for people. Even so, the impact of people in organizations varies. For example, service industries such as healthcare and education, by and large, depend heavily on the technical and social skills that their members possess. Traditionally, other industries such as mining, agriculture, car production and engineering, while valuing personal skills, may in fact employ fewer people, more machines, and be more reliant on the technical capabilities of staff and technology-directed systems at all levels of the organizations. However, this traditional clear demarcation is rapidly changing (Hilton 2008), so that even traditionally scientific- and technology-based occupations in future will require more 'soft skills'. Additionally, in the next 20 years, healthcare will expand enormously. By 2025 it is predicted that healthcare providers will be caring for an older, wiser and more complex clientele and that healthcare will also have the largest workforce of any organization in the western world (e.g. Buerhaus et al. 2008). Thus, for healthcare at least, developing the people in these organizations would seem not only to have some merit as a rational strategy to promote change, but also to be absolutely vital to the general mission of healthcare. The study of nurses learning new communication skills, described in the next section (Heaven et al. 2006), demonstrates quite clearly that approaching the development of faculty in a more inclusive manner has advantages. But it also makes it more taxing because it needs to take into account a wider range of factors.

Another feature of faculty development is that the choice of the faculty development program is usually determined by the individual, typically from a smorgasbord of offerings prepared by the institution. That menu can be modern and adventurous, or classic and refined. In either case, this has utility for the individual; they develop skills, have time for reflection, and can pursue their personal goals. But in doing so, they may develop skills that are well matched to the organization's goals and profile, and/or outgrow the organization's role and mandate, and be reluctant, or unable, to function within it. From the organization's point of view, they will be 'lost' to the system and organizational change will be less likely as a result. Hence the second strategy for success, which takes the first strategy a step forward, is that: **Faculty development needs to be forward looking and directly linked to, or at least cognizant of and responsive to, organizational goals if it is to assist in promoting organizational change**. In the example we gave earlier of delivering better feedback to students, the development activity was presaged by information that linked it directly to institutional as well as individual goals.

Where faculty development is placed in an organization, how it is funded and governed, its structures and its staffing are therefore vitally important. If 'the University' needs change, it is unlikely that a faculty development unit that is primarily focused on a faculty or department (e.g. the Medical Education Unit) will be able to deliver it. This is not because it could not achieve the required programs, but because it would not be guided and driven by the appropriate power-brokers and supported in its mission at an appropriate level. From the counter perspective, if a faculty or divisional unit took on such a role, it would probably be seen as not being sufficiently focused on the needs of its faculty members. In practical terms, for organizational change, the Vice Chancellor or President (or whoever is the most powerful stakeholder in the organization) needs to show visible enthusiasm for the development program, and offer encouragement and support to those who undertake it.

6.6   What Happens to Faculty Members Who Have Been 'Developed'?

Paradoxically, organizations that have invested in faculty development for their staff can be unreceptive to, or even inhibit, change that might otherwise result from the faculty development activities. For example, in a well-designed randomized controlled trial, 61 clinical nurse specialists received workshops with either new patient-centered communication skills training, followed by clinical supervision, or communication skills training alone (Heaven et al. 2006). The authors first measured the impact of the workshops with simulated patient encounters, and there were clear immediate impacts on skills, which were, in fact, developed equally well by both groups. The researchers then followed the nurses in their real-patient encounters, at baseline before, and then twice after the intervention. The results showed that only those who experienced the additional supervision showed *any* evidence of continued transfer of the workshop-learned skills to the workplace. The study was groundbreaking in that it not only showed that clinical supervision had an effect; it also demonstrated that 'without such support in the workplace, clinical nurse specialists find it virtually impossible to provide optimal support for their patients and find integration of new learning extremely difficult' (p. 323). An almost identical process was charted in psychiatry nursing by White and Winstanley (2010). These studies underline the fact that just training someone to take on a more complex role will not guarantee that this role will be developed in the workplace, unless it is accepted by co-workers, and championed, directed and supported by a supervision process.

In a prescient paper, Shanley (2004), writing from the nurse education perspective, critiques the deficiencies of many faculty development programs in relation to organizational change. She identifies that a 'sophisticated and learner-centered staff development program will have little effect if the learner has to return to a workplace where managers, supervisors, and peers do not support implementation of the new learning…' (p. 84). She also raises a number of other issues that confirm the frequent tensions between existing systems, procedures and protocols, and new learning. She presages the Van Roermund et al. (2011) study's findings (see below) about new work practices that are not encouraged because things have always been done in 'a different way'. Shanley also highlights the negative impact that underlying conflict or lack of direction and cohesion within the organization can have on the outcomes of faculty development programs. The 'characteristics' of organizationally responsive faculty development that Shanley goes on to identify in the article have much in common with the 'strategies for success' that are described here.

A related phenomenon was also detected by a recent study of how general practitioners (GPs) in the Netherlands see themselves as teachers. These GPs had been engaged in some faculty development on a new competency framework for educators in general practice (Van Roermund et al. 2011). The authors described how two major factors appeared to have had the greatest influence on implementation of this new educational framework. The first was 'identification'. This process took place post-faculty development and involved the faculty development recipients identifying or characterizing themselves in relation to the new framework; they effectively asked 'what type of professional/teacher/person am I?' The authors used the metaphor of a mirror to describe this process. When teachers looked into the new mirror provided by the faculty development experience, they truly believed they could do better and engaged with enhancing their competencies. However, they nevertheless held on to the beliefs and methods they had learned through experience. In this situation, the faculty development activity did not automatically lead to acceptance of the new model of teaching or to expression of the desired outcomes. The second factor was the organizational culture. As soon as a new staff member was appointed, existing experienced mentors engaged in a socialization process that shaped their new colleague's professional development as a teacher. In this type of environment, the new teacher not only learnt 'how to teach' (irrespective of what the faculty development process might have been), but they were also 'initiated into the do's and don'ts of teaching in the local departmental culture' (Van Roermund et al. 2011, p. 6). This phenomenon has been recognized by researchers such as Billet (1995), as the inherent 'power' of work-based learning and culture to trump other more traditional, propositional and procedural forms of learning: craft holding sway over concepts.

These analyses tell us a great deal about the need to pay attention to an organization's characteristics when developing individuals to work more effectively in that organization. Faculty development needs to address the workforce needs, but also the leadership and middle management perspectives in an organization. In universities and faculties of health, which are often required to respond rapidly to change, there is huge inertia compared to organizations that exist in the competitive or volatile market place and have to change on a regular basis to survive (Ernst and Young 2012).

This brings us to the third strategy for success: **When designing development activities for organizational change, it is necessary to address the elements in the organization, or in the participants' institutions, that can foster or impede the work of those that have undertaken the development process.**

One way of doing this, of course, is to engage the participants, and those who may represent potent barriers to change in the development process, by asking them who or what will help them to change their practice or might hinder it; in other words, how will their new skills fit into their existing organization and what support will they need or receive? In one of my early forays into faculty development in the early 1980s, colleagues and I designed a 2–3 day program on teaching skills for medical registrars to use in the clinical context. We reasoned that it would be important to engage the registrars' seniors, the consultants, in this process. We therefore offered a 1-day orientation course to the consultants to show them what their registrars would be doing. This turned out to be so effective that a year later we had to start a course for the consultants as well.

Another way of managing the process is to enable the participants to deal with their own organizations in a more effective way. This highlights the importance of faculty developers or participants in programs spending some time getting to know their organization, the participants in the program and how they work in their own environment.

6.7 What Does Research Tell Us About Faculty Development as an Organizational Change Agent?

Faculty development is also challenged because most research and evaluations of its impact (see Chap. 17 for examples) have used self-reports from faculty or individual behavioral change as outcome measures, and not indices of the extent of ensuing organizational development (Towle 1998). In a recent systematic review of the impact of 'resident-as-teacher' programs, only 2 of the 29 studies that met the inclusion criteria addressed organizational change as an outcome (Hill et al. 2009), and notably both of these were undertaken in the early 1990s. Of course, faculty development frequently results in some organizational change, and most faculty developers have observed, and long exploited, this feature (Elton 1998; Hatton and Bullimore 1993; Mennin and Kaufman 1989).

Nevertheless, it is likely that many organizational outcomes have remained unreported in the literature, even in education journals, let alone in those reporting organizational change. This limits our understanding of how effective faculty development can be at this level. Moreover, the organizational benefits of faculty development can be almost completely overshadowed by concurrent political, social and economic changes. For example, in the 1980s, a new faculty development initiative at St Bartholomew's ('Bart's') Hospital Medical School, comprising a week-long course on teaching and assessment, resulted in a small, well-motivated, cadre of highly trained faculty who, with some support from educational professionals, went on to radically change the undergraduate medical curriculum from a highly traditional subject-based model to a community-oriented, integrated and student-directed one. However, the major changes that took place were often attributed to the contiguous reorganization of hospitals and medical schools in the London area that dominated the front page of the daily London papers for months (Waddington 2003). Teasing out the relative impacts of all these influences would have taken an extensive and probably unachievable research program. Critical co-dependencies between the various drivers for change would have been huge confounders in the investigation.

Generally, the research effort required to monitor all the impacts of faculty development is substantial. Historically, such research has not been within the remit of units set up to manage faculty development (O'Sullivan and Irby 2011, Chap. 18). Consequently, as a whole, faculty development programs have been evaluated only over the short term and, commonly, at an individual level. Many have also not been in a position to scope their longer term impacts, either because of a dearth of research skills or a lack of appropriate funding; it is difficult to persuade institutions to fund follow-up outcome studies 5–10 years after the program has run its course.

This leads to a consideration of how faculty development can best lead to change. The first three strategies in our quest for organizational change are really focused on where faculty development needs to start, not where it needs to go.

6.8 How Does Faculty Development Challenge the Organization?

A good deal of faculty development that occurs appropriately in health professions education is frequently also responsible for confronting university staff and administrations with uncomfortable educational and social justice issues. For example, faculty development programs that target cultural competence often invoke challenges to the way in which indigenous or immigrant students are customarily dealt with. Achieving increased access by low socio-economic status groups to higher education through programs that allow less academically successful students entry (see Langlands 2005) sometimes involves changing the mindset of academic institutions wedded to high academic achievement and elitist models of academic progress. In the same vein, equality of access programs for students in medical and other healthcare disciplines (see GMC 2010), for which there has been associated faculty development, have challenged the accepted university standards for singular merit-based entry criteria (e.g. a certain grade point average in the USA, or 3 A grades in the national 'A level' school examinations in the UK). This has led to some faculties being identified as mavericks within the larger institutional context. Thus, 'faculty requirements' and 'university needs' may not be aligned, let alone those between individuals and the parent organization. This can cause tension and leads to the fourth strategy for success in exploiting faculty development to accomplish organizational change: **Faculty development programs must possess attributes and enshrine values that are shared, or at least tolerated, by the organizations and the faculty members that use them.** However they must also be prepared to manage and successfully reconcile, or at least balance, the tensions that arise when these values are not shared, or indeed clash.

Currently, faculty development in most organizations is not linked to strategic organizational issues, but to concepts of best practice in teaching, research, and management. So it is legitimate to discuss what, if any, organizational changes have come about as the result of faculty development initiatives.

6.9 How Does Faculty Development Promote Organizational Change?

There are few published studies of faculty development that seem to aim for, or report, organizational change. Faculty development is the method of choice to attempt to change staff practice by most health professions educational organizations: professional groups and associations, universities, and postgraduate colleges. As the article by Heaven et al. (2006) suggested, faculty development is often used to generate new clinical practice. It is also virtually the only framework used to change educational practice, even though the engagement with faculty development by the vast majority of teachers in higher and professional education is relatively infrequent. Many academics and practicing health professionals also attend conferences to develop their knowledge and skills, but this can frequently be less related to institutional priorities and more to discipline or methodological issues. Nonetheless, uptake rates of faculty development opportunities provided by institutions are universally low. Consequently, perhaps we should not be surprised to find that faculty development does not currently have a huge demonstrable impact at an organizational level.

There has also been an extensive and continued debate about the extent to which organizations can learn. Antonacopoulou (2006), in a review of several studies from this literature, makes some salient points. First, she suggests that the concept of the 'learning organization' (Argyris and Schön 1978) is flawed by the fact that organizations do not have brains. However recent conceptions, such as the notion of a community of practice (Lave and Wenger 1991), position the responsibility for organizational change within a group, locally and culturally determined, exercising organizational control functions. This immediately reinforces the same issues we have previously discussed: isolated individuals having been successful in developing themselves (or being developed) into change agents cannot necessarily effect substantial organizational development, even in a relatively small part of the organization. Antonacopoulou (2006) further discusses how, in the banking sector, an organization's approach to self-development and/or learning can have significant effects on the middle managers' capacity to change organizational practice. She identifies that in organizations in which respect for learning and encouragement to learn is genuine, managers are more likely to be self-reliant, more likely to pursue goals that will widen their employability, and more likely to seek the respective development more often. By contrast, managers who learn in order to satisfy the organization's requirements effectively do not learn at all, they 'merely play by the rules of the political game' (p. 465). In this respect, universities paradoxically seem to have taken an almost opposite path. The academic culture values self-development above most other things, as long as it reflects the academic values of freedom of thought, quality research and impactful publications. So, courses on statistical methods to improve research quality outnumber, by the tens or hundreds, courses on teaching and learning. Courses on managing a department and changing a culture to be more research-productive occur with some frequency; however, they are usually taught in a theory-free context. That is, our understanding about how some strategies work is very limited, and although there are often practical hints and rules of thumb, no real theoretical guidelines may exist. Also, in this process, individuals make choices from a menu of courses that is provided by other individuals with specific interests rather than as a collective (community of practice) decision to self-develop skills in certain areas. The chances of this approach having an impact on the organization are small. Let's take work on leadership as an example.

Steinert et al. (2012) reviewed the literature on faculty development programs aimed at leadership. They aimed to synthesize existing evidence addressing the effects of faculty development interventions designed to improve leadership abilities on the knowledge, attitudes, and skills of faculty members in medicine and on their institutions. Scrutiny of 48 articles, describing 41 studies of 35 interventions, showed limited changes in organizational practice. The authors also identified that although there was evidence of some organizational impact through implementation of specific educational innovations, changes in organizational practice were infrequently examined. In the small number of studies that did include this dimension, there were reported organizational benefits such as a shift to mission-based budgeting, an improved profile for education and scholarship in promotion and tenure decisions, implementation of specific educational innovations, increased collaboration, and creation of new leadership development programs. Thus, either because of lack of research power, or because of little attention to institutional outcomes, we know very little about how faculty development can generate a leadership culture. Currently, in Australia, a government agency, Health Workforce Australia, is promoting a framework called 'LEADS' to address leadership issues in healthcare reform (Health Workforce Australia 2012) and is offering leadership fellowships to individuals to use in the workplace and act as change stimulators.

In universities, the major effects of successful faculty development at the organizational level seem to be when a faculty development course is so well received by an organization and evaluated highly by participants that it becomes part of the institution's activities. This has happened several times, as reported in the literature (e.g. Litzelman et al. 1994; Roberts et al. 1994). However, it is likely that many more such 'adoptions' have been accomplished without making it into print.

Yet, we might ask, does adoption into the activities rank highly as an organizational change? Other hallmarks of organizational change might be expected in 'true' or transformational change, such as reference to continued development of faculty members or recognition of objectives contained in faculty development programs that become part of the mission and goals of the institution. Or perhaps transfer to another context would rank as even higher organizational impact. For example, Johansson et al. (2009) successfully disseminated, into a Swedish setting, a Californian-based faculty development model for residents that the originating institution had adopted.

But some programs seem to be energizing change quite effectively. The Foundation for Advancement of International Medical Education and Research (FAIMER) asked whether its International Fellowship Program was having an impact on leadership and institutional change respectively (Burdick et al. 2010, 2012; Friedman et al. Chap. 15). FAIMER uses a project-based approach to its programs; fellows who come from a wide variety of countries and healthcare contexts must devise a local project, describe why the project is important, what will be achieved, the methods, timeline, and budget, as well as how they will evaluate the success of the project. Notably, projects are required to have written support from their institutional leadership.

Findings from the first study (Burdick et al. 2010) suggested that the high engagement experience of the FAIMER model offering integration of education and leadership/management tools gave participants skills and capabilities that could be utilized across national contexts and result in a global network of interdependent leaders. A similar process is being used also in the Australasian College for Emergency Medicine's Mentoring Champions Program – designed to strengthen an individual's capacity to mentor others and lead the implementation of a mentoring program across the workplace (Australasian College for Emergency Medicine 2012).

The second study of FAIMER fellows investigated the degree and mode of impact of the fellowship projects. Across the 435 projects analyzed, the vast majority addressed one or more of the following areas: educational methods, curriculum change, program evaluation, student assessment, and alignment of educational content with local healthcare needs. Overall 62 % of these projects achieved (self-reported) high institutional impact. Burdick et al. (2012) suggest that one explanation for the relatively high incidence of organizational impact may be effective project mentoring and their demanding fellow selection process. This process includes the essential requirement of support for the project by the leadership of the fellow's home institution before the project commences. Such a requirement is a key feature of many change management theories (Grant and Gale 1989), and faculty development may be no exception to this.

The insistence by FAIMER on getting engagement between fellows and their institutions before the faculty development is delivered may turn out to be a key factor in a project's capacity to engender institutional change on a wide front. So, reflecting this in the steps for success would suggest that the fifth strategy should be as follows: **Faculty development facilitators and faculty development participants should engage with their respective institutional leadership *before* the faculty development takes place to negotiate the scope of potential desired outcomes and to gain institutional support and/or commitment.** This might be easiest when both facilitators and participants work in the same organization. But the international and cross-cultural success of the FAIMER fellowship program suggests that it is also worth the effort even if they work independently, and it may be beneficial to have an external, and potentially more objective, perspective.

In addition to this legitimization stage, achieving a wide impact may depend on other skills that are not traditionally the focus of faculty development programs. Some illuminating research throws light on what skills might be needed in this complex setting. Lieff and Albert (2012) studied 16 medical education leaders' approaches to what they do and how they learn and influence change. They found that these leaders operated in four major 'domains' of activity; intrapersonal, interpersonal, organizational (e.g. creating a shared vision), and systemic. In relation to the organizational context it was salient to discover that, among many other activities:

> Much of their (leaders') attention was given to understanding the role of individuals and the culture in the facilitation of change. This resulted in developing a diversity of efforts at diffusing organizational resistance as well as shifting attitudes and culture (Lieff and Albert 2012, p. 315).

Examples like this emphasize that if organizational change is desired from a faculty development program, it should perhaps give champions the skills and the institutional support to study how the essential pieces, the structures and the people, fit together, and where the pockets of resistance might come from.

These authors also found that the leaders in their study took an external systemic perspective and that:

> Political navigation of individuals, processes and structures of their academic contexts was essential for their success. They oriented themselves by deliberately engaging with certain groups in order to learn about the politics, power, culture and issues (Lieff and Albert 2012, p. 315).

Although such skills may come naturally to some people, or be developed as the result of their career paths, there is no reason to believe that occupying an academic or professional career would necessarily provide such skills, anymore than it would be to assume the same about teaching and assessment skills. So faculty development focused on organizational change should contain an element of politics, social theory and strategic planning.

One of the most wide ranging and intensive faculty development programs to have been launched in the last decade involves the attempts to eradicate error and improve patient safety. It is difficult to know whether this could be characterized as totally 'faculty development' as opposed to continuing professional development but, in the main, in Australia at least, there has been collaboration between the university and health care sectors that has produced many faculty development initiatives. Greenfield et al. (2011) documented the progress of one area of this development – interprofessional learning (IPL) towards better patient safety. Specifically, the researchers looked at which factors shaped the development and organizational impact of interprofessional improvement initiatives, created through collaborative action research, in one politically autonomous health organization. This organization provided healthcare to a population of nearly 500,000 people, encompassing three domains: a health service, incorporating 5,000 managers, clinicians and policymakers; an academic nexus involving 400 health academics in university settings; and 71 professional associations with an estimated 300 staff. Over a 2-year period, participants devised more than 111 interprofessional improvement projects including the development of an IPL focused approach to health professions preceptorship, to achieve a shared approach to learning and practice for student clinical placements. Three researchers analyzed ethnographic data relating to the 111 initiatives to identify factors that promoted or inhibited their development and impact on the organization. The analysis showed that of the 111 initiatives, 76 progressed beyond the initial proposal and/or discussion. The degree of success was variable between the three domains. Very few of the projects that were aimed at the interface between one domain and another made an impact, and little impact was made within the professional association domain, even though participants in all domains had identified that such activity was highly important.

This is of great concern because a very great many faculty development projects operate at these margins. For example, universities train registered health professionals to teach and assess students using faculty development approaches. Medical schools and postgraduate colleges accredit work sites for training suitability often achieved through a briefly visiting accreditation panel or paper based exercises, without real social engagement. In Greenfield's (2011) study, success *within* health and academic domains was relatively high; more than 50 % of projects made an organizational impact. Out of the 111 projects, 27 were formally sanctioned within the organization. Six determinants of maximal impact were identified:

- Site receptivity, which echoes the features identified earlier in the Heaven et al. (2006) study on communications skills.
- Team cohesion, which related to the strength and determination of the team involved in each initiative.
- Leadership, which concerned the presence of a champion at the head of, or supervising, the team who could articulate concrete aims for initiatives in

ways that resonated with the professional and organizational concerns of their colleagues.

- Impact on healthcare relations, which was about team processes.
- Impact on quality and safety issues, which highlighted the visibility of the initiative's agenda toward the aim of patient safety.
- The degree of integration into or legitimization by the institution.

There has traditionally been tension in health care organizations between providers (doctors, nurses) and managers (administrators) (e.g. Davies et al. 2003). A major faculty development initiative in many countries, but particularly in the UK, has been the attempt to get more doctors involved in health care management. This has not been altogether a successful program. Ham et al. (2011) researched the activities of doctors who became chief executives of National Health Service organizations. Most had left a clinical role to bring organizational and service improvement to patients. Although these doctors were positive about their roles, they nevertheless described themselves as 'keen amateurs' who identified that they needed structured support to become skilled management professionals. In a way, the connection between these executives and the nurses in Heaven et al.'s (2006) study is easy to see; putting people with certain new skill sets into roles is one thing; making them effective in that role is another. This allows us to identify two further 'strategies for success' in faculty development for organizational change. The first of these is that: **Faculty development must include a focus on those complex skills necessary for the participants in the program to impartially and sensitively observe, engage, and persuade their colleagues back in the workplace.**

In a sense, this resonates with the reality television series that immerse undercover bosses in their own organizations, or those that train up apprentices for chief executive status. These shows, while trite, clearly show how important those skills, not normally regarded as academic ones, really are; selling as opposed to explaining, promoting as opposed to evaluating, and engaging in menial as opposed to intellectual tasks. Hence, the final strategy would be as follows: **Faculty development must recognize the range of the additional contextual factors in the field, and identify and enhance the capacity of the developed professionals to deal with these factors.**

This strategy is also crucial if the faculty development program is being run on behalf of another organization. It also implies that, as far as organizational change is concerned, generic courses are likely to be less successful than those tailored to an organization's needs, structure and culture.

6.10   Conclusion

We have identified seven strategies for success at the organizational level if institutions are going to achieve positive organizational change themselves as a result of faculty development. Of course there are probably many more to be tried, but the literature base for this area is widespread, multi-disciplinary, not always reported in the kind of journals health professionals tend to read, and has a wide conceptual scope. In this chapter, we have just scratched the surface of this literature in attempting to bring together a contemporary and relevant set of strategies.

The main criticism to be leveled at faculty development programs in this context is that they often are not, or at least are not seen to be, aimed at long term institutional transformation of the kind that might be required to engage with major challenges: the need, for example, to provide a learning culture in health care organizations or value work-readiness in academic ones (Newton et al. 2009, 2011). To be useful as organizational change agents, faculty development programs also need to be designed, supported and promoted in ways that, at a minimum, reflect organizational values and goals. The explanation of why a program is being developed should be identified in the program's rationale and reflect the institution's main values, whether it is teaching, research, or a balanced combination of the two.

Such constraints will impact how activities are funded. Academic and health organizations should present these programs as delivering what they need, and make explicit why they need it. Then perhaps we would see units that run these activities flourish. In addition, perhaps if programs explicitly embraced academic values in their preparation and design (be they evidence-based, visibly anchored in real world problems, and diligently monitored, as FAIMER does), they would be better received and more successful.

6.11   Key Messages

Faculty development for organizational change:

- Must be defined for, and promoted to, an institution's members in a manner that clearly connects with its capacity to contribute to organizational change.
- Needs to be forward looking and directly linked to, or at least cognizant of and responsive to, organizational goals if it is to assist in promoting organizational change.
- Should address the elements in the organization, or in the participants' institutions, that can foster or impede the work of those that have undertaken the development process.
- Must possess attributes and enshrine values that are shared, or at least tolerated, by the organizations and faculty members that use them.
- Should enable facilitators and participants to engage with their respective institutional leadership *before* the faculty development takes place to negotiate the scope of potential desired outcomes.
- Must include a focus on those complex skills necessary for the participants in the program to impartially and sensitively observe, engage, and persuade their colleagues back in the workplace.
- Must recognize the range of the additional contextual factors in the field, and identify and enhance the capacity of the developed professionals to deal with these factors.

Acknowledgements The author wishes to acknowledge the gracious help and stimulating ideas of Clare and Jane Conway and Mary Lawson in the preparation and proofing of this chapter.

References

1st International Conference on Faculty Development in the Health Professions. (2011). Retrieved January 29th, 2013, from http://www.facultydevelopment2011.com

ACEM (Australasian College for Emergency Medicine). (2012). *Mentoring Champions Program.* Retrieved February 14th, 2012, from http://www.acem.org.au/sitedocument.aspx?docId=1268

Allen, D. L. (1990). Faculty development. *Journal of Dental Education, 54*(5), 266–267.

Antonacopoulou, E. P. (2006). The relationship between individual and organizational learning: New evidence from managerial learning practices. *Management Learning, 37*(4), 455–473.

Argyris, C. & Schön, D. A. (1978). *Organizational learning: A theory of action perspective.* New York, NY: Addison-Wesley.

Brew, A. & The Society for Research into Higher Education. (1995). *Directions in staff development.* Bristol, PA: Open University Press.

Billett, S. (1995). Workplace learning: Its potential and limitations. *Education and Training, 37*(5), 20–27.

Buerhaus, P. I., Staiger, D. O., & Auerbach, D. I. (2008). *The future of the nursing workforce in the United States: Data, trends and implications.* Boston, MA: Jones & Bartlett.

Burdick, W. P., Diserens, D., Friedman, S. R., Morahan, P. S., Kalishman, S., Eklund, M. A., et al. (2010). Measuring the effects of an international health professions faculty development fellowship: The FAIMER Institute. *Medical Teacher, 32*(5), 414–421.

Burdick, W. P., Friedman, S. R., & Diserens, D. (2012). Faculty development projects for international health professions educators: Vehicles for institutional change? *Medical Teacher, 34*(1), 38–44.

Davies, H. T. O., Hodges, C. L., & Rundall, T. G. (2003). Views of doctors and managers on the doctor-manager relationship in the NHS. *BMJ, 326*(7390), 626–628.

Davis, D., O'Brien, M., Freemantle, N., Wolf, F., Mazmanian, P., & Taylor-Vaisey, A. (1999). Impact of formal continuing medical education: Do conferences, workshops, rounds, and other traditional continuing education activities change physician behavior or health care outcomes? *JAMA, 282*(9), 867–874.

Elton, L. (1987). *Teaching in higher education: Appraisal and training.* London, UK: Kogan Page.

Elton, L. (1998). Staff development and the quality of teaching. In B. C. Jolly & L. Rees (Eds.), *Medical education in the millennium,* (pp. 199–204). Oxford, UK: Oxford University Press.

Ernst & Young. (2012). University of the future: A thousand year old industry on the cusp of profound change. Retrieved November 26th, 2012, from http://www.ey.com/Publication/vwLUAssets/University_of_the_future/$FILE/University_of_the_future_2012.pdf

General Medical Council. (2010). *Widening access into the medical profession.* Retrieved January 29th, 2013, from http://www.gmc-uk.org/Widening_Access_to_Medical_Education_1.0.pdf_25397210.pdf

Grant, J. & Gale, R. (1989). Changing medical education. *Medical Education, 23*(3), 252–257.

Greenfield, D., Nugus, P., Travaglia, J., & Braithwaite, J. (2011). Factors that shape the development of interprofessional improvement initiatives in health organisations. *BMJ Quality and Safety, 20*(4), 332–337.

Ham, C., Clark, J., Spurgeon, P., Dickinson, H., & Armit, K. (2011). Doctors who become chief executives in the NHS: From keen amateurs to skilled professionals. *Journal of The Royal Society of Medicine, 104*(3), 113–119.

Handy, C. B. (1999). *Understanding organizations, (4th Ed.).* London, UK: Penguin.

Hatton, P. & Bullimore, D. (1993). The role of staff development in changing environment: Experience from the University of Leeds. In Angela Towle (Ed.), Ch. 1, Section A, *Effecting change through staff development: Change in medical education (Sharing ideas 2)*, (pp. 33–38). London, UK: The King's Fund.

HWA (Health Workforce Australia). (2012). *Health LEADS Australia, Draft Australian Leadership Framework*. Retrieved January 29th, 2013, from http://www.hwaleadershipframework.net.au/about

Heaven, C., Clegg, J., & Maguire, P. (2006). Transfer of communication skills training from workshop to workplace: The impact of clinical supervision. *Patient Education and Counseling, 60*(3), 313–325.

Hill, A. G., Yu, T. C., Barrow, M., & Hattie, J. (2009). A systematic review of resident-as-teacher programmes. *Medical Education, 43*(12), 1129–1140.

Hilton, M. (2008). Skills for work in the 21st century: What does the research tell us? *Academy of Management: Perspectives, 22*(4), 63–78.

Johansson, J., Skeff, K., & Stratos, G. (2009). Clinical teaching improvement: The transportability of the Stanford Faculty Development Program. *Medical Teacher, 31*(8), e377–e382.

Jolly, B. C. (2002). Faculty development for curricular implementation. In G. R. Norman, C. P. M. van der Vleuten, & D. I. Newble (Eds.), *International handbook of research in medical education, Vol. 1*, (pp. 945–967). Dordrecht, NL: Kluwer Academic Publishers.

Khan, N., Khan, M. S., Dasgupta, P., & Ahmed, K. (2013). The surgeon as educator: Fundamentals of faculty training in surgical specialties. *BJU International, 111*(1), 171–178.

Langlands, Sir A. (2005). The gateways to the professions report. London, UK: Department for Education and Skills. Retrieved January 29th, 2013, from http://www.bis.gov.uk/assets/biscore/corporate/migratedd/publications/g/gateways_to_the_professions_report.pdf

Laprise, R. & Thivierge, R. L. (2012). Using speed dating sessions to foster collaboration in continuing interdisciplinary education. *Journal of Continuing Education in the Health Professions, 32*(1), 24–30.

Lave, J. & Wenger, E. (1991). *Situated learning: Legitimate peripheral participation*. Cambridge, UK: Cambridge University Press.

Lieff, S. & Albert, M. (2012). What do we do? Practices and learning strategies of medical education leaders. *Medical Teacher, 34*(4), 312–319.

Litzelman, D. K., Stratos, G. A., & Skeff, K. M. (1994). The effect of a clinical teaching retreat on residents' teaching skills. *Academic Medicine, 69*(5), 433–434.

Marinac, J. S., & Gerkovich, M. M. (2012). Outcomes from a mentored research boot camp: Focused Investigator Training (FIT) Program. *Pharmacotherapy, 32*(9), 792–798.

Mennin, S. P. & Kaufman, A. (1989). The change process and medical education. *Medical Teacher, 11*(1), 9–16.

Meyers, D. (2012). *Australian Universities: A portrait of decline*. AUPOD (e-Book). Available from: http://www.australianuniversities.id.au/Australian_Universities-A_Portrait_of_Decline.pdf

Muurlink, O. & Matas, C. P. (2011). From romance to rocket science: Speed dating in higher education. *Higher Education Research & Development, 30*(6), 751–764.

Newton, J. M., Billett, S., Jolly, B., & Ockerby, C. M. (2009). Lost in translation: Barriers to learning in health professional clinical education. *Learning in Health and Social Care, 8*(4), 315–327.

Newton, J. M., Billett, S., Jolly, B., & Ockerby, C. M. (2011). Preparing nurses and engaging preceptors. In S. Billett & A. Henderson (Eds.), *Developing learning professionals: Integrating experiences in university and practice settings*. Dordrecht, NL: Springer.

Onsman, A. (2009). *Carrots and sticks: Mandating teaching accreditation in higher education*. AARE 2009 International Education Research Conference: Canberra, Australia. Retrieved September 29th, 2012, from http://monash.academia.edu/AndrysOnsman/Papers/943519/Carrots_and_sticks_mandating_teaching_accreditation_in_Higher_Education

O'Sullivan, P. S. & Irby, D. M. (2011). Reframing research on faculty development. *Academic Medicine, 86*(4), 421–428.

Roberts, K. B., DeWitt, T. G., Goldberg, R. L., & Scheiner, A. P. (1994). A programme to develop residents as teachers. *Archives of Pediatrics & Adolescent Medicine, 148*(4), 405–410.

Rust, C. (2011). The professional development of faculty in the UK. *In Y. Dong (Ed.), Developing coordinately and growing together: Proceedings of the 2011 International Conference on Faculty Development.* Changchun, CN: Northeast Normal University Press. Available from: http://www.academia.edu/1019080/The_professional_development_of_faculty_in_the_UK

Shanley, C. (2004). Extending the role of nurses in staff development by combining an organizational change perspective with an individual learner perspective. *Journal for Nurses in Staff Development, 20*(2), 83–89.

Steinert, Y. (2010). Developing medical educators: A journey, not a destination. In Tim Swanwick (Ed.), *Understanding medical education: Evidence, theory and practice,* (pp. 403–418). Edinburgh, UK: The Association for the Study of Medical Education.

Steinert, Y., Naismith, L., & Mann, K. (2012). Faculty development initiatives designed to promote leadership in medical education. A BEME systematic review: BEME Guide No. 19. *Medical Teacher, 34*(6), 483–503.

Towle, A. (1998). Staff development in UK medical schools. In B.C. Jolly & L. Rees (Eds.), *Medical education in the millennium,* (pp. 205–210). Oxford, UK: Oxford University Press.

UK Department for Education and Employment. (1999). Learning to succeed: A new framework for post-16 learning. London, UK: Department for Education and Employment.

Van Roermund, T. C. M., Tromp, F., Scherpbier, A. J. J. A., Bottema, B. J. A. M., & Bueving, H. J. (2011). Teachers' ideas versus experts' descriptions of 'the good teacher' in postgraduate medical education: Implications for implementation. A qualitative study. *BMC Medical Education, 11*, 42.

Waddington, K. (2003). *Medical education at St. Bartholomew's Hospital, 1123–1995.* Suffolk, UK: Boydell Press.

White, E. & Winstanley, J. (2010). Clinical supervision: Outsider reports of a research-driven implementation programme in Queensland, Australia. *Journal of Nursing Management, 18*(6), 689–696.

Wildavsky, B. (2010). The great brain race: How global universities are reshaping the world. Princeton, NJ: Princeton University Press.

Wilkerson, L. & Irby, D. M. (1998). Strategies for improving teaching practices: A comprehensive approach to faculty development. *Academic Medicine, 73*(4), 387–396.

Part III
Approaches to Faculty Development

Chapter 7
Learning from Experience: From Workplace Learning to Communities of Practice

Yvonne Steinert

7.1 Introduction

Although the majority of faculty development activities consist of workshops and seminars, fellowships, and other longitudinal programs (Steinert et al. 2006), much of faculty development occurs in the workplace; in fact, many faculty members learn about teaching, leadership, and scholarship 'on the job'. For example, when teachers work together to develop new curricula or assess student progress, they are learning from experience; when chairs of departments meet together to discuss the joys and challenges of mentoring junior faculty, they are engaged in 'on the job' professional development that builds capacity and helps to meet organizational priorities; when researchers develop a new grant or prepare a novel experiment for presentation, they are engaged in workplace learning. In a recent study (Steinert 2012), 12 faculty members described the process by which they became medical educators and highlighted the following variables as critical to their development: the interest and desire to teach; the value of 'doing' medical education and learning as a result of specific job responsibilities; the value of mentors and role models; the benefits of belonging to a community of like-minded individuals; participating in formal (structured) faculty development opportunities; and pursuing an advanced degree. Faculty members in this study also highlighted the value of authentic experiences in the workplace. Although this study specifically examined the role of faculty members as educators, we could postulate that the value of learning on the job and belonging to a community of practice is also relevant in developing faculty members' other roles.

The goal of this chapter is to highlight the role that learning from experience can play in the development of health professionals. Although workplace learning

Y. Steinert, Ph.D. (✉)
Centre for Medical Education and Department of Family Medicine,
Faculty of Medicine, McGill University, Montreal, QC, Canada
e-mail: yvonne.steinert@mcgill.ca

Y. Steinert (ed.), *Faculty Development in the Health Professions: A Focus on Research and Practice*, Innovation and Change in Professional Education 11, DOI 10.1007/978-94-007-7612-8_7, © Springer Science+Business Media Dordrecht 2014

(or work-based learning as it is sometimes called) has been described as a strategy to promote professional development in higher education and other contexts (e.g. Billett 1996; Eraut 2004a; Raelin 1997), it has largely been ignored in the faculty development literature in the health professions (Cook 2009; Steinert 2010a, c). As DuFour (2004) has noted, 'the traditional notion that regarded staff development as an occasional event that occurred off the school site has gradually given way to the idea that the best staff development happens in the workplace rather than in a workshop' (p. 63).

This observation is consistent with the view expressed in Chap. 1 that 'professionals learn in a way that shapes their practice, from a diverse range of professional development activities' (Webster-Wright 2009, p. 705) and that we should move away from the notion of *developing* faculty to ongoing professional *learning*. This perspective also reminds us that we may have inadvertently created a false dichotomy between working and learning. In this chapter, we will discuss the role that learning from experience can play in the development of faculty members and suggest that it is time to refocus our attention on the workplace. More specifically, we will discuss the tenets of workplace learning and some of its key components, including role modeling, reflection, and learning from peers. Other aspects of learning from experience, such as repetition, rehearsal, practice, and feedback, will not be the focus of this chapter. However, we will explore the link between workplace learning and communities of practice, the role of such communities in promoting faculty development, and the need for organizational/institutional support to enable learning in the workplace.

7.2 Workplace Learning

Health professionals learn in the workplace. In fact, 'it is in the everyday workplace – where faculty members conduct their clinical, research and teaching activities, and interact with faculty, colleagues and students – that learning most often takes place' (Steinert 2010b, p. 407). Although this form of learning has not received significant attention in the faculty development literature in the health professions, its importance has been described in higher education, management and human resource development (Boud and Garrick 2001), undergraduate medical education (Dornan et al. 2007), and postgraduate medical education (Swanwick 2005, 2008). Swanwick and McKimm (Chap. 3) also highlighted its importance for leadership development.

7.2.1 What Is Workplace Learning?

There is no one definition or theory of learning in the workplace. Rather, the literature provides a range of conceptual approaches and empirical findings (Cheetham and Chivers 2001). For the purpose of this discussion, workplace learning will be defined as 'learning *for* work, learning *at* work, and learning *from* work' (Swanwick 2008, p. 341), with an emphasis on observation, participation, and expert guidance in an authentic environment (Billett 1994). According to Boud and Garrick (2001), the goals of workplace learning vary considerably and can include the improvement of performance for the benefit of the *organization* (i.e. the team or the enterprise), the improvement of learning for the benefit of the *learner*, and the improvement of learning as a *social investment* (i.e. for citizenship or social responsibility). However, fundamental to the notion of workplace learning is a view of learning as a socially mediated constructive process (Billett 1996), the value of 'participation in work' as a catalyst for learning (Billett 2004), and the complexity of this process in an ever-changing environment. Retallick (1999) has described a number of features of workplace learning that distinguish it from other forms of professional learning: 'it is task-focused, collaborative, and often grows out of an experience or problem for which there is no known knowledge base' (p. 34). Workplace learning also occurs in a political and economic context (Retallick 1999) in which the notion of learning and work may not always be compatible.

How then does learning in the workplace occur? Eraut (2004a) describes four types of work activity that give rise to the acquisition of knowledge and skill: participation in group activities (including team work); working alongside others (and gaining a new perspective from colleagues); tackling challenging tasks (which can increase confidence and problem solving abilities); and working with clients (or patients). Awareness of these different opportunities, which do not rely on the transmission of facts or expertise, can help faculty members and faculty developers begin to think about facilitating learning in the workplace. Eraut (2005) also identifies three main factors which influence learning in this setting: those deriving from the organization of work; those deriving from relationships at work; and those deriving from the agency of the individual and those who help him or her. This classification can provide health professionals with an additional road map for analysis and change.

In another context, Billett (1996) proposes a learning curriculum for workplace learning which accounts for the 'constructive nature of learning through problem-solving' (p. 53) and consists of two key components: activities and guidance. From this perspective, we need to *sequence* workplace activities that are of increasing complexity and, in so doing, permit the learner to experience more responsible goals and tasks, and *create a pathway* that affords learners the opportunity to access the outcomes of their work activities so that they will understand what they have achieved. For example, a faculty member might first learn about clinical teaching with one student at the bedside, and then with guidance from a colleague, work with a more heterogeneous group of students and residents. Feedback from the learners will also help to inform future actions. Alternatively, another faculty member might first design a practicum for nursing students before taking on the leadership of a clinical placement. Clearly, the sequencing of activities and the delineation of learning pathways to achieve specific goals are critical factors in the development of faculty members. The process of engagement is another essential component in this learning pathway, and as Swanwick (2005) has suggested, without individual engagement, learning may be superficial or, at worst, non-existent. Engagement is also dependent upon the congruence between the individual's interests and values with those of the workplace (Billett 2002).

Learning in the workplace offers a number of advantages: the value of authentic activities (which enable goal-directed learning and problem-solving), close (or proximal) guidance by colleagues in achieving relevant goals and moving from peripheral tasks to complex activities, interaction with 'expert others' (who also serve as role models for problem-solving), and engagement in tasks (which promotes reinforcement of knowledge and skill) (Billett 1995). Taking advantage of these opportunities, and overcoming some of the common limitations (e.g. the possible construction of inappropriate knowledge, reluctance of experts to provide guidance or sharing of knowledge, and limited access to appropriate expertise), remains a challenge.

7.2.2 What Is Learned in the Workplace?

In examining what is learned in the workplace, Eraut (2004b) identifies the following possibilities: task performance (e.g. collaborative work); awareness and understanding (e.g. of priorities and strategic issues); personal development; team work; role performance (e.g. leadership; accountability); academic knowledge and skills; decision-making and problem-solving; and judgment. This typology, based on Eraut's research in a number of settings, could be used as a way of helping faculty members to identify their own learning goals and outcomes in the workplace. In an interesting study of novice teachers in the health professions, Cook (2009) used these descriptors and observed that workplace learning primarily involved personal development, task and role performance, and awareness and understanding (of clinical teaching), in addition to experience, observation, reflection, and feedback. As Cook (2009) noted, the novice teachers in this study learned both the 'means' and 'ends' of teaching through their everyday practice (p. e612).

7.2.3 How Can Learning in the Workplace Be Enhanced?

Billett (2002) has suggested that participatory practices in the workplace are central to learning and include: engaging in work activities that are novel; securing appropriate guidance from experienced colleagues; and being able to practice critical tasks. He also highlights the interaction between the 'affordances and constraints' of the work setting (Billett 2004, p. 312) and the 'agency and biography' of the individual participant. That is, the work environment imposes certain norms and expectations (often in the interest of its own continuity and survival) regarding who can benefit from specific opportunities; at the same time, the individual can choose when he or she wants to engage – and in what way. Awareness of both organizational factors (e.g. in the hospital, the community or the university) and individual factors (e.g. learning goals and preferences) is key to enhancing workplace learning. So is the notion of expert guidance. For example, Billett (2002) stresses the value of *intentional*, guided learning strategies in the workplace and identifies different levels of guidance which may be required for optimal learning, dividing them into 'proximal (close) and distal (distant) forms of guidance'. Proximal guidance refers to guidance from a colleague or expert that enables joint problem solving and mirrors many facets of cognitive apprenticeship (Collins et al. 1989), including modeling, coaching, scaffolding, and fading. In this case, the 'learner' (i.e. a faculty member) remains in the 'driver's seat' and can determine the choice and sequencing of activities. On the other hand, distal guidance is less direct, providing 'clues and cues' based on social influences, cultural norms, the physical environment, and institutional practices. Distal guidance can suggest ways of problem solving in a much less direct fashion; however, it can be equally powerful in the learning process. Although proximal guidance is preferred by most professionals, both forms of guidance influence faculty members' behaviors.

7.2.3.1   Making Learning Visible

Based on research in higher education, it would be worthwhile to help health professionals see their everyday experiences as 'learning experiences' and be encouraged to reflect with colleagues and students on learning that has occurred in the clinical or the classroom setting (Steinert 2010a). Interestingly, Eraut (2004a) uses the term 'informal learning' to describe learning in the workplace. As he postulates, the use of 'informal' recognizes the 'social significance of learning from other people, but implies greater scope for individual agency than socialization' (p. 247). It also draws attention to the learning that takes place during or between professional tasks, sometimes even without the individual being aware of what is being learned. Ironically, this can be viewed as both a strength and weakness of workplace learning. Informal learning is largely invisible, either because much of it is taken for granted or not recognized as learning (Eraut 2004a), and it is our responsibility to make the invisible visible, through ongoing reflection and dialogue. We must also remember that this type of learning need not be serendipitous (Swanwick 2005); rather, informal learning can be 'planned' or 'emergent' (Megginson 1996), and we must take advantage of what occurs in our everyday environment.

7.2.3.2   Adopting a Workplace Pedagogy

The notion of a 'workplace pedagogy' (Billett 2002) has great appeal. It brings together notions of teaching and learning for faculty members and helps to explain how cultural, social, and situational factors interact with the individual's interests, preferences, and capacities (Billett 2002). A pedagogy for the workplace consists of more than intentional, guided learning at work, and as faculty members, we need to examine participatory practices (e.g. engaging in workplace activities; seeking guidance; accessing valued practices) and be cognizant of the fact that 'access' is not always equitable. As Billett (2002) has stated, 'workplace pedagogy needs to account for how workplaces *invite* access to activities and guidance and how individuals *elect* to participate in what the workplace affords' (p. 27). This framework suggests that we need to carefully examine how intentional and indirect guidance can be accessed in the workplace, how workplaces facilitate participation and guidance, and how individuals choose to engage in learning in the workplace. The strength of workplace learning lies in the notion of guided participation while performing authentic activities; as a result, we should try to maximize these learning opportunities for all health professionals.

7.3   Role Modeling as a Key Feature of Workplace Learning

Learning through role modeling, by observing colleagues and other team members, is a key feature of workplace learning (MacDougall and Drummond 2005). Although this complex method of learning has been frequently described in the training of health professionals (e.g. Cruess et al. 2008; Jochemsen-van der Leeuw et al. 2013; Kenny et al. 2003), it is rarely discussed as a method of faculty development. And yet, we can all remember moments when we observed colleagues in action and were impressed by either what they said or how they behaved in a particular situation. In multiple ways, role modeling is a powerful process by which faculty members can learn about the various aspects of their many roles.

Learning from role models occurs through observation and reflection and, as Epstein et al. (1998) noted, is a mix of both conscious and unconscious activities. While most health professionals are aware of the conscious observation of behaviors in others, much of what we learn through this process is incorporated into our daily lives without conscious awareness. As a result, becoming aware of this unconscious process can be a first step in making the most of role modeling's learning potential. As noted by Mann (Chap. 12), the process of role modeling is rooted in Bandura's (1986) theory of social learning and consists of four inter-related processes: attention, retention, reproduction, and motivation. Awareness of these processes, which are influenced by environmental, behavioral, and personal factors (Jochemsen-van der Leeuw et al. 2013), can help faculty members benefit from what occurs naturally. It is also important to note that role modeling, and observational learning which underlies this process, can be quite informal (and spontaneous) or more structured (and deliberate) (Steinert 2010a). Making this process more intentional, and valuing its contribution to ongoing professional development, would be a worthwhile first step.

In addition, learning from role models is a complex process, especially as we cannot assume what the role model is intending to demonstrate, even if we share similar backgrounds and interests. As a result, dialogue about what is being observed is important, and both the observer and the one being observed should be encouraged to talk and reflect on what is occurring – either in the moment or at a later time.

Mann (Chap. 12) outlines how faculty members can be more mindful and explicit in their role modeling with students across the continuum. In looking at role modeling as a strategy for faculty development, we must also become aware of its power as a method for personal learning and professional growth. In addition, we need to become more aware of what we are observing, reflect on our observations (either alone or with colleagues), and be willing to discuss what we have seen in a safe environment. Role modeling has previously been described as central to 'character formation' (Kenny et al. 2003), professional identity (Reuler and Nardone 1994), and the acquisition of professional behaviors (Cruess et al. 2008; Jochemsen-van der Leeuw et al. 2013) for students across the health professions. Its role in the formation of faculty members' identity and behaviors is yet to be determined. The impact of negative role modeling must also be explored and, as faculty members, we should be mindful of what we emulate. Lastly, we should be aware of the critical role of the institution (and the environment) in facilitating role modeling as a component of professional learning, especially as the influence of the 'hidden curriculum' (Hafferty 1998) on role modeling can be profound (Cruess et al. 2008). Moving forward, faculty developers should not only help faculty members take advantage of this powerful method of learning, they should also strive to change the workplace environment in which role modeling takes place. By working together with colleagues in making this implicit strategy more explicit, we can help to promote role modeling as a valued instrument in the process of change.

7.4 The Role of Reflection

Learning through reflection on experience is 'a key process in understanding how learning actually occurs in the workplace' (Retallick 1999, p. 34). Health professionals' ability to think critically and engage in reflection has long been considered an important factor in the improvement of clinical performance (Epstein 1999; Mamede and Schmidt 2004). Would it then not stand to reason that reflection could improve health professionals' skills and behaviors as faculty members?

Although many interpretations of reflection exist, the following definition will help to guide this discussion:

> Reflection is the process of stepping back from an experience to ponder, carefully and persistently, its meaning to the self through the development of inferences; learning is the creation of meaning from past or current events that serve as a guide for the future (Daudelin 1996, p. 39).

The notion of reflection has its roots in the work of Dewey (1933), who conceptualized reflective thought as a five-stage process (in Mamede and Schmidt 2004, p. 1302–1303):

1. A state of doubt, perplexity or uncertainty due to an emerging difficulty in understanding an event or solving a problem.
2. Definition of the difficulty by thoroughly understanding the nature of the problem.

3. Occurrence of a suggested explanation or possible solution for the problem, through inductive reasoning.
4. Rational elaboration of ideas produced through abstract, deductive thought focusing on their implications.
5. Testing resulting hypotheses by overt or imaginative action.

In looking at these stages through the lens of a teacher/educator, leader/manager or researcher/scholar, we can easily see how this could apply. A 'state of doubt or perplexity' is not uncommon in the life of a faculty member.

Building on the work of Dewey, Schön (1983) suggested the notion of reflective practice, which he viewed as consisting of two kinds of reflective activity: 'reflection *in* action', which refers to a spontaneous reaction (i.e. 'thinking on your feet') and 'reflection *on* action', which refers to thinking of a situation after it has happened. The former, which is frequently described as a subliminal process of which the participant is only partially aware, is usually triggered by recognition that 'something does not seem right' (Hewson 1991). This type of reflection also allows a faculty member to mentally reconstruct the experience, paying particular attention to context. Reflection *on* action forms a bridge between the re-lived situation and knowledge retrieved from internal memory or other external sources. While the development of the capacity to reflect 'in' and 'on' action has become an important feature of clinical practice, 'reflection *for* action' (Lachman and Pawlina 2006), which involves planning for the next step, forms an additional avenue for improvement. Moreover, although the concept of reflective practice fits in well with attempts to understand the development of professional expertise (Mamede and Schmidt 2004), it has remained relatively unexplored – and undervalued – in faculty development.

Mann (Chap. 12) reviews a number of underlying concepts and principles related to reflection and reflective practice. Essential to the context of workplace learning is the importance of being aware of different stages of reflection, learning to reflect, and acknowledging the role of reflection in professional development (or learning) in the workplace. According to Retallick (1999), reflection may progress through four stages: articulation of a problem or concern; analysis of the problem by probing for information or asking questions; generation of hypotheses that address the problem and development of tentative theories and solutions; and learning by testing hypotheses and theories in the workplace. Knowledge of these stages may help a researcher think about challenges in his lab or the supervision of graduate students, just as it may be of value to a course coordinator or unit head. Boud et al. (1985) provide another framework, consisting of three elements that are critical to the reflective process and can enhance workplace learning. They include:

- *Returning to experience* – which refers to the recollection of salient events, the replaying of the initial experience in the mind of the learner, or the recounting to others of the key features of the experience.
- *Attending to feelings* – which includes utilizing positive feelings and removing negative feelings, both of which are needed for learning to occur.
- *Re-evaluating experience* – which is clearly the most important and is often not completed if the other two phases are ignored. Re-evaluation involves a

re-examination of the original experience in light of the learner's goals, associating new knowledge with that which is already processed, and integrating new knowledge into the learner's conceptual framework.

This conceptualization may also be helpful to individual faculty members or faculty developers who would like to help improve the reflective abilities of their colleagues. As Raelin (1997) observed, 'since higher level reflection may not occur naturally, educational opportunities need to be provided within the workplace to provoke critical reflection' (p. 567). In addition to creating a work environment that supports reflection, such opportunities can include the use of reflective exercises, narrative writing and storytelling, appreciative inquiry, and the analysis of critical incidents (Branch et al. 2009; Higgins et al. 2011; Mann Chap. 12; Sandars 2009). Faculty members and faculty developers would be wise to consider these triggers for reflection, especially if we decide to not leave learning to chance.

In multiple ways, reflection can contribute as much to learning as experience itself (Raelin 1997), for reflective learning can help to make the implicit explicit and promote professional growth by changing perspectives, uncovering attitudes, and linking knowledge and skills to faculty members' professional values (Higgins et al. 2011). As Lachman and Pawlina (2006) observed, 'the process of reflection and its basis of critical thinking allows for the integration of theoretical concepts into practice, increased learning through experience, enhanced critical thinking and judgment in complex situations' (p. 460).

7.5 Learning from Peers

As stated at the outset, learning from peers in the workplace is formally recognized as a strategy for personal growth and development in the education and business literature. It is also a common strategy in the clinical arena, as health professionals learn from each other in both formal (e.g. rounds) and informal (e.g. in the hallway) settings. Surprisingly, however, learning from peers has not traditionally been viewed as an approach to faculty development in the health professions, and it is only recently beginning to emerge in this literature (McLeod and Steinert 2009). However, learning from peers is closely related to the notions of role modeling (as peers are often the role models) and reflection (as discussion with peers can prompt critical thinking) and can take on different forms.

Earlier in this chapter, we discussed Billett's (1996) notion of guidance from peers (and experts), much of which occurs spontaneously in an unstructured fashion. Boillat and Elizov (Chap. 8) also describe the value of peer coaching and mentoring – both in the workplace and in more formal contexts. As these authors describe, peer coaching is a form of workplace learning and commonly involves observation and feedback; it can also include consultation around specific issues or challenges and can help to enhance faculty members' performance in their diverse roles. In multiple ways, peer coaching is well-suited to the health professions as it is problem-based and built upon trust and collegiality. It is also 'learner-centered,' relying on collaborative expertise and joint decision-making. In an interesting monograph, Claridge and Lewis (2005) state that 'coaching is about enabling a learner to develop in the best way for them at the time' (p. 1) and describe a number of principles of coaching for effective learning that is relevant to workplace learning. These include the central role of the 'learner' in moving the process forward, the fundamental importance of the relationship between peers (built on trust and respect), the value of curiosity-driven questions with a focus on appreciative inquiry (rather than a deficit-based approach), and an emphasis on outcome and action. This approach has numerous advantages and can easily be adopted by faculty members and faculty developers to enhance the process of learning from peers.

Most of the literature on peer coaching and feedback in the workplace relates to the improvement of teaching effectiveness (Bennett et al. 2012; Brown and Ward-Griffin 1994). In a variation on this theme, McLeod et al. (2013) examined the value of peer assessment of lecturing skills. To accomplish the task, the authors invited faculty members to videotape their lectures and then critique their performance with a small group of peers. Feedback on this activity highlighted the benefits of peer review, including increased reflection, a renewed sense of collegiality, exposure to new ideas, and an opportunity for skill acquisition. The value of reflection was also highlighted in one of the participants' remarks: 'it is helpful to see yourself through the eyes of others' (McLeod et al. 2013, p. e1048). In fact, the notion of seeing yourself through the eyes of a peer is probably the single most powerful aspect of learning in this context.

Peer mentoring has also been highlighted as an important component of workplace learning, especially in the promotion of research capacity in the health professions (McCloughen et al. 2006; Paul et al. 2002; Records and Emerson 2003; Santucci et al. 2008). In this context, a sense of trust, collegial support, common goals, critical inquiry, and shared experiences can lead to successful relationships. Chapter 8 outlines a number of mentoring models that exist in the literature. Suffice it to say that we should recognize mentoring as an important learning strategy in workplace learning (Carter and Francis 2001), for it offers many advantages, including the mitigation of professional isolation while promoting an understanding of organizational norms and values. Moreover, as with peer coaching, it can help to contextualize learning, promote reflection, and foster collaborative inquiry and practice.

7.6 From Workplace Learning to Communities of Practice

Learning in the workplace often leads to the development of a community of practice. However, although these two concepts are distinct, they are both grounded in social constructivism and the belief that social participation is the basis of learning. Critical reflection and dialogue are also considered essential to both (Herbers et al. 2011). Communities of practice, which have been described in many fields, vary in nature. Some are quite formal in their organization, while others are more fluid and dynamic. Irrespective of the structure, however, it has been suggested that members are brought together by engaging in common activities and by what they learn through this mutual engagement (Wenger 1998).

Barab et al. (2002) define a community of practice as a 'persistent, sustaining, social network of individuals who share and develop an overlapping knowledge base, set of beliefs, values, history and experiences focused on a common practice and/or mutual enterprise' (p. 495). To elaborate on this definition, a community of practice involves three defining components: a domain, a community, and a practice (Wenger 1998). That is, a community of practice refers to a group of individuals with a shared *domain* of interests and concerns. These individuals have a clear commitment to the domain, value their collective experience, and learn from each other. Members of a community of practice also engage in joint activities and discussions and share information. They develop relationships among themselves and view interaction (and a sense of *community*) as critical to their success. Members of the community are also practitioners, and they work to develop a shared repertoire of resources, experiences, and tools to solve problems and promote scholarship and change (Herbers et al. 2011). Based on this perspective, *practice* refers to what community members do to advance a set of shared goals, and in this context, this can refer to health professionals' work in education, leadership or research.

Lave and Wenger (1991) suggest that the success of a community of practice depends on five factors: the existence and sharing by the community of a common goal; the existence and use of knowledge to achieve that goal; the nature and importance of relationships formed among community members; the relationships between the community and those outside it; and the relationship between the work of the community and the value of the activity. In his later work, Wenger (1998) adds the notion that achieving the shared goals of the community requires a shared repertoire of common resources, including language, stories, and practices. Interestingly, this list of 'indicators' can be helpful to individual faculty members who are wondering if their workplace might be a community of practice and to faculty developers who would like to help nurture their potential.

To facilitate this process, Wenger et al. (2002) describe a number of principles that can help to build a community of practice. These principles, outlined in Chap. 14 as well, include the following: design for evolution; open a dialogue between inside and outside perspectives; invite different levels of participation; develop both public and private community space; focus on value; combine familiarity and excitement; and create a rhythm for the community. Clearly, these design principles are not recipes for success; they do, however, provide a framework for developing a community of practice.

This discussion would be incomplete if we did not address the concept of legitimate peripheral participation, which is closely tied to learning and development in a community of practice. This social practice, which combines 'learning by doing' and apprenticeship into a single theoretical perspective, is the process by which a novice becomes an expert. According to Lave and Wenger (1991), learners begin by practicing legitimately on the periphery of a community and slowly move towards full participation (as they negotiate their own place within that community); in so doing, they develop expertise and 'know how'. That is, they move from 'newcomer to old-timer' (Swanwick 2008), and in the process, learn to 'talk-the-talk' and 'walk-the-walk'. Learning in the clinical environment has recently been recognized as a process of legitimate peripheral participation (Egan and Jaye 2009) that is fundamental to the development of professional identity for students at all levels of the continuum. Would this process not also be a critical factor in the development of faculty members' identity and the acquisition of expertise in the many facets of being a faculty member?

Few articles have specifically examined the role of communities of practice in faculty development. In one study, Herbers et al. (2011) report on the experience of four faculty members who tried to improve their teaching practices and enhance their graduate programs in education by belonging to a community of practice. Not surprisingly, critical reflection and dialogue were fundamental to the learning process, viewed as a transformative process by the authors and the participants. In another report, Sherer et al. (2003) describe the development of an online community of practice of college teachers through a faculty development portal and cite several benefits to participation, including the opportunity to access educational materials and enhance knowledge of teaching through collaboration with colleagues. The emerging potential of online communities is also discussed by Cook (Chap. 11). In the context of the health professions, Sherbino et al. (2010) relay the benefits of a national clinician educator program (e.g. improved educational problem solving; development of new projects) through the lens of a community of practice, and Jippes et al. (2013) demonstrate how social networks (in a community) can enhance the adoption of an educational innovation.

Although communities of practice can develop in the workplace, they can also emerge as a result of structured (or formal) faculty development programs, usually longitudinal in nature. For example, a number of longitudinal programs (e.g. Teaching Scholars Programs) have led to the development of a community of practice (e.g. Gruppen et al. 2006, Chap. 10; Moses et al. 2009; Steinert and McLeod 2006). In a similar vein, Lown et al. (2009) reported that fellowship participants commented on the value of support from a community of peers and mentors and perceived this sense of collegiality as a 'ticket of admission' to an academic career. Moreover, although the creation of a community was not an intended outcome in this program, belonging to a network of peers who shared similar goals and values was viewed as an unexpected benefit. This finding was also observed in a faculty development program for physicians in a longitudinal mentoring program for undergraduate students (Steinert et al. 2010) as well as in the rehabilitation sciences and nursing (Li et al. 2009). Despite these findings, it is surprising that faculty developers have not made this goal more explicit in the design and delivery of their educational activities. It would also be worthwhile to examine the role that Academies of Medical Educators (Bligh and Brice 2007; Cooke et al. 2003; Irby et al. 2004; Searle et al. 2010) and Centres (or Departments) of Medical Education (Davis et al. 2005), communities of practice in varying degrees, can play in the development of faculty members.

According to Wenger (1998), social participation within the community is the key to informal learning. It is 'embedded in the practices and relationships of the workplace and helps to create identity and meaning' (Boud and Middleton 2003, p. 194). As faculty members and faculty developers, we face an array of possibilities to make this learning count.

7.7   The Role of the Organization

The workplace (or organizational setting) clearly plays a role in facilitating both intended and unexpected learning experiences. Workplace 'affordances' (labeled as such by Billett 1994) vary from setting to setting and from group to group, and health professional leaders need to examine the workplace itself to assess whether it promotes – or hinders – a spirit of inquiry and learning. For example, Evans et al. (2006) used the concept of 'expansive' and 'restrictive' environments to describe the extent to which they facilitate learning. Expansive environments include close collaboration and opportunities for networking outside the immediate environment and, in the process, facilitate professional development. Building on this notion, Fuller and Unwin (2003) found that 'successful' workplaces demonstrated a number of common characteristics, of which some were related to the configuration of formal and informal learning; other attributes related to allowing participation in multiple communities of practice, the development of what they called a 'participative memory', and the provision of access to learning opportunities. Recognition of the 'learner' (or in this case, the faculty member) – and the value of learning within the organization – was also described as a key ingredient to successful apprenticeships in the workplace. Other factors that can affect learning in the workplace include: the allocation and structuring of work; expectations of individual roles, performance, and progress; the facilitation of encounters and relationships with people in the workplace; and continuity and support, over an extended period of time (Eraut 2005). As faculty members and faculty developers, we must be aware of the factors that can promote learning in the workplace, strive to overcome perceived barriers, and acknowledge success.

7.8   Challenges Moving Forward

Boud and Middleton (2003) suggest that informal learning (in the workplace) is often not acknowledged as learning within organizations as it is viewed as 'part of the job'. Others have described workplace learning as *ad hoc* or incidental (Billett 1994), and not part of professional development. However, from our perspective, there is value in rendering informal learning (in the workplace) as visible as possible. How do we do this? What barriers must we overcome to achieve this goal?

In discussing the question of how teachers' workplace learning can receive recognition as a legitimate form of professional development, or be accredited by universities and other professional bodies, Retallick (1999) suggests that professional learning portfolios can play an important role. In fact, he argues that a portfolio can contribute to enhanced educational effectiveness, a renewed professional culture of teaching and learning, and ongoing development. He also states that the 'systematic documentation of workplace learning could become a normal part of teachers' work… [and] play an important part in developing the scholarship of teaching' (p. 49). Although Retallick (1999) and other authors focus on the educational role of faculty members, this suggestion can apply to all faculty roles, as a portfolio can easily be used to document personal and professional growth as a leader and scholar. It is clear that professional learning does occur in the workplace, that faculty members can provide evidence of, and make sound judgments about, the quality of their learning, and that workplace learning does not only mean *experience*, but also refers to the *learning* which results from that experience (Retallick 1999). We must now find ways to credential this learning. At the same time, the challenge for faculty developers is to understand how faculty members learn in the workplace, discover ways of enhancing – and optimizing – this learning, and find the means to more effectively utilize this learning within the organizational context.

In summary, it is important to not leave workplace learning to chance. Enhancing role modeling and reflection, as stated earlier, is one option. There is also merit in ensuring that learning on the job is not haphazard and that we work with departments, divisions or other designated units to ascertain whether ongoing professional development in the workplace can achieve its desired outcomes and increase faculty members' individual abilities and collective capacity (DuFour 2004). In addition, it would be worthwhile to explore whether workplace learning can enable faculty members to apply their new knowledge to a change in behavior, focus on results rather than activities, and demonstrate a sustained commitment to achieving mutually beneficial goals.

7.9 Conclusion

The goal of this chapter has been to highlight the role of workplace learning and its key elements of role modeling, reflection, and learning from peers in an attempt to help us begin to recognize, acknowledge, and validate naturally occurring events as a form of learning and faculty development. Moreover, although the primary goal of this chapter has been the professional growth and development of the individual faculty member in the workplace, we should remember that the development of individuals can lead to more productive workplaces (Bierema 1996).

Health professionals encounter numerous competing demands and priorities in the workplace and often experience a tension between their multiple responsibilities (e.g. clinical demands versus educational needs). As faculty members and faculty developers, we need to distinguish between learning episodes (in which learning is the main objective) and those in which work is primary (and learning may be an unrecognized by-product). We may also wish to re-consider the value of apprenticeships in faculty development, for as Wenger (1998) has said, 'learning cannot be designed. Ultimately, it belongs to the realm of experience and practice… Learning happens, design or no design' (p. 225).

7.10   Key Messages

- Health professionals learn about their multiple roles in the workplace.
- Workplace learning requires authentic experiences, individual engagement, intentional guidance, and organizational support.
- Role modeling, reflection, and learning from peers are essential components of workplace learning.
- Workplace learning can lead to a community of practice, which in turn can promote ongoing professional learning.
- Faculty members and faculty developers should try to intentionally recognize and validate workplace learning and communities of practice as venues for faculty development.

References

Bandura, A. (1986). *Social foundations of thought and action: A social cognitive theory.* Englewood Cliffs, NJ: Prentice-Hall.

Barab, S. A., Barnett, M., & Squire, K. (2002). Developing an empirical account of a community of practice: Characterizing the essential tensions. *The Journal of the Learning Sciences, 11*(4), 489–542.

Bennett, P. N., Parker, S., & Smigiel, H. (2012). Paired peer review of university classroom teaching in a school of nursing and midwifery. *Nurse Education Today, 32*(6), 665–668.

Bierema, L. L. (1996). Development of the individual leads to more productive workplaces. *New Directions for Adult and Continuing Education, 1996*(72), 21–28.

Billett, S. (1994). Situating learning in the workplace - Having another look at apprenticeships. *Industrial and Commercial Training, 26*(11), 9–16.

Billett, S. (1995). Workplace learning: Its potential and limitations. *Education and Training, 37*(5), 20–27.

Billett, S. (1996). Towards a model of workplace learning: The learning curriculum. *Studies in Continuing Education, 18*(1), 43–58.

Billett, S. (2002). Toward a workplace pedagogy: Guidance, participation, and engagement. *Adult Education Quarterly, 53*(1), 27–43.

Billett, S. (2004). Workplace participatory practices: Conceptualising workplaces as learning environments. *Journal of Workplace Learning, 16*(5–6), 312–324.

Bligh, J. & Brice, J. (2007). The Academy of Medical Educators: A professional home for medical educators in the UK. *Medical Education, 41*(7), 625–627.

Boud, D. & Garrick, J. (2001). *Understanding learning at work.* London, UK: Routledge.

Boud, D., Keogh, R., & Walker, D. (1985). *Reflection: Turning experience into learning.* New York, NY: Nichols Publishing Company.

Boud, D. & Middleton, H. (2003). Learning from others at work: Communities of practice and informal learning. *Journal of Workplace Learning, 15*(5), 194–202.

Branch, W. T. Jr., Frankel, R., Gracey, C. F., Haidet, P. M., Weissmann, P. F., Cantey, P., et al. (2009). A good clinician and a caring person: Longitudinal faculty development and the enhancement of the human dimensions of care. *Academic Medicine, 84*(1), 117–125.

Brown, B. & Ward-Griffin, C. (1994). The use of peer evaluation in promoting nursing faculty teaching effectiveness: A review of the literature. *Nurse Education Today, 14*(4), 299–305.

Carter, M. & Francis, R. (2001). Mentoring and beginning teachers' workplace learning. *Asia-Pacific Journal of Teacher Education, 29*(3), 249–262.

Cheetham, G. & Chivers, G. (2001). How professionals learn in practice: An investigation of informal learning amongst people working in professions. *Journal of European Industrial Training, 25*(5), 247–292.

Claridge, M. T. & Lewis, T. (2005). *Coaching for effective learning: A practical guide for teachers in health and social care*. Abingdon, UK: Radcliffe Publishing Ltd.

Collins, A., Brown, J. S., & Newman, S. E. (1989). Cognitive apprenticeship: Teaching the crafts of reading, writing and mathematics. In L.B. Resnick (Ed.), *Knowing, learning, and instruction: Essays in honor of Robert Glaser*. Hillsdale, NJ: Erlbaum.

Cook, V. (2009). Mapping the work-based learning of novice teachers: Charting some rich terrain. *Medical Teacher, 31*(12), e608–e614.

Cooke, M., Irby, D. M., & Debas, H. T. (2003). The UCSF Academy of Medical Educators. *Academic Medicine, 78*(7), 666–672.

Cruess, S. R., Cruess, R. L., & Steinert, Y. (2008). Role modelling: Making the most of a powerful teaching strategy. *BMJ, 336*(7646), 718–721.

Daudelin, M. W. (1996). Learning from experience through reflection. *Organizational Dynamics, 24*(3), 36–48.

Davis, M. H., Karunathilake, I., & Harden, R. M. (2005). AMEE Education Guide No. 28: The development and role of departments of medical education. *Medical Teacher, 27*(8), 665–675.

Dewey, J. (1933). *How we think*. Boston, MA: Heath.

Dornan, T., Boshuizen, H., King, N., & Scherpbier, A. (2007). Experience-based learning: A model linking the processes and outcomes of medical students' workplace learning. *Medical Education, 41*(1), 84–91.

DuFour, R. (2004). Leading edge: The best staff development is in the workplace, not in a workshop. *Journal of Staff Development, 25*(2), 63–64.

Egan, T. & Jaye, C. (2009). Communities of clinical practice: The social organization of clinical learning. *Health, 13*(1), 107–125.

Epstein, R. M. (1999). Mindful practice. *JAMA, 282*(9), 833–839.

Epstein, R. M., Cole, D. R., Gawinski, B. A., Piotrowski-Lee, S., Ruddy, N. B. (1998). How students learn from community-based preceptors. *Archives of Family Medicine, 7*(2), 149–154.

Eraut, M. (2004a). Informal learning in the workplace. *Studies in Continuing Education, 26*(2), 247–273.

Eraut, M. (2004b). Transfer of knowledge between education and workplace settings. In H. Rainbird, A. Fuller, A. Munro (Eds.), *Workplace learning in context*, (pp. 201–221). London, UK: Routledge.

Eraut, M. (2005). Continuity of learning. *Learning in Health and Social Care, 4*(1), 1–6.

Evans, K., Hodkinson, P., Rainbird, H., & Unwin, L. (2006). *Improving workplace learning*. London, UK: Routledge.

Fuller, A. & Unwin, L. (2003). Learning as apprentices in the contemporary UK workplace: Creating and managing expansive and restrictive participation. *Journal of Education and Work, 16*(4), 407–426.

Gruppen, L. D., Simpson, D., Searle, N. S., Robins, L., Irby, D. M., & Mullan, P. B. (2006). Educational fellowship programs: Common themes and overarching issues. *Academic Medicine, 81*(11), 990–994.

Hafferty, F. W. (1998). Beyond curriculum reform: Confronting medicine's hidden curriculum. *Academic Medicine, 73*(4), 403–407.

Herbers, M. S., Antelo, A., Ettling, D., & Buck, M. A. (2011). Improving teaching through a community of practice. *Journal of Transformative Education, 9*(2), 89–108.

Hewson, M. G. (1991). Reflection in clinical teaching: An analysis of reflection-on-action and its implications for staffing residents. *Medical Teacher, 13*(3), 227–231.

Higgins, S., Bernstein, L., Manning, K., Schneider, J., Kho, A., Brownfield, E., et al. (2011). Through the looking glass: How reflective learning influences the development of young faculty members. *Teaching and Learning in Medicine, 23*(3), 238–243.

Irby, D. M., Cooke, M., Lowenstein, D., & Richards, B. (2004). The academy movement: A structural approach to reinvigorating the educational mission. *Academic Medicine, 79*(8), 729–736.

Jippes, E., Steinert, Y., Pols, J., Achterkamp, M. C., van Engelen, J. M., & Brand P. L. (2013). How do social networks and faculty development courses affect clinical supervisors' adoption of a medical education innovation? An exploratory study. *Academic Medicine, 88*(3), 398–404.

Jochemsen-van der Leeuw, H. G., van Dijk, N., van Etten-Jamaludin, F. S., & Wieringa-de Waard, M. (2013). The attributes of the clinical trainer as a role model: A systematic review. *Academic Medicine, 88*(1), 26–34.

Kenny, N. P., Mann, K. V., & MacLeod, H. (2003). Role modeling in physicians' professional formation: Reconsidering an essential but untapped educational strategy. *Academic Medicine, 78*(12), 1203–1210.

Lachman, N. & Pawlina, W. (2006). Integrating professionalism in early medical education: The theory and application of reflective practice in the anatomy curriculum. *Clinical Anatomy, 19*(5), 456–460.

Lave, J. & Wenger, E. (1991). *Situated learning: Legitimate peripheral participation.* New York, NY: Cambridge University Press.

Li, L. C., Grimshaw, J. M., Nielsen, C., Judd, M., Coyte, P. C., & Graham, I. D. (2009). Use of communities of practice in business and health care sectors: A systematic review. *Implementation Science, 4*, 27.

Lown, B. A., Newman, L. R., & Hatem, C. J. (2009). The personal and professional impact of a fellowship in medical education. *Academic Medicine, 84*(8), 1089–1097.

MacDougall, J. & Drummond, M. J. (2005). The development of medical teachers: An enquiry into the learning histories of 10 experienced medical teachers. *Medical Education, 39*(12), 1213–1220.

Mamede, S. & Schmidt, H. G. (2004). The structure of reflective practice in medicine. *Medical Education, 38*(12), 1302–1308.

McCloughen, A., O'Brien, L., & Jackson, D. (2006). Positioning mentorship within Australian nursing contexts: A literature review. *Contemporary Nurse, 23*(1), 120–134.

McLeod, P. J. & Steinert, Y. (2009). Peer coaching as an approach to faculty development. *Medical Teacher, 31*(12), 1043–1044.

McLeod, P. J., Steinert, Y., Capek, R., Chalk, C., Brawer, J., Ruhe, V., et al. (2013). Peer review: An effective approach to cultivating lecturing virtuosity. *Medical Teacher, 35*(4), e1046–e1051.

Megginson, D. (1996). Planned and emergent learning: Consequences for development. *Management Learning, 27*(4), 411–428.

Moses, A. S., Skinner, D. H., Hicks, E., & O'Sullivan P. S. (2009). Developing an educator network: The effect of a teaching scholars program in the health professions on networking and productivity. *Teaching and Learning in Medicine, 21*(3), 175–179.

Paul, S., Stein, F., Ottenbacher, K. J., & Liu, Y. (2002). The role of mentoring on research productivity among occupational therapy faculty. *Occupational Therapy International, 9*(1), 24–40.

Raelin, J. A. (1997). A model of work-based learning. *Organization Science, 8*(6), 563–578.

Records, K. & Emerson, R. J. (2003). Mentoring for research skill development. *Journal of Nursing Education, 42*(12), 553–557.

Retallick, J. (1999). Teachers' workplace learning: Towards legitimation and accreditation. *Teachers and Teaching: Theory and Practice, 5*(1), 33–50.

Reuler, J. B. & Nardone, D. A. (1994). Role modeling in medical education. *The Western Journal of Medicine, 160*(4), 335–337.

Sandars, J. (2009). The use of reflection in medical education: AMEE Guide No. 44. *Medical Teacher, 31*(8), 685–695.

Santucci, A. K., Lingler, J. H., Schmidt, K. L., Nolan, B. A. D., Thatcher, D., & Polk, D. E. (2008). Peer-mentored research development meeting: A model for successful peer mentoring among junior level researchers. *Academic Psychiatry, 32*(6), 493–497.

Schön, D. A. (1983). *The reflective practitioner: How professionals think in action.* New York, NY: Basic Books.

Searle, N. S., Thompson, B. M., Friedland, J. A., Lomax, J. W., Drutz, J. E., Coburn, M., et al. (2010). The prevalence and practice of academies of medical educators: A survey of U.S. medical schools. *Academic Medicine, 85*(1), 48–56.

Sherbino, J., Snell, L., Dath, D., Dojeiji, S., Abbott, C., & Frank, J. R. (2010). A national clinician-educator program: A model of an effective community of practice. *Medical Education Online, 15*, Art. 5356.

Sherer, P. D., Shea, T. P., & Kristensen, E. (2003). Online communities of practice: A catalyst for faculty development. *Innovative Higher Education, 27*(3), 183–194.

Steinert, Y. (2010a). Becoming a better teacher: From intuition to intent. In J. Ende (Ed.), *Theory and practice of teaching medicine,* (pp. 73–93). Philadelphia, PA: American College of Physicians.

Steinert, Y. (2010b). Developing medical educators: A journey not a destination. In T. Swanwick (Ed.), *Understanding medical education: Evidence, theory and practice,* (pp. 403–418). Edinburgh, UK: Association for the Study of Medical Education.

Steinert, Y. (2010c). Faculty development: From workshops to communities of practice. *Medical Teacher, 32*(5), 425–428.

Steinert, Y. (2012). Faculty development: On becoming a medical educator. *Medical Teacher, 34*(1), 74–76.

Steinert, Y., Boudreau, J. D., Boillat, M., Slapcoff, B., Dawson, D., Briggs, A., et al. (2010). The Osler Fellowship: An apprenticeship for medical educators. *Academic Medicine, 85*(7), 1242–1249.

Steinert, Y., Mann, K., Centeno, A., Dolmans, D., Spencer, J., Gelula, M., et al. (2006). A systematic review of faculty development initiatives designed to improve teaching effectiveness in medical education: BEME Guide No. 8. *Medical Teacher, 28*(6), 497–526.

Steinert, Y. & McLeod, P. J. (2006). From novice to informed educator: The Teaching Scholars Program for Educators in the Health Sciences. *Academic Medicine, 81*(11), 969–974.

Swanwick, T. (2005). Informal learning in postgraduate medical education: From cognitivism to 'culturism'. *Medical Education, 39*(8), 859–865.

Swanwick, T. (2008). See one, do one, then what? Faculty development in postgraduate medical education. *Postgraduate Medical Journal, 84*(993), 339–343.

Webster-Wright, A. (2009). Reframing professional development through understanding authentic professional learning. *Review of Educational Research, 79*(2), 702–739.

Wenger, E. (1998). *Communities of practice: Learning, meaning, and identity.* New York, NY: Cambridge University Press.

Wenger, E., McDermott, R., & Snyder, W. M. (2002). *Cultivating communities of practice.* Boston, MA: Harvard Business School Press.

Chapter 8
Peer Coaching and Mentorship

Miriam Boillat and Michelle Elizov

8.1 Introduction

As our understanding of the processes of learning and change has evolved, the paradigm of faculty development has also changed in both its focus and scope of activities. Faculty development is now accepted to be more than the improvement of teaching skills and can include personal growth, work-life balance and career development. It encompasses the broad development of many academic roles, some of which may be better developed by activities that incorporate notions of self-directed learning, collaborative peer relationships, reflection and work-based learning (Steinert 2011). Support for new approaches to faculty development is found in two reviews of faculty development initiatives in medical education (McLean et al. 2008; Steinert et al. 2006). Key features of effective faculty development highlighted in these reviews include the role of experiential and authentic learning, the value of feedback, the importance of peers as role models and as providers of collegial support, and the value of extended programs. The conceptual framework developed by Steinert (2010), where peer coaching is described as a more formal, individualized form of faculty development, and mentorship as a means of enhancing any faculty development strategy, lends further support. Faculty development should encompass both formal and informal approaches, and should provide opportunities for individual and group reflection. Common goals, collegiality and shared reflection are important components of faculty development that is work-based and integrated within communities of practice (Steinert 2010).

M. Boillat, MD, CCFP, FCFP (✉)
Centre for Medical Education and Department of Family Medicine,
Faculty of Medicine, McGill University, Montreal, QC, Canada
e-mail: miriam.boillat@mcgill.ca

M. Elizov, MD, FRCPC, MHPE
Centre for Medical Education and Department of Medicine,
Faculty of Medicine, McGill University, Montreal, QC, Canada
e-mail: michelle.elizov@mcgill.ca

Y. Steinert (ed.), *Faculty Development in the Health Professions: A Focus on Research and Practice*, Innovation and Change in Professional Education 11, DOI 10.1007/978-94-007-7612-8_8, © Springer Science+Business Media Dordrecht 2014

Peer coaching and mentorship share at their core unique strengths that align with these concepts of effective faculty development. They are highly personalized approaches that are learner-centered, thus meeting individual faculty needs. Their relational nature requires a level of collegiality, trust and commitment to both the process and to the individuals involved that is beyond what one might expect in traditional faculty development activities. Additionally, the need for honest reflection when using these approaches has the potential to increase self-awareness and facilitate lasting change. Because both these approaches encourage the admission of uncertainty and fallibility, they require a safe environment that optimally develops in a longitudinal fashion. Peer coaching and mentorship both emphasize experiential and authentic learning. The educational principles and theories that inform them include situated learning (Lave and Wenger 1991), experiential learning (Kolb 1984), principles of adult learning (Knowles 1973), and transformative learning (Mezirow 1991).

As peer coaching and mentorship share many features, they are sometimes used interchangeably; however, key differences should be highlighted. *Peer coaching* often focuses on tasks or skills to be developed. It is immediately practical and exploits daily learning opportunities. It is a form of work-based learning and commonly involves observation of teaching and feedback. It is also useful for other teaching activities such as developing course objectives or preparing tests and assignments. Peer coaching is not limited, however, to improving teaching skills, and can be used in leadership development or to support other faculty roles. Peer coaching often involves reciprocal learning between faculty members with similar levels of experience and expertise. On the other hand, *mentorship* has more of an 'abstract' quality in that it is often removed in either place or time from daily events. Mentoring relationships may involve a greater sense of depth, caring and emotional bonding because they address issues such as personal work-life balance and career development. Mentors also provide guidance instrumental to effective functioning within an organization and advocate on behalf of their mentees for resources and support necessary for the fulfillment of the mentees' goals (Allen et al. 2009).

This chapter will provide definitions of peer coaching and mentorship which will frame the subsequent description of these faculty development strategies. A number of different models of peer coaching and mentorship will be reviewed and the benefits and challenges of each will be discussed. General principles for the implementation of these strategies in faculty development will be outlined. In closing, we will suggest future directions for research and summarize key messages regarding the utilization of these promising faculty development strategies for the health professions.

8.2   Definition of Terms

8.2.1   Peer Coaching

There is lack of consensus in the literature about the precise definition of peer coaching (D'Abate et al. 2003). Peer coaching was initially developed to improve teaching skills in classroom settings. However, it is also useful to support and develop other faculty roles and skills such as leader, manager or researcher (McLeod and Steinert 2009). In business and management, peer coaching to improve performance in the workplace, and coaching for leadership (often referred to as *executive coaching*), have been used for a number of years (Joo 2005). Peer coaching may involve coaching by a more experienced individual or by a peer with a similar level of experience. It may be *reciprocal*, with two partners serving as coach to each other, or it may be *one-way*, with one partner serving as coach and the other receiving the coaching. Peer coaching may also occur in small groups. In the educational context, Huston and Weaver (2008) define peer coaching as 'a collegial process whereby two faculty members voluntarily work together to improve or expand their approaches to teaching' (p. 7). Peer coaching can be considered a *peer learning partnership*, described by Eisen (2000) as a 'voluntary, reciprocal helping relationship between individuals of comparable status who share a common or closely related learning/development objective' (p. 5).

Peer coaching as a faculty development approach is well suited for the health professions. It depends on a trusting collegial relationship and promotes shared reflection. It generally involves learning with a colleague in one's own context. At its core, peer coaching involves *peer feedback*, which itself has been identified as a key component of effective faculty development programs (Steinert et al. 2006).

Three phases have been described in peer coaching for *teaching skill development*: (1) pre-observation discussion to clarify personal learning objectives, context, expectations and process; (2) direct observation by the peer coach; and (3) post-observation debriefing session when observations are shared, constructive feedback is provided, and shared reflection and discussion occur (Flynn et al. 1994).

Peer coaching should be distinguished from consultation with an expert. The latter can be of great value as well, though it does not tap into the unique opportunity for growth when individuals learn together through discussion, observation of specific skills, feedback and reflection. It is also important to differentiate peer coaching as a *faculty development* initiative, from *summative peer review*, which has been described as a component of performance review for the purpose of evaluation and promotion (Bernstein et al. 2000). Although both approaches share some common elements (observation of teaching, intent to improve teaching practices), in its essence, peer coaching is voluntary, confidential, formative and based on the self-identified needs of the recipient of the coaching.

The length of peer coaching programs described in the literature is variable, and it may take place once or be longitudinal over time (Eisen 2001; Fry and Morris 2004; O'Keefe et al. 2009). When longitudinal, peer coaching relationships often change according to evolving needs (Huston and Weaver 2008).

8.2.2   Mentorship

The literature abounds with definitions of mentor or mentorship. Some of these describe characteristics of good mentors or mentoring relationships, while others describe the strategies or roles employed within the mentoring relationship

(Blixen et al. 2007; Rose et al. 2005; Smith and Zsohar 2007; Tobin 2004). A landmark study from business defined mentorship as '…a relationship with a person who took a personal interest in your career and who guided or sponsored you…' (Roche 1979, p. 15). Despite varying definitions of mentorship, the essence is a *relationship*, and those that attempt to define the relationship itself often describe some or all of the following important elements (Bland et al. 2009; Eby et al. 2010; Jackson et al. 2003; Johnson 2007; Kram 1983):

- An *interpersonal connection*, sometimes described as a 'click' or a 'fit' that is felt to be most effective and satisfying.
- The *development and evolution of the relationship over time* passing through specific phases: initiation, cultivation, separation and redefinition (Kram 1983).
- The need for a *defined purpose*, noting that this purpose may change over time as it is frequently determined by both the life phase and career phase of the mentee.
- The *broad purpose* being to help the mentee develop or acquire the skills, the competencies and the relationships needed to be successful and satisfied in their personal and professional lives.
- A *collaborative learning relationship* with each person benefitting from the experience to varying degrees.

An additional component, developing a *reflective* practice, cannot be underestimated. Reflection in medicine, as described by Schön (1983), is commonly understood to mean self-reflection on one's own experience and this is extremely important for mentees to do. However, reflecting on the experience of *others*, in this case the mentor, can also be extremely valuable, particularly in certain higher stakes situations such as making career decisions or finding work-life balance, potentially avoiding erroneous or ill-timed decisions that can have far-reaching and long-lasting consequences.

While these elements are not exclusive to mentoring relationships, it is their combination that leads to the working definition of mentorship that will be used in this chapter.

This section would be incomplete if the attributes of both the mentor and the mentee that contribute to the relationship's success are not considered. The characteristics of ideal mentors do not change and these have been well described in the literature (Sambunjak et al. 2010). These can be divided into personal, relational and professional characteristics. The personal ones include being altruistic, patient, trustworthy, reliable and motivating. The relational ones include being compatible, sincerely dedicated to developing an important relationship with the mentee, able to assist the mentee in identifying their strengths, and developing and reaching specific goals. The professional characteristics include being experienced, knowledgeable and well-respected.

Sambunjak et al. (2010) also described the findings of several studies that examined the characteristics of good mentees and found that good mentees are those that take initiative in the relationship and are committed to its success. They are passionate about achieving their own success and are proactive and willing to learn. They come prepared for meetings with their mentor, complete assigned tasks, and honestly respond to feedback. Importantly, they are also self-reflective and have the courage to make effective changes.

8.3   Peer Coaching as a Strategy for Faculty Development

First described in the education literature as a process for professional development primarily in the classroom setting, Flynn et al. (1994) adapted peer coaching to the clinical setting and reported on its use as a method for personalized faculty development in that context. Hekelman et al. (1994) described the following goals for peer coaching: to help clinician teachers recognize and improve teaching behaviors and practices; to develop the ability to adapt teaching strategies to meet the needs of individual students; and to evolve into a community of peer coaches who work together to enhance teaching.

Effective faculty development should result in positive changes in practice. Peel (2005) argues that peer coaching is transformative in nature because it relies on active engagement by the professional and on critical reflection. A comprehensive approach to faculty development should include activities that enhance the reflective capacity of faculty members and that emphasize learning from experience and from peers (Wilkerson and Irby 1998). Peer coaching does just that.

We will describe four models of peer coaching and the contexts in which they have been used. We will consider their strengths and limitations, as well as their similarities and differences. Finally, we will highlight some recommendations for the successful implementation of a peer coaching program.

8.3.1   Peer Coaching Models

The first two models of peer coaching are situated in a general educational context but can be readily adapted to the health professions. The third model uses peer coaching for teaching improvement in the clinical setting, and the fourth emphasizes a multi-disciplinary application of peer coaching across the health professions and focuses on broad teaching responsibilities.

8.3.1.1   Teaching Partners Program (TPP)

The Teaching Partners Program is a faculty development program for teaching enhancement that involved 12 community colleges in Connecticut (Eisen 2001). The program was 1 year in length and participation was voluntary. Participants came from different disciplines and selected their teaching partners with assistance only as needed. Thus, some partners knew each other well, while others started the program as strangers. There were a total of 120 participants over 5 years. Mandatory attendance at three workshops providing group training on the TPP was required before starting the program. The partnerships were reciprocal: each partner spent a semester as the observer and then switched in the next semester to be the one observed. Most observations and feedback sessions occurred on a weekly basis. Each participant was asked to set personal learning goals for the observations and feedback sessions. The program included three components: (1) in-class observations and surveys of each other's students; (2) feedback sessions to discuss and explore alternate teaching approaches; and (3) reflective written reports of their experiences each semester. The program was evaluated using a qualitative case study design. During in-depth interviews, when participants were asked to define their learning, most described some kind of *change*: change in practices, change in self and change in perspective. They felt the changes resulted from what they learned through peer feedback, modeling, student feedback gathered by the partner, peer-supported experimentation, joint reflection and self-reflection. They felt the key facilitator of learning and change was the peer relationship, in particular its authenticity and trustworthiness, the non-evaluative nature of the feedback, the non-hierarchical status of the partners, and the duration and intensity of the partnership. Eisen (2001) concludes by stating that 'peer learning partnerships may be particularly well-suited for established professionals who have expertise to share in return for support with their own professional growth goals' (p. 41) and by noting that it is consistent with the principles of collaboration and teamwork.

Health professionals can benefit from this novel form of professional development that draws upon shared expertise, authentic work-based learning, peer relationships and non-evaluative feedback.

8.3.1.2 Peer Coaching: Professional Development for Experienced Faculty

This peer coaching program was created at Seattle University in 2005 (Huston and Weaver 2008). It resulted from a number of requests by faculty members for classroom observations that exceeded the capacity of the faculty development office. Ten senior faculty members from five colleges and ten different departments known for their exemplary teaching were selected as peer coaches. Preparatory workshops were conducted to introduce the coaches to the practice of peer coaching. The coaches were first partnered *with each other* and asked to engage in reciprocal peer coaching, taking turns coaching and being coached over a period of 4 months. At the end of this period, they were offered the possibility to serve as coaches for other faculty members who were requesting in-class observations of their teaching. Eight of the ten agreed to continue coaching. The success of this program included the ability to recruit, train, and retain senior teachers as peer coaches. These senior teachers received 4-months of intensive 'faculty development' through an experience of reciprocal coaching, which prepared them to become peer coaches for others. The coaches in this program were *senior* faculty members. The authors describe the effectiveness of this program in meeting the professional development needs of this unique group by allowing them to: (1) converse with colleagues; (2) admit limitations or lack of knowledge in a safe and confidential environment; (3) analyze real-life problems in a sophisticated manner; (4) share teaching practices and make teaching visible to others; (5) see how others teach; (6) decrease isolation and increase collegial relations; (7) give back to the community by helping less experienced faculty improve teaching; and (8) link scholarship and teaching. The challenges of this program were primarily logistic in nature: finding dates and times for the senior faculty members to get together, and developing an efficient system to subsequently connect coaches with teachers in a timely fashion. The authors conclude by saying:

> Finally, if campuses are dedicated to providing faculty development throughout the career-span of the faculty they support, providing additional opportunities for experienced faculty members is a must. We believe peer coaching is an appropriate and meaningful investment in the ongoing development of this important group (Huston and Weaver 2008, p. 18).

Experienced health professionals may be particularly well-suited for, and willing to engage in, a faculty development program like this that prepares them to take on the role of a senior coach for a less experienced faculty member. In fact, the role of senior coach may provide serendipitous professional development opportunities for experienced health professionals as it allows them to share best practices, reflect on common challenges, find solutions to problems, and see how others teach.

8.3.1.3 Physician Peer Coaching Program (PPCP)

This model focuses on peer coaching in the clinical context (Sekerka and Chao 2003). The Physician Peer Coaching Program was started in the Department of Family Medicine at the Case Western Reserve University in 1991. PPCP trains preceptors as coaches so they can help other preceptors with ambulatory teaching practices. It is based on the following principles: voluntary participation by both the coaches and the preceptors being coached; intentional training of the coaches; collaboration and parity of colleagues (coaches and preceptors); shared identification of goals; focused observation of teaching; non-evaluative feedback and ongoing coach support. The PPCP is a one-way model of peer coaching, with one partner doing the coaching and the other being coached. Using an inductive qualitative method, the coaches' experiences (n=26) were analyzed and both coaches and preceptors were asked to evaluate the coaching session. The authors found that peer coaching contributes to professional development by encouraging time for reflection and for learning; it also positively influences the coach as well as the preceptor who receives the coaching.

Reflection plays an important role in health professions education. Sandars (2009) says that 'guided reflection, with supportive challenge from a mentor or facilitator, is important so that underlying assumptions can be challenged and new perspectives considered' (p. 685). Peer coaching structures a conversation with the aim of promoting self-awareness and joint reflection. Thus, it is not surprising that peer coaching shows benefit to the coach as well as to the person being coached.

8.3.1.4 The Colleague Development Program

In 2006, the Faculty of Health Sciences at the University of Adelaide in Australia developed and implemented a faculty-wide multi-disciplinary program of peer observation of teaching (O'Keefe et al. 2009). The program was designed to provide opportunities to develop teaching skills, to explore innovative teaching and/or assessment techniques and to receive constructive feedback and suggestions for improvement within the context of a collegial partnership. Participation was voluntary. Due to the varied disciplinary backgrounds of the participants, it was hoped that the program would promote collegiality across the six schools of the Faculty of Health Sciences. The program was conducted over 8 weeks and participants were asked to complete the following components: (1) identification of personal learning objectives; (2) identification of a colleague to serve as peer coach; (3) discussion of objectives, challenges and context with the peer coach; (4) observation of teaching; (5) discussion and feedback; (6) review of the written report provided by the peer coach that included mutually agreed outcomes, documentation of good practice and suggestions for improvement; and (7) attendance at the program debriefing and evaluation meeting. Two interactive seminars were offered in the first week of the program that provided instruction on how to identify personal learning objectives and how to give effective feedback. Teaching activities around which peer observation partnerships could occur included direct observation of teaching, review of video-recorded teaching or review of course documentation such as curriculum design or assessment documentation. Reciprocal partnerships were encouraged but were not obligatory. The program was evaluated through an anonymous written survey of participants' expectations at the introductory seminar and an anonymous questionnaire and focus group discussion upon completion of the program. Twenty-three of the forty-two enrolled faculty members completed the study. For many participants, the partner was from the same school. Approximately half had a reciprocal relationship. Direct observation of teaching was the most popular form of teaching activity, and although the majority of observations involved the minimum requirement of one teaching session, some colleagues did multiple observations. The average time commitment over the 8-week program was 10 h. Four themes emerged from the focus groups: an appreciation for the opportunity to discuss teaching challenges and experiences, the value of meeting teachers' individual needs, a greater sense of connectedness, and suggestions for improving the program in the future. Strengths of the program included: flexibility, non-evaluative formative feedback based on the teacher's learning objectives, its multidisciplinary nature, and selection of the peer coach by the teacher. Unfortunately, only a small number of teachers participated in the program in the first year and approximately half completed the program. Although the program was faculty-wide, most partnerships were from within the same school. Overall, the authors felt the program was a success and concluded that participants in the Colleague Development Program reported 'increased confidence in teaching, confirmation of good practice, exposure to new ideas, a feeling of institutional support and a greater sense of collegiality' (O'Keefe et al. 2009, p. 1064).

Most clinical settings involve teams of health professionals working together. Interprofessional peer coaching provides an ideal opportunity to promote collegiality and to model interprofessional collaboration and communication.

All four models of peer coaching for faculty development that we have described allow for personalized coaching based on the teacher's individual needs in a specific setting. They engage feedback from colleagues in a constructive and formative manner. This feedback provides insights and perspectives that go beyond the feedback and evaluation normally received from students. The above models also rest on the power of shared reflection and self-reflection. Through reflection, teachers are encouraged to question what they do, how they do it, and how they might do it differently. Cole et al. (2004) state that 'reflective activities, when combined with skills practice, may result in more durable change than would skill acquisition alone, because they can produce new insights and motivation for change' (p. 470). Another similarity in the models described is the self-identification of the learning objectives by the teachers which serves to engage the teachers in the process. All programs include an introductory workshop or seminar which provides training on personal goal-setting and the principles of feedback. They all depend on a collaborative, supportive and safe environment which is a key feature of peer coaching.

There are some differences in the four models that deserve to be highlighted: (1) the reciprocity of the partnership is not always present or even encouraged. A disadvantage of a one-way partnership is the potential loss of the sense of shared learning; (2) in one of the models, experienced faculty with exemplary teaching are chosen to serve as coaches. It is difficult in this situation to avoid the power relationship that may emerge; (3) the teacher being coached does not always choose the observing peer coach which can lead to diminished buy-in by the teacher, poor chemistry between the partners, and less trust and honesty in giving feedback; and (4) the length and intensity of the peer coaching relationship vary among models.

While each model has advantages and disadvantages, we believe that there are unique strengths to peer coaching when it is a non-hierarchical and reciprocal partnership between two colleagues of similar experience and expertise, and is longitudinal over several months.

8.3.2 General Principles

8.3.2.1 Peer Coaching as a Faculty Development Strategy

Peer coaching is a dynamic and flexible faculty development approach that depends on a collaborative and supportive relationship between peers. It is based on identification by the faculty member of *personal learning needs* based on real-life experiences and challenges, and provides the opportunity to work with a colleague to find strategies and solutions. This often results in a deep and trusting longitudinal partnership with a colleague. The faculty member being coached may feel less intimidated when working with a peer coach with a similar level of experience and expertise. On the other hand, some faculty members may prefer to be observed and to receive feedback by an 'expert' rather than by an 'equal' peer. Both the faculty member being coached and the peer coach benefit from shared reflection and enhanced self-assessment (Bell 2001; Sekerka and Chao 2003). Peer coaching is an approach that can also adapt and respond to the evolution and growth of faculty members as they work together to improve their skills.

Peer coaching is not for everyone and may feel threatening to some. In a recent study by Peyre et al. (2011), the majority of faculty members indicated interest in a program of peer observation, but a few cited not wanting to be watched as a reason for not participating.

The following guidelines should be considered when implementing a peer coaching program (Huston and Weaver 2008; Siddiqui et al. 2007):

- The program should ensure a safe, collegial environment where confidentiality is respected.
- The aim of the peer coaching program should be for development and improvement, and thus formative in nature.
- The goals should be set by the colleague being coached and shared with the coach.
- The context of the person being coached should be reviewed before the observation occurs and mutual expectations should be clarified and discussed.
- Whenever possible, the experience should be one of shared learning both for the coach and for the person being coached.
- Sufficient allocation of time is also needed for participants, and their participation should be encouraged, recognized and rewarded in some way.

Peer coaching is an individualized faculty development approach that is well suited to enhance the development of health professionals. Although commonly used to improve teaching skills, it can be adapted for other faculty roles such as leadership and management skills. For example, Henochowicz and Hetherington (2006) conducted a literature review that described different models of leadership coaching for health care leaders. They found that coaching was an effective but underutilized tool for leadership development in the health professions. Peer coaching reduces isolation, increases collegiality, promotes shared practices, enhances reflection, and encourages new strategies and approaches in a safe and supportive environment. It can be applied in a cross-disciplinary or similar-discipline fashion. Huston and Weaver (2008) comment that cross-disciplinary coaching *broadens* the conversations and encourages exchange around common issues. Similar-discipline coaching *deepens* the conversations by allowing colleagues with a good understanding of the other's contexts to help each other to improve. Finally, peer coaching focuses on change and on application of new learning in the workplace. It creates a sense of accountability for change between peer coaches. And although peer coaching requires time, is resource intensive, and may be more difficult to implement than a one-time activity, the long term impact of such a program is promising.

8.3.2.2 Faculty Development for Peer Coaching

Introductory training in the form of preparatory workshops or seminars on peer coaching is essential to its success (Claridge and Lewis 2005). Tee et al. (2009), in a study looking at the academic coaching role to enhance student learning, describe how coaches were prepared for their role by attending a faculty development program that focused on skill development and a shared understanding of the role. Because much of the success of peer coaching relies on peer to peer feedback, consideration should also be given to training coaches in the principles and practice of giving feedback effectively. The underlying principles that enhance the quality of feedback include establishing a respectful learning environment, communicating clear objectives for the feedback session, beginning with self-assessment, basing feedback on observation and promoting reflection (Ramani and Krackov 2012).

8.4 Mentorship as a Strategy for Faculty Development

In this section we will describe the various mentoring models that exist, and the faculty development contexts in which they have been, and can be, used. Drawing from the relevant literature, general indications for the effective use of mentoring as a faculty development strategy will be developed. This literature is still relatively sparse and will therefore be complemented by literature from outside the health professions.

As has been described earlier in this chapter, faculty development in its broadest sense is the development of all the skills, competencies and relationships that a person needs in order to be a satisfied and successful member of the faculty. Explicitly, this requires the development of more than just teaching and research skills, though these are clearly important. It requires, for example, that the faculty member identify and pursue goals meaningful to them, while appreciating the very real functional and organizational limitations that impact on those very goals. It requires that the faculty member find personal and professional balance allowing them to weather disappointments, overcome obstacles, and find satisfaction in their successes. It also requires the faculty member to build and maintain the relationships they need to not only actively pursue their goals but also to feel supported as they immerse themselves in the culture of their professional environment. (See Chap. 5 for a more detailed discussion of faculty development for career development.)

These are not new concepts, and they have been explored, along with evidence of their effectiveness, in business and academia (Merriam 1983). Within the health professions, the nursing literature is more robust in its examination of mentoring and its benefits, but mentorship specifically as a faculty development strategy in this broad sense has not been systematically examined. The development of these kinds of skills, competencies and relationships are not easily, or necessarily appropriately, achieved in the lectures, courses or workshops classically associated with the term 'faculty development'. However, mentorship can be an ideal faculty development strategy for these more personal and interpersonal skills and competencies because of the equally personal and interpersonal nature of the mentoring relationship, its mentee-centered focus and the reflective practice it encourages. Mentorship can provide the instrumental and psychosocial support needed for faculty development that goes beyond the traditional instructional needs (Sambunjak et al. 2006).

8.4.1 Mentoring Models

As described by Bland et al. (2009), there are three main models of mentorship: the traditional dyadic mentoring relationship, peer mentoring and group mentoring, and while the basic structure of these models may differ, the key elements of the relationships within them, as outlined in the definition section, are retained. These elements include the interpersonal connection, the evolution of the relationship over time, the need for a defined purpose, the collaborative learning environment within the relationship, and the importance of a reflective practice.

In this chapter, we will collapse the three models described by Bland et al. (2009) into two main models: dyadic and group mentoring. Peer mentoring and the more traditional hierarchical mentoring structure can be viewed as characterizing the nature of the interpersonal relationship, and as such can be subsets of both the dyadic and group mentoring models.

8.4.1.1 Dyadic Mentoring Models

The traditional, hierarchical dyadic relationship is the one most classically associated with mentoring. It is a relationship between two people, in which the mentor is usually more senior than the mentee and has the advantage of experience that can be incorporated into the guidance provided. Because of their more senior position, the mentor can often effectively advocate for their mentee, protect their mentee from excessive time demands, and provide networking opportunities that are so invaluable (Johnson 2002). A faculty member could, and probably should, have multiple mentors of this traditional kind as each mentor can provide either a different perspective, or can focus on different areas of the mentee's needs depending on the mentor's individual strengths and achievements (de Janasz and Sullivan 2004).

Descriptions and some elements of evaluation of formal traditional dyadic mentoring programs exist the literature (Mark et al. 2001; Tracy et al. 2004); however, only a few describe these as intentionally part of a wider faculty development program, and fewer still have evaluated outcomes. In an article by Morzinski et al. (1996), a formal mentoring program as part of a 2-year faculty development program was described. The mentoring aspect was incorporated to help address three core areas of professional academic skills identified as being critical to the success of faculty members. These skills, as described by Bland (1990), were: (1) knowing how to manage one's career; (2) understanding the values, norms and expectations of academic medicine; and (3) developing and maintaining a productive network of colleagues. The program included a formal matching and orientation process, planned mentor-mentee pair activities, and larger group activities. The authors found that the program had overall moderate to high effect on the participants' development of their professional academic skills, and felt that these findings supported previous reports of the effectiveness of mentoring as a broader professional development strategy.

Another study by Balmer et al. (2011) described a traditional dyadic mentorship within a 3-year faculty development program specifically designed to help pediatricians develop their educational scholarship skills. The assigned mentor was focused on helping the participant develop their educational project, and had a very functional role, almost akin to a research supervisor. The study found that though the participants began with just the traditional dyadic relationship with their project mentor, over time they typically developed a network of senior mentors as their project needs evolved. Additionally, while the project mentors were meant to assist the participants in completing their scholarly projects, many became mentors in a broader sense, providing support, advocating for their mentees, and providing networking opportunities and career advice. This study again shows that while mentorship may initially be formed around a specific need, when the relationship works well, it can also become a strategy for developing many non-instructional skills required by faculty in order to become successful and satisfied in their careers.

Significant challenges exist with the traditional dyadic mentoring relationship, often related to potentially negative interpersonal interactions and power differential issues (Connor et al. 2000; Johnson 2007; Pololi et al. 2002). As a result, mentorship between peers has emerged as an interesting alternative. Peer mentorship has been described as a process whereby two or more people at a similar professional stage enter a more equal relationship in that all parties provide and receive support and guidance from each other drawing on relevant experiences and knowledge. Each person can then be both mentee and mentor at different times depending on the expressed needs. This differs from the traditional dyadic model wherein the mentor draws on their greater experience and expertise to guide and advise the mentee. In the study by Balmer et al. (2011), participants in the program also developed peer mentoring relationships as important informal support systems which complemented the more formally established traditional mentoring relationships. The authors concluded that 'the complex reality of these relationships challenges the application of traditional mentoring models and suggests unique considerations in developing mentoring programs...' (p. 85), lending support to the notion of peer mentoring as valid and useful. The non-hierarchical nature of this type of mentorship can allow for an exchange that is not constrained by the sense of vulnerability inherent in relationships wherein a significant power differential (actual or perceived) exists.

8.4.1.2 Group Mentoring Models

In this model, a group of people are mentored at the same time with a single mentor acting as both mentor and group facilitator. In the more hierarchical approach, the mentor/facilitator is separate from the group and is a more experienced or senior colleague who can draw upon their experience to guide discussions. In the peer group mentoring approach, either discussions are led by consensus, or each member of the group acts as a facilitator at different times (Bland et al. 2009). The line between *traditional hierarchical* and *peer* group mentoring approaches is blurred when peer mentorship evolves within a group initially led by a single senior mentor and members of the group recognize that they can learn and be guided by each other and not just by the senior mentor.

Several authors describe programs that have used these methods as faculty development strategies. Connor et al. (2000) describe the development of a network of senior doctors who used peer mentorship to assist each other in their personal and professional development. While the initial program was designed to specifically teach senior doctors practical mentoring skills, what evolved was the development of a network of senior physicians who would call upon each other as peers and co-mentors for personal and professional issues. A second program, described by Pololi et al. (2002), illustrated the benefits of a facilitated group mentorship program wherein intra-group peer mentorship also evolved. The Collaborative Mentoring Program was a program that aimed to 'provide a framework for professional development, emotional support, career planning, and the enhancement of personal awareness and skills important for a successful career in academic medicine.' (p. 378). While the participants clearly benefitted from the structured activities and mentorship provided by the mentors/facilitators, they also described their peers as having attributes consistent with those of a mentor, and very much valued the peer mentorship in their development process.

While group mentoring models were developed to address some of the challenges with the dyadic mentoring model such as recruiting and training of sufficient numbers of effective and implicated mentors, and the significant time demands required of the mentors in the dyadic model (Johnson 2007; Pololi et al. 2002), they are not without their own challenges. The issues of recruitment, training and time requirements remain when mentors for groups are needed, though fewer are needed overall as a single mentor can be responsible for several mentees. In group mentoring using a more senior mentor/facilitator, issues related to a hierarchical structure and power differentials again exist, but the value of learning from a senior mentor's experience is lost when using a peer group mentoring structure. Additional potential challenges can exist when group members have differing needs and when group dynamics are suboptimal. Not all groups will 'click' and evolve to develop the trust and respect for this process to be most effective and beneficial, similar to dyadic relationships.

8.4.1.3 Dyadic vs. Group Mentoring Models

No single model seems to be 'the best' when it comes to mentorship in faculty development. The selection of a model would depend on the identified needs as well as the resources available, and models can be blended or modified. Ideally, a faculty member would have both a traditional dyadic mentoring relationship to benefit from a very personalized focus with an experienced mentor, as well as some form of peer mentorship, either as a dyad or within a group, for the support and collegial networking that are so vital. While Balmer et al. (2011) described how peer group mentorship evolved as an unintended, but positive, outcome of a program initially designed using only a traditional hierarchical dyadic mentoring model, one could envision the development of a program where both models would be part of the structure from the outset. This blended model could then capitalize on all the best that mentorship as a faculty development strategy has to offer.

8.4.1.4 Formal and Informal Mentoring Formats

A traditional view of the mentoring relationship is that it is an informal process where two people with common interests simply find each other and develop a relationship (Kram 1983). The importance of the personality fit and match of interests and goals cannot be underestimated in the success of a mentoring relationship, and forms the basis of informal processes. The reality, however, is that many people who would benefit from having a mentor, including women and minorities (Johnson 2007; Ragins 1989; Sambunjak et al. 2006), do not find a suitable match. It may also be that individuals who are less able to network or self-promote, and who would derive great benefit from having a mentor, will have difficulty finding a mentor through informal processes. Additionally, finding even one mentor can often be challenging given the time commitment required and the need for a good fit of goals and personalities, and certainly finding several on an informal basis becomes even harder.

As a result, some academic centers have developed formal mentoring programs that ensure that each new faculty member has a mentor. Some programs achieve this by creating a database of potential mentors or by facilitating introductions to potential mentors while still letting new faculty initiate and develop their own mentoring relationships. Others, such as those described in the section above (Balmer et al. 2011; Morzinski et al. 1996; Pololi et al. 2002), assign matches through structured mentoring programs. While these programs may improve participation rates and the studies described have shown good outcomes, they demand far more resources (human and financial) than informal processes, and they may ultimately still be unsuccessful if the match between mentor and mentee is suboptimal.

Just as a blending of mentoring models may be appropriate depending on circumstances, a blending of formal and informal mentoring formats may also be ideal. A program wherein all faculty are provided a mentor in some way (formal), but where matches can be re-assigned without stigma or fear of reprisal if the 'fit' is missing or needs change (informal), would be optimal, although this would require significant belief in the validity and utility of the process by all parties.

8.4.2 General Principles

8.4.2.1 Mentorship as a Faculty Development Strategy

Mentorship cannot, and should not, be the sole faculty development strategy employed. However, from the studies described above, it can be seen that mentorship can complement the more traditional faculty development teaching necessary for the acquisition of practical or technical skills related to a faculty member's roles in areas such as instruction and research. Mentorship can be very effective in the development of personal and professional skills and competencies that require significant introspection and personal reflection to achieve, or are highly relational and interpersonal in nature. It implies the development of the faculty member in a broader sense, taking the faculty member as a whole person whose personal and professional lives are intertwined and inseparable, and for whom the development of skills in either sphere can impact positively, both in terms of increased success and satisfaction and less stress and burnout.

8.4.2.2 Faculty Development for Mentorship

Regardless of the mentoring format or model used, mentoring as an effective faculty development strategy requires both effective mentors and effective mentees. Scant literature exists describing programs designed to train people to become betters mentors and fewer still have assessed outcomes. Johnson et al. (2010) describe the Mentor Development Program designed to train health science researchers to be effective research mentors and discuss evaluation methods. Connor et al. (2000) evaluated a program designed to train senior physicians in mentoring skills, and found that not only did those physicians feel they developed mentoring skills, they also benefitted from becoming part of a network of senior doctors and engaging in their own personal and professional development. This suggests that, at least for the mentors, faculty development to improve mentoring skills can be both useful and appreciated. To our knowledge, no studies exist describing or evaluating faculty development activities designed to help people become better mentees, though as described earlier, there is literature that describes the characteristics of good mentees.

8.5 Implications for Research

Peer coaching and mentoring have only been described as faculty development activities in the health professions in the relatively recent past. Therefore, there are many avenues for further exploration and we will highlight four of these:

1. The interplay between peer coaching and mentorship as formative faculty development strategies and their use in the process of academic promotion could be explored. As faculties put more emphasis on mentoring as a *required* academic activity, and on the use of peer coaching for *summative peer review* for promotion, the safe and honest atmosphere so essential to the success of these strategies and to buy-in by faculty may be compromised. On the other hand, making these approaches part of the promotion process may lend more legitimacy to these approaches and enhance their use.
2. There is a need to evaluate faculty development outcomes at the higher levels of Kirkpatrick's (1994) model of evaluation (Steinert et al. 2006). This is particularly important as both peer coaching and mentorship are resource intensive activities and support for them would depend on evidence of tangible outcomes beyond satisfaction.
3. The growing emphasis on the interprofessional nature of the clinical environment and the importance of *learning together* can be further explored within the context of peer coaching and mentorship as novel faculty development strategies. Research looking at the impact of these approaches on teamwork is needed. We suspect that faculty participation in interprofessional peer coaching and/or mentorship may well enhance the communication, collaboration and collegiality so essential to effective clinical teams.
4. Exploring more explicitly blended models of mentoring is needed to capitalize on the benefits of having a more experienced senior mentor, as well as the benefits of the support and collegial networking that comes from peer mentorship.

8.6 Conclusion

As we better understand how faculty learn and change, the value of peer coaching and mentorship as effective faculty development strategies in the appropriate contexts becomes evident. Health professions organizations need to recognize a broader definition of faculty development that includes all the personal and professional skills needed for success in the various roles that faculty members play. The power in these strategies lies in their highly relational quality and in the self and shared reflective practices that they encourage and develop. They are truly learner-centered in their essence, as faculty members self-identify their learning needs and determine their level of engagement. The dynamic nature of these processes can adapt and respond to the changing needs of faculty members. They are highly personal forms of faculty development and we feel that the resultant sense of accountability in addition to enhanced reflective capacity will lead to greater long term change. Although they are both time and human-resource intensive, when they work well, we believe they can create self-sustaining communities of practice where faculty members feel committed to each other and to learning, improving and growing together.

8.7 Key Messages

- Peer coaching and mentorship show promise as novel faculty development strategies in the health professions.
- Their effective use rests on an acceptance of a broad definition of faculty development, one that supports multiple faculty roles (including roles beyond teaching) and both personal and professional skills.
- Peer coaching and mentorship are relational and reflective in their essence, and evolve with changing faculty needs.
- Although peer coaching and mentorship are resource-intensive, they involve a greater sense of commitment and accountability, which may result in more sustained change over time.
- Intentional and structured faculty development to train effective peer coaches and mentors is essential.

References

Allen, T. D., Finkelstein, L. M., & Poteet, M. L. (2009). *Designing workplace mentoring programs: An evidence-based approach*. Oxford, UK: Wiley-Blackwell.

Balmer, D., D'Alessandro, D., Risko, W., & Gusic, M. E. (2011). How mentoring relationships evolve: A longitudinal study of academic pediatricians in a physician educator faculty development program. *Journal of Continuing Education in the Health Professions, 31*(2), 81–86.

Bell, M. (2001). Supported reflective practice: A programme of peer observation and feedback for academic teaching development. *International Journal for Academic Development, 6*(1), 29–39.

Bernstein, D. J., Jonson, J., & Smith, K. (2000). An examination of the implementation of peer review of teaching. *New Directions for Teaching and Learning, 2000*(83), 73–86.

Bland, C. J. (1990). *Successful faculty in academic medicine: Essential skills and how to acquire them*. New York, NY: Springer Publishing.

Bland, C. J., Taylor, A. L., Shollen, S. L., Weber-Main, A. M., & Mulcahy, P. A. (2009). *Faculty success through mentoring: A guide for mentors, mentees, and leaders*. Lanham, MD: Rowman & Littlefield.

Blixen, C. E., Papp, K. K., Hull, A. L., Rudick, R. A., & Bramstedt, K. A. (2007). Developing a mentorship program for clinical researchers. *Journal of Continuing Education in the Health Professions, 27*(2), 86–93.

Claridge, M. T. & Lewis, T. (2005). *Coaching for effective learning: A practical guide for teachers in health and social care*. Oxford, UK: Radcliffe Publishing.

Cole, K. A., Barker, L. R., Kolodner, K., Williamson, P., Wright, S. M., & Kern, D. E. (2004). Faculty development in teaching skills: An intensive longitudinal model. *Academic Medicine, 79*(5), 469–480.

Connor, M. P., Bynoe, A. G., Redfern, N., Pokora, J., & Clarke, J. (2000). Developing senior doctors as mentors: A form of continuing professional development. Report of an initiative to develop a network of senior doctors as mentors: 1994–99. *Medical Education, 34*(9), 747–753.

D'Abate, C. P., Eddy, E. R., & Tannenbaum, S. I. (2003). What's in a name? A literature-based approach to understanding mentoring, coaching, and other constructs that describe developmental interactions. *Human Resource Development Review, 2*(4), 360–384.

de Janasz, S. C. & Sullivan, S. E. (2004). Multiple mentoring in academe: Developing the professorial network. *Journal of Vocational Behavior, 64*(2), 263–283.

Eby, L. T., Rhodes, J. E., & Allen, T. D. (2010). Definition and evolution of mentoring. In T. D. Allen, & L. T. Eby (Eds.), *The Blackwell handbook of mentoring: A multiple perspectives approach,* (pp. 7–20). West Sussex, UK: Blackwell Publishing.

Eisen, M. J. (2000). Peer learning partnerships: Promoting reflective practice through reciprocal learning. *Inquiry: Critical Thinking Across the Disciplines, 19*(3), 5–19.

Eisen, M. J. (2001). Peer-based professional development viewed through the lens of transformative learning. *Holistic Nursing Practice, 16*(1), 30–42.

Flynn, S. P., Bedinghaus, J., Snyder, C., & Hekelman, F. (1994). Peer coaching in clinical teaching: A case report. *Family Medicine, 26*(9), 569–570.

Fry, H. & Morris, C. (2004). Peer observation of clinical teaching. *Medical Education, 38*(5), 560–561.

Hekelman, F. P., Flynn, S. P., Glover, P. B., Galazka, S. S., & Phillips Jr., J. A. (1994). Peer coaching in clinical teaching: Formative assessment of a case. *Evaluation & the Health Professions, 17*(3), 366–381.

Henochowicz, S. & Hetherington, D. (2006). Leadership coaching in health care. *Leadership and Organization Development Journal, 27*(3), 183–189.

Huston, T. & Weaver, C. L. (2008). Peer coaching: Professional development for experienced faculty. *Innovative Higher Education, 33*(1), 5–20.

Jackson, V. A., Palepu, A., Szalacha, L., Caswell, C., Carr, P. L., & Inui, T. (2003). 'Having the right chemistry': A qualitative study of mentoring in academic medicine. *Academic Medicine, 78*(3), 328–334.

Johnson, M. O., Subak, L. L., Brown, J. S., Lee, K. A., & Feldman, M. D. (2010). An innovative program to train health sciences researchers to be effective clinical and translational research mentors. *Academic Medicine, 85*(3), 484–489.

Johnson, W. B. (2002). The intentional mentor: Strategies and guidelines for the practice of mentoring. *Professional Psychology: Research and Practice, 33*(1), 88–96.

Johnson, W. B. (2007). *On being a mentor: A guide for higher education faculty.* Mahwah, NJ: Lawrence Erlbaum Associates.

Joo, B. K. (2005). Executive coaching: A conceptual framework from an integrative review of practice and research. *Human Resource Development Review, 4*(4) 462–488.

Kirkpatrick, D. L. (1994). *Evaluating training programs: The four levels.* San Francisco, CA: Berrett-Koehler Publishers.

Knowles, M. S. (1973). *The adult learner: A neglected species.* Houston, TX: Gulf Publishing Company.

Kolb, D. A. (1984). *Experiential learning: Experiences as the source of learning and development.* Englewood Cliffs, NJ: Prentice-Hall.

Kram, K. E. (1983). Phases of the mentor relationship. *Academy of Management Journal, 26*(4), 608–625.

Lave, J. & Wenger, E. (1991). *Situated learning: Legitimate peripheral participation.* New York, NY: Cambridge University Press.

Mark, S., Link, H., Morahan, P. S., Pololi, L., Reznik, V., & Tropez-Sims, S. (2001). Innovative mentoring programs to promote gender equity in academic medicine. *Academic Medicine, 76*(1), 39–42.

McLean, M., Cilliers, F., & Van Wyk, J. M. (2008). Faculty development: Yesterday, today and tomorrow. *Medical Teacher, 30*(6), 555–584.

McLeod, P. J. & Steinert, Y. (2009). Peer coaching as an approach to faculty development. *Medical Teacher, 31*(12), 1043–1044.

Merriam, S. (1983). Mentors and protégés: A critical review of the literature. *Adult Education Quarterly, 33*(3), 161–173.

Mezirow, J. (1991). *Transformative dimensions of adult learning.* San Francisco, CA: Jossey-Bass.

Morzinski, J. A., Diehr, S., Bower, D. J., & Simpson, D. E. (1996). A descriptive, cross-sectional study of formal mentoring for faculty. *Family Medicine, 28*(6), 434–438.

O'Keefe M., Lecouteur, A., Miller, J., & McGowan, U. (2009). The Colleague Development Program: A multidisciplinary program of peer observation partnerships. *Medical Teacher, 31*(12), 1060–1065.

Peel, D. (2005). Peer observation as a transformatory tool? *Teaching in Higher Education, 10*(4), 489–504.

Peyre, S. E., Frankl, S. E., Thorndike, M., & Breen, E. M. (2011). Observation of clinical teaching: Interest in a faculty development program for surgeons. *Journal of Surgical Education, 68*(5), 372–376.

Pololi, L. H., Knight, S. M., Dennis, K., & Frankel, R. M. (2002). Helping medical school faculty realize their dreams: An innovative, collaborative mentoring program. *Academic Medicine, 77*(5), 377–384.

Ragins, B. R. (1989). Barriers to mentoring: The female manager's dilemma. *Human Relations, 42*(1), 1–22.

Ramani, S. & Krackov, S. K. (2012). Twelve tips for giving feedback effectively in the clinical environment. *Medical Teacher, 34*(10), 787–791.

Roche, G. R. (1979). Much ado about mentors. *Harvard Business Review, 57*(1), 14–28.

Rose, G. L., Rukstalis, M. R., & Schuckit, M. A. (2005). Informal mentoring between faculty and medical students. *Academic Medicine, 80*(4), 344–348.

Sambunjak, D., Straus, S. E., & Marusic, A. (2006). Mentoring in academic medicine: A systematic review. *Journal of the American Medical Association, 296*(9), 1103–1115.

Sambunjak, D., Straus, S. E., & Marusic, A. (2010). A systematic review of qualitative research on the meaning and characteristics of mentoring in academic medicine. *Journal of General Internal Medicine, 25*(1), 72–78.

Sandars, J. (2009). The use of reflection in medical education: AMEE Guide No. 44. *Medical Teacher, 31*(8), 685–695.

Schön, D. A. (1983). *The reflective practitioner: How professionals think in action.* New York, NY: Basic Books.

Sekerka, L. E. & Chao, J. (2003). Peer coaching as a technique to foster professional development in clinical ambulatory settings. *Journal of Continuing Education in the Health Professions, 23*(1), 30–37.

Siddiqui, Z. S., Jonas-Dwyer, D., & Carr, S. E. (2007). Twelve tips for peer observation of teaching. *Medical Teacher, 29*(4), 297–300.

Smith, J. A. & Zsohar, H. (2007). Essentials of neophyte mentorship in relation to the faculty shortage. *Journal of Nursing Education, 46*(4), 184–186.

Steinert, Y. (2010). Faculty development: From workshops to communities of practice. *Medical Teacher, 32*(5), 425–428.

Steinert, Y. (2011). Commentary: Faculty development: The road less traveled. *Academic Medicine, 86*(4), 409–411.

Steinert, Y., Mann, K., Centeno, A., Dolmans, D., Spencer, J., Gelula, M., et al. (2006). A systematic review of faculty development initiatives designed to improve teaching effectiveness in medical education: BEME Guide No. 8. *Medical Teacher, 28*(6), 497–526.

Tee, S. R., Jowett, R. M., & Bechelet-Carter, C. (2009). Evaluation study to ascertain the impact of the clinical academic coaching role for enhancing student learning experience within a clinical masters education programme. *Nurse Education in Practice, 9*(6), 377–382.

Tobin, M. J. (2004). Mentoring: Seven roles and some specifics. *American Journal of Respiratory and Critical Care Medicine, 170*(2), 114–117.

Tracy, E. E., Jagsi, R., Starr, R., & Tarbell, N. J. (2004). Outcomes of a pilot faculty mentoring program. *American Journal of Obstetrics and Gynecology, 191*(6), 1846–1850.

Wilkerson, L. & Irby, D. M. (1998). Strategies for improving teaching practices: A comprehensive approach to faculty development. *Academic Medicine, 73*(4), 387–396.

Chapter 9
Workshops and Seminars: Enhancing Effectiveness

Willem de Grave, Anneke Zanting, Désirée D. Mansvelder-Longayroux, and Willemina M. Molenaar

9.1 Introduction

Workshops and seminars are among the mainstays of faculty development programs in the health professions. They can vary in duration, modality and content, and can include topics such as education and research as well as career and leadership development (Steinert 2011). In the educational sphere, workshops and seminars may include instructional development and other teaching responsibilities, such as curriculum planning and evaluation, stimulating and managing curricular change, and promoting educational improvement at the organizational level (Wilkerson and Irby 1998). Depending on specific goals, workshops and seminars can target individuals, groups or entire organizations. This modality holds strong appeal for most participants because face-to-face delivery of professional development, and collegial exchanges among participants and facilitators, can encourage deep learning

W. de Grave, Ph.D.
Department of Educational Development and Research, Faculty of Health,
Medicine and Life Sciences, University of Maastricht, Maastricht, The Netherlands
e-mail: w.degrave@maastrichtuniversity.nl

A. Zanting, Ph.D.
Centre for Education and Training, Ikazia Hospital Rotterdam, Rotterdam, The Netherlands
e-mail: a.zanting@ikazia.nl

D.D. Mansvelder-Longayroux, Ph.D.
Faculty Development Programmes, Centre for Innovation in Medical Education,
Leiden University Medical Centre, Leiden, The Netherlands
e-mail: d.d.mansvelder-longayroux@lumc.nl

W.M. Molenaar, MD, Ph.D. (✉)
Institute for Medical Education, University of Groningen and University Medical Center
Groningen, Groningen, The Netherlands
e-mail: w.m.molenaar@umcg.nl

Y. Steinert (ed.), *Faculty Development in the Health Professions: A Focus on Research and Practice*, Innovation and Change in Professional Education 11, DOI 10.1007/978-94-007-7612-8_9, © Springer Science+Business Media Dordrecht 2014

and change (Byham 2008). Additional appeal stems from their relatively short duration, which allows teachers to fit them into their busy schedules, as well as their formal nature, which ensures their visibility and credibility within the organization.

Traditionally, faculty members' learning was largely *informal*, including 'learning on the job' and learning through 'trial and error', with or without support by senior colleagues. More recent faculty development programs have shifted towards more *formal* learning, which according to Eraut (2000) is characterized by a higher intention to learn (as compared to informal learning). Formal learning is characterized by a prescribed learning framework, an organized learning event or package, the presence of a designated teacher or trainer, the award of a qualification or credit, and the external specification of outcomes. Clearly, neither formal nor informal learning can fulfill all the needs of faculty members, and a mix is likely to be most effective (Steinert 2011; Wilkerson and Irby 1998). In fact, for optimal effectiveness, the selection of formats should be based on reliable evidence (Blumberg 2011; O'Sullivan and Irby 2011). As a result, the notion of Best Evidence Medical Education (BEME) as 'the implementation, by teachers in their practice, of methods and approaches to education based on the best evidence available' (Harden et al. 1999, p. 553) can be transferred to faculty development as well. However, many faculty developers are 'experts by experience'. Their professional and educational backgrounds vary widely and many have had little or no training for their role as faculty developers. As a consequence, they are often guided by professional and personal insights and experiences rather than by empirical evidence of available methods and formats. Therefore, our goal in this chapter is to encourage faculty developers to adopt a more critical stance when selecting and developing activities and formats by asking questions such as the following (Clark 2010; Yardley and Dornan 2012): What are the features of this particular method? What is the evidence to support its use? How valid is this evidence? For what purpose, for whom, and when is this method appropriate? How does this method or format fit with our understanding of teacher learning?

This chapter focuses on workshops and seminars, formal learning activities of short duration. We view these as valuable contributions to the gamut of faculty development activities in addition to those which are described in other chapters of this book. After defining these two formats, we will briefly review the literature on the evidence of effectiveness of faculty development, in general, and of workshops and seminars, in particular. We will also formulate recommendations to enhance their effectiveness. Subsequently, we will propose a framework for a new approach to the design of workshops and seminars, based on theories about learning for teachers which combine learning outcomes, learning activities and instructional methods. To illustrate these principles, we will provide an example of a workshop and a seminar, using this framework. Although both examples focus on the enhancement of instructional effectiveness, workshops and seminars can be used to address other faculty roles (e.g. leadership and research) as well. We will then discuss transfer of acquired knowledge, skills and attitudes to daily practice; the final section will focus on challenges and opportunities for the future.

9.2 Defining Workshops and Seminars

The terms workshop, seminar and short course are often used interchangeably. As the terminology used for such faculty development activities is not always well defined, the intended meaning varies widely, depending on the developer's intentions and the facilitator's knowledge, skills and familiarity with the format (Clark 2010). In addition, evaluation studies often fail to provide a detailed description of the activity they are evaluating (Amundsen and Wilson 2012; Steinert et al. 2006; Stes et al. 2010). Compounding the confusion is the wide variation in outcomes and context. In this chapter, we will focus on workshops and seminars (or short series of seminars), representing well-known and frequently used formats for faculty development. However, much of what is discussed here also applies to other modular formats, such as short courses and training sessions.

Workshops generally have two different emphases: the acquisition of knowledge and skills, and the stimulation of changes in attitudes and behavior (Brooks-Harris and Stock-Ward 1999; Sork 1984; Steinert et al. 2006). In the 1970s, due to prevalent behavioral learning theories, workshops focused on behavioral change that could be facilitated by instruction, practice and feedback. During the 1980s, influenced by cognitive learning theories, workshops started to address the knowledge, beliefs and attitudes that underlie desirable behaviors (Wilkerson and Irby 1998). Despite their rich variety in content and focus, characteristics common to workshops include a limited time investment (usually between a half and 2 days) from both participants and the organization, a small group (usually less than 20) of active participants, and a facilitator (Brooks-Harris and Stock-Ward 1999; Grossman and Salas 2011; Sork 1984; Steinert et al. 2008).

Seminars (or short series of seminars) tend to focus on a single, primarily cognitive topic, usually aimed at expanding the participants' knowledge base (e.g. for education in the health professions). A seminar is usually facilitated by an expert, while participants acquire and share knowledge by interacting with each other and with the facilitator. In practice, seminars may vary on numerous dimensions (Schmitt 2011; Steinert et al. 2006; Stes et al. 2010) such as the intended outcomes, the role of the facilitator, the composition, size and experience level of the group, the duration, scheduling and number of sessions, and the use of instructional design principles. For an appropriate understanding of the effects of a seminar, a clear description of these dimensions is indispensable. When active learning methods are utilized in a seminar, the distinction between seminar and workshop can easily become blurred.

In this chapter, we will refrain from strict definitions of formats; rather, we will focus on the process of faculty development *design* in order to reach desirable learning outcomes and transfer to daily practice.

9.3   Evidence for Effectiveness of Workshops and Seminars

Reviews of programs for professional development in higher education, in general, and in health professions education, in particular, offer useful insights into the effectiveness of faculty development programs and activities. Steinert et al. (2006) concluded that, in general, health professionals were not only highly satisfied with faculty development programs, but they also reported and demonstrated improvement of their teaching skills and behaviors. Both Steinert et al. (2006) and Stes et al. (2010) found evidence that, compared to one-time events, longitudinal interventions are more effective in achieving behavior changes. Remarkably similar conclusions were drawn from several reviews (Davis et al. 1999; Flottorp 2008; Forsetlund et al. 2009) focusing on the effects of formal continuing medical education on professional practice and health care outcomes. These also showed that educational interventions may improve professional practice and health care outcomes, especially when the latter are perceived as serious. As in the educational setting, the effects on professional behavior appeared stronger when (mixed) interactive methods were used, especially the practicing of skills (Davis et al. 1999); educational meetings were not found to be effective in influencing complex behavior.

Steinert et al. (2006) presented evidence that *workshops* can contribute to changing teachers' attitudes, skills and behavior and can enhance teachers' motivation, self-awareness and enthusiasm. Participants also reported that workshops are helpful, relevant and useful and that they improved their knowledge and skills and enhanced application of newly acquired skills to their teaching practices. Based on these results, Steinert et al. (2006) deduced five important characteristics of effective faculty development workshops: the use of experiential learning; the provision of feedback; effective peer and colleague relationships; the application of principles of teaching and learning; and the use of multiple instructional methods. These findings are supported by evidence cited by Wilkerson and Irby (1998) who state that teachers' knowledge, skills and attitudes can be enhanced by workshops of long duration and by two or more types of interventions, followed by practice. *Seminars* (especially a series of seminars) have proven to be particularly effective with respect to acquiring knowledge and changing awareness and attitudes about teaching. Steinert et al. 2006 concluded that participants are usually satisfied with this modality and consider seminars to be useful for having a positive impact on: awareness of teaching issues, teaching methods and theory; motivation and attitude towards teaching; acquisition of new knowledge about teaching and related skills; and stimulating cooperation between teachers. This pattern of outcomes is in line with the results of a recent qualitative study about the effects of a seminar for new faculty (Behar-Horenstein et al. 2008) which reported the acquisition of new knowledge, intent to change, and increased awareness of educational topics (in this order of importance), but only a few perceived changes in actual teacher behavior. Research on seminars or similar learning methods in different contexts, such as undergraduate education and continuing medical education (CME), suggests that the following dimensions can explain the positive outcomes of seminars: interactivity and the quality of the interaction in small groups; the use of multiple methods of small group learning; the limited number of participants and stability of the group composition; the focus on cases and the application of the acquired knowledge; the role of the facilitator and adequate preparation for the seminar; and the scheduling of sufficient time between meetings (Davis and Davis 2010; Spruijt et al. 2012). The emphasis on interaction, the duration of the seminar series, and the stability of group composition are likely essential in bringing about attitude change.

Reviews have also indicated a need to describe the *design* of faculty development practices. Guskey (2003) argued that describing good practices for a specific context can result in new insights for effective faculty development initiatives. Amundsen and Wilson (2012) recommended detailed descriptions of professional development practices and their outcomes in relation to the objectives and format of the design. They stated that these descriptions should focus on learning outcomes and processes. Bakkenes et al. (2010) identified the importance of a conceptual framework encompassing theories of teachers' learning for designing professional development activities. They also noted that the learning processes of teachers are rarely described, even though the success or failure of educational innovations relies heavily on their efforts.

Based on the above, we recommend two ways to improve the effectiveness of workshops and seminars: to describe the activities in detail, in relation to their learning objectives and design; and to ground faculty development activities in a theoretical framework of teacher learning. In the next section, we propose a new framework which can serve as a guideline for the design of faculty development activities such as workshops and seminars based on these recommendations.

9.4   A New Framework for the Development of Workshops and Seminars

When taking part in faculty development programs, faculty members adopt the role of learners, and in line with the literature on adult learning (Cercone 2008), we expect them to actively construct their own knowledge by undertaking learning activities. We have therefore chosen to apply the theory of Vermunt and Verloop (1999), which takes students' learning activities as the starting point, to the design of faculty development workshops and seminars. This theory, which is based on empirical research on university students' learning, has recently also been applied to teacher learning (Bakkenes et al. 2010; Mansvelder-Longayroux et al. 2007; Vermunt and Endedijk 2011; Zanting et al. 2001). In the context of faculty development workshops and seminars, the challenge is to actively engage faculty members in learning activities. Learning activities can be observable, overt activities such as reading a book or article and making a summary, taking part in a discussion with peers, teachers or facilitators, or working together on assignments or projects. At the same time, if the participants are engaged, important, but invisible, mental activities can occur. These include relating new knowledge to prior knowledge, selecting relevant information from a text or presentation, or critically processing an author's conclusion (Vermunt and Endedijk 2011; Vermunt and Verloop 1999). From this perspective, learning activities during the process of learning largely determine the quality of the learning outcomes and, thus, whether or not the learning objectives are achieved. Therefore, the design of faculty development activities should begin with defining the learning objectives (i.e. what is to be learned). The objectives should, in turn, determine the choice of teaching methods and the types of activities to be used (i.e. how this content can best be learned) (Steinert 1992).

In this section, we provide a framework to guide workshop design based on combinations of desired learning outcomes and related learning activities. The framework consists of three main elements: (1) learning outcomes; (2) learning activities; and (3) instructional methods to elicit specific learning activities.

We distinguish two learning outcomes on a cognitive level, that is, changes in knowledge and beliefs (awareness, confirmed or new ideas) and intent to practice (to try or continue to use new practices, or to continue using current practices) and one learning outcome on a behavioral level, that is, changes in skills and behavior (Bakkenes et al. 2010). We also distinguish three types of learning activities to describe the learning process: (1) cognitive learning activities; (2) affective learning activities; and (3) regulative or metacognitive activities. Cognitive learning activities are those mental activities that learners use to process information, leading to changes in knowledge and beliefs, (e.g. by relating or structuring information). In contrast to affective and regulative learning activities, different cognitive learning activities are required for different learning outcomes. Cognitive learning activities and related learning outcomes and instructional methods are described in Table 9.1.

Affective activities include focusing attention, self-motivation and coping with feelings of uncertainty, boredom or distraction. Regulative or metacognitive activities are mental activities by which learners monitor, adjust and evaluate their cognitive and affective learning activities. For example, learners can facilitate their own learning process by starting to question which knowledge, skills and/or attitudes should be acquired. Subsequently, they can select the appropriate learning strategy to achieve their learning goals (e.g. to acquire knowledge of leadership styles, studying books and articles is adequate; to experience various leadership styles, a workshop with role playing might be appropriate; to apply a new leadership style, another strategy might be required, including coaching on the job). Examples of these activities are described in Tables 9.2 and 9.3; instructional methods to stimulate these activities are also described.

9.5 Case Examples

9.5.1 A Teach-the-Teacher Workshop

To illustrate the use of learning activities, we describe a 2-day, small group (8–12 participants) workshop for clinical teachers who supervise students and residents. This workshop is given at the Erasmus University Medical Center, in Rotterdam, the

Table 9.1 Learning outcomes, *cognitive learning activities* and instructional methods

Learning outcomes	Cognitive learning activities	Instructional methods to facilitate cognitive learning activities
	Learners…	The facilitator…
Changes in knowledge and beliefs	…analyze and concretize their knowledge and beliefs	…stimulates participants to articulate their knowledge and beliefs by questioning, mind concept mapping, responding to a statement, etc.
		…provides cases or scenarios to make participants aware of the limitations of their knowledge and beliefs
	…apply theoretical knowledge	…presents learning and teaching theories, stimulates participants to study these theories and elaborate on them by generating examples
	…relate their own knowledge and beliefs to those of others and to theories	…instructs participants to look for similarities and differences between their own knowledge and beliefs, those of others and existing theories
	…critically appraise different viewpoints and draw conclusions for their own actions and theory of practice	…stimulates participants to make a choice from the different viewpoints or to combine them
Changes in skills and behavior	…observe examples	…or other participants demonstrate (new) skills and behaviors; other methods may be used as well, such as video, role play, simulation
		…creates cases or simulations in which participants' skills and behavior are lacking
	…elicit underlying ideas and principles	…discusses the skills demonstrated, including the underlying choices that were made
	…experiment/practice	…invites participants to demonstrate their (adapted) skills while other participants observe
	…evaluate	…gives feedback and invites the other participants and others, such as an actor involved in role plays, to give feedback: what went well, what can be improved and how?
Intentions for practice	…learners relate the outcomes of new behavior and skills practiced during the workshop to their teaching practice	…stimulates participants to discuss their daily behavior and specify their commitments to change
		…discusses opportunities and threats for application in practice with the participants
	…critically appraise whether the new skills and behavior are useful and attainable in practice	…formulates intentions to stimulate participants to apply new practices or go back to old practices
		…stimulates participants to reflect on/evaluate the effects of new practices

Table 9.2 *Affective learning activities* and instructional methods

Affective learning activities	Instructional methods to create a promoting, affective climate
Learners...	*The facilitator...*
...express their motivation and expectations	...discusses the participants' learning needs and integrates these in the program of the workshop
	...outlines the objectives of the workshop and their relevance, and asks participants to formulate personal learning goals
	...gives participants tasks they can handle
	...relates the content to teaching practice to generate interest
...concentrate and exert efforts	...uses various teaching methods and breaks
	...activates participants by questioning them and involving them in discussions
	...gives participants challenging tasks and assignments
...attribute and judge themselves	...creates opportunities to observe other participants, to experiment, and to give and receive feedback
...appraise	...emphasizes the relevance of the workshop objectives and tasks for personal development and practice
...deal with emotions	...enhances self- confidence through encouragement to explore new ideas and practices
	...gives feedback that emphasizes what participants are doing well,
	... ensures that the feedback is task-oriented, specific, useful and gives tips for improvement
	...creates a safe learning environment in which participants can experience success, take risks, dare to experiment, and be willing to 'fail'

Table 9.3 *Regulative learning activities* and instructional methods

Regulative learning activities	Instructional methods to facilitate regulation of learning
Learners...	*The facilitator...*
...orient themselves and plan	...first activates prior knowledge and experiences by questioning, short presentations, and discussions about teaching concepts and critical incidents
	...subsequently introduces the content, learning objectives and tasks of the workshop
...monitor, test and diagnose	...lets participants present elaborated tasks and assignments to each other
	...gives feedback
...adjust	...encourages participants to search for difficulties and solutions for experienced problems, on their own or with others
...evaluate/reflect	...allows participants to evaluate whether the (personal) learning objectives are realized or not
	...generate suggestions for future improvement

Netherlands, but is comparable in content and methods to the so-called 'Teach the Teacher' workshops given at other Dutch medical centers (Busari et al. 2006). The 2 days are scheduled 2 weeks apart to allow participants to apply new knowledge, ideas, and skills learned in the first day to their teaching practice. Learning objectives include acquiring and adjusting (new) knowledge and beliefs (e.g. active and adult learning), acquiring and adjusting skills (e.g. observing, giving feedback and assessing) and translating new skills to daily practice (e.g. innovations in supervision). The first day starts with an affective learning activity; in a plenary session, participants describe their expectations and personal learning objectives. At the end of this activity the facilitator asks the participants to reflect on it. Usually, the participants report that they are more motivated to learn after having formulated their own learning needs and goals, even if their attendance at the workshop was compulsory. The facilitator then explains that this was the purpose of the exercise and indicates that participants may use the same approach when they are teaching themselves. To further increase the participants' internal motivation, the facilitator incorporates the participants' learning objectives in the program, whenever possible.

Changes in knowledge, ideas and skills are encouraged by asking the participants to watch a video showing a clinician supervising a student or resident. Participants are then asked to identify strong points and areas for improvement in the scenario, thereby articulating their own knowledge and beliefs about supervision. By doing this in a group, different conceptions of supervision are elicited and compared. Participants experienced this mutual exchange of ideas as valuable and as a helpful tool to develop or adjust their own beliefs about supervision. In the last part of this exercise, the facilitator introduces adult learning and participants reflect on the application of this framework to the video and their own knowledge and beliefs. In this way, participants are stimulated to undertake various cognitive learning activities aimed at (re)constructing their knowledge about teaching, such as relating and processing information and ideas and applying theoretical knowledge. Subsequently, participants practice component skills of supervision, such as observing, giving feedback and assessing. At the end of the first day, the participants record their main learning outcomes, remaining questions and specific actions for practice. In doing so, they apply regulative learning activities such as evaluating, reflecting, orienting and planning.

Participants evaluated this workshop as useful for developing or adjusting ideas about 'good' supervision and attributed success to the interaction between the participants as well as between the facilitator and the participants. They stated that their greatest challenge was to apply their learning outcomes and intentions in daily practice. They also indicated that splitting the workshops into 2 days during 2 weeks gave them the opportunity and the incentive to practise in the workplace.

9.5.2 A Seminar Series on the Integration of Technology Tools in a Problem-Based Learning Curriculum

We will illustrate the basic principles of seminar design by describing a seminar that focused on the integration of technology tools in a problem-based learning curriculum at the Faculty of Health, Medicine, and Life Sciences, Maastricht University. The seminar consisted of a series of six 1 h lunchtime sessions targeting a group of

12 experienced teachers from different disciplines. The meeting schedule and content of the seminars was prepared in advance, in consultation with the participants. The main aim of the seminar was to achieve more in depth evidence-based knowledge about effective integration of technology into the curriculum and to positively change teachers' attitudes towards the use of technology in education. All sessions were supported by expert resources in an electronic learning environment. Participants were expected to prepare for each meeting by studying selected resources and watching demonstrations of each technological tool. Each meeting focused on a specific tool such as blogs, wiki's, audio response tools, collaborative working tools, social bookmarking and social networking. The meeting began with affective learning activities which included reflecting on perceptions and (possible) experiences with the technological tool and discussions of the text accompanying each tool. A technological expert provided explanations, presented information found on the internet, and/or demonstrated the use of the tool. The participants had the opportunity to ask questions about the tools and participate in a discussion. The expert moderated this discussion, by summarizing, asking questions and taking notes. Prior theoretical knowledge, personal opinions and prior experience with the technological tool were activated, used and compared in the discussion. After this initial phase of discussion, participants discussed the practical educational relevance and possible application and conditions for implementation of the tool. In this way, the participants made use of a diversity of cognitive learning activities to acquire in-depth understanding and knowledge about the tool and possibly change their attitudes about it. At the end of the session, participants assessed the learning goals and developed action plans to experiment with, or implement, the technological tool in education. In this way, they regulated their learning activities by means of evaluation, reflection and planning. After the session, different experts supported the participants in these activities to stimulate transfer of learning to actual behavior.

9.6 Factors Affecting Transfer of Training from Workshops and Seminars to Educational Practice

The impact of faculty development on the learning of students and residents is highly dependent on the ability of faculty members to transfer their newly acquired knowledge, skills and attitudes to their teaching practices. In 1988, Baldwin and Ford introduced a model to study transfer of training and described key factors related to training inputs, training outputs and conditions of transfer. Since then, many studies and reviews have been published (Blume et al. 2010; Burke and Hutchins 2007; Grossman and Salas 2011) and have identified a wealth of factors that can possibly influence the level and maintenance of transfer of training to the workplace. However, not all results are unequivocal, and the relationships between the factors are complex and may depend on the organizational context as well as on the definitions and measurements of transfer (Blume et al. 2010; Burke and Hutchins 2007). Therefore, Grossman and Salas (2011) selected factors from the

Table 9.4 Factors related to training transfer, based on Grossman and Salas (2011)

Training inputs	Positive relationships with…
Trainee characteristics	
Cognitive ability	Processing, retaining, generalizing skills
Self-efficacy	Confidence and persistence in application of acquired skills; generalizing and maintenance of skills
Motivation to learn and transfer	Facilitation of transfer
Perceived utility of training	Application of acquired skills
Training design	
Behavioral modeling	Facilitation of transfer
Error management	Facilitation of transfer
Realistic training environments	Facilitation of transfer
Work environment	
Transfer climate	Application of acquired skills
Support	Transfer
Opportunity to perform	Success of transfer
Follow-up	Facilitation of transfer

available literature which have a strong relationship to transfer and used these to provide guidance for evidence-based training programs. They slightly adapted the original model of Baldwin and Ford (1988) and restricted their analysis to factors related to the training inputs, grouped in three categories (see Table 9.4). We will use this guide to identify factors that have to be considered in order to enhance the transfer of training when designing and executing workshops and seminars for faculty development.

The most obvious of the three categories in Table 9.4 appears to be the *training design*. Workshops are close to ideal in providing realistic environments for participants to practice various strategies and learn from their own and others' errors, 'risk free'. The effectiveness may be further improved if follow-up meetings, in which experiences from the work situation can be discussed and/or replayed in role plays, are organized. The challenge for the designers and facilitators is to create a safe atmosphere and environment that sufficiently resembles the work situation of all participants, defining clear objectives, providing relevant content and giving feedback (Carnes 2010). The challenge for the organization as a whole is to give the learners opportunities to practice their newly acquired skills in authentic situations. In the category *trainee characteristics*, motivation to learn, motivation to transfer, and perceived utility form a cluster of related factors. These factors may be positively influenced if a careful needs assessment is performed preceding (or at the start of) the workshop or seminar, a practice that currently appears to be neglected (Burke and Hutchins 2007). A (pending) change in the educational environment, such as a new teaching philosophy or curriculum change, may create a sense of urgency that can be seized as an opportunity to train highly motivated learners for a new educational working environment. The category of the *work environment* is largely beyond the domain of educational workshops and seminars. However, workshops and seminars may contribute to a bottom-up change in the work climate by a change in attitude of the participants (e.g. a culture of giving feedback), and the development of organization-wide networks and communities of learning (Steinert et al. 2006). In addition, other faculty development activities, such as leadership and career development workshops and seminars, may induce a change in the work climate as well (Burke and Hutchins 2007; Steinert 2011).

9.7 Opportunities and Challenges for the Future of Workshops and Seminars

The theory and evidence used in this chapter to describe and design workshops and seminars (or a series of seminars), as well as knowledge about factors influencing the transfer of training, can increase the learning potential of these approaches and stimulate thinking about the relationship of workshops and seminars to other approaches for faculty development. It is also an opportunity to design faculty development programs where there is a mix of more formal approaches, such as workshops and seminar series, and more informal approaches, such as work-based learning. In addition, workshops can be combined with coaching, making these different approaches complementary. It would also be worthwhile to find an optimal mix of these approaches in more longitudinal faculty development programs.

The generally short duration of faculty development activities such as workshops and seminars can limit their effectiveness for certain outcomes, particularly with respect to those related to attitudinal and behavioral change. When attitudinal change or new approaches for teaching are involved, time and attention to group dynamics is mandatory. On the other hand, because of their brevity, these formats can also be used flexibly in different faculty development activities and very often 'just in time'. Thus, although the risk may be less effectiveness, workshops and seminars provide an opportunity for flexibility in different faculty development contexts, which can also enhance their effectiveness.

Another characteristic of workshops and seminars which determines their effectiveness, but also heightens their risks and opportunities, is the small group context, where interaction and active and experiential learning methods make the difference. A risk is that workshops and seminar series sometimes decrease the emphasis on interaction and active learning methods. As an example, seminars can sometimes be reduced to one-way presentations with little or no interaction with the audience. The challenge is therefore to create high quality interaction, incorporating active learning in these approaches.

The facilitator in these formats plays a key role in their effective use, and attention must be paid to the professional development of the facilitators to make these formats work (O'Sullivan and Irby 2011). A train-the-trainer model which is theory and evidence-based can be of help (Pearce et al. 2012).

Another challenge is to explore new uses of the above discussed formats, not only for instructional development, but also for leadership and/or organizational development.

Workshops can play a role in the adoption, implementation and dissemination of educational innovations. These new formats should be used and adapted in the context of faculty development.

9.8 Conclusion

Workshops and seminars (or a series of seminars) have proven to be effective and remain the dominant approach to faculty development. History has shown us that these approaches have evolved and have been adapted to different circumstances. In fact, workshops and seminars are fixtures in an ever changing landscape that is shaped by new insights (e.g. learning theories) and new developments (e.g. technology). The main challenge is to optimize the learning potential of these approaches. In this chapter, we have provided some suggestions and recommendations for the use and the design of these formats in enhancing the personal and professional development and growth of faculty members.

9.9 Key Messages

- Incorporate theory and evidence in the description and design of workshops and seminars. Specifically, define the goals, identify the required learning activities, and select the appropriate instructional design.
- Experiment with and study the integration and effects of workshops and seminars in more longitudinal approaches to faculty development.
- Experiment with new uses of workshops and seminar series in different contexts, including leadership and organizational development, and assess their effectiveness.

References

Amundsen, C. & Wilson, M. (2012). Are we asking the right questions? A conceptual review of the educational development literature in higher education. *Review of Educational Research, 82*(1), 90–126.

Bakkenes, I., Vermunt, J. D., & Wubbels, T. (2010). Teacher learning in the context of educational innovation: Learning activities and learning outcomes of experienced teachers. *Learning and Instruction, 20*(6), 533–548.

Baldwin, T. T. & Ford, J. K. (1988). Transfer of training: A review and directions for future research. *Personnel Psychology, 41*(1), 63–105.

Behar-Horenstein, L. S., Schneider-Mitchell, G., & Graff, R. (2008). Faculty perceptions of a professional development seminar. *Journal of Dental Education, 72*(4), 472–483.

Blumberg, P. (2011). Making evidence-based practice an essential aspect of teaching. *Journal of Faculty Development, 25*(3), 27–32.

Blume, B. D., Ford, J. K., Baldwin, T. T., & Huang, J. L. (2010). Transfer of training: A meta-analytic review. *Journal of Management, 36*(4), 1065–1105.

Brooks-Harris, J. E. & Stock-Ward, S. R. (1999). *Workshops: Designing and facilitating experiential learning*. Thousand Oaks, CA: Sage Publications, Inc.

Burke, L. A. & Hutchins, H. M. (2007). Training transfer: An integrative literature review. *Human Resource Development Review, 6*(3), 263–296.

Busari, J. O., Scherpbier, A. J. J. A., van der Vleuten, C. P. M., Essed, G. G. M., Rojer, R. (2006). A description of a validated effective teacher-training workshop for medical residents. *Medical Education Online, 11*(15). Available from: http://med-ed-online.net/index.php/meo/article/view/4591/4770

Byham, W. C. (2008). Luminary perspective: Face-to-face delivery - as important as ever. In Elaine Biech (Ed.), *ASTD handbook for workplace learning professionals,* (pp. 295–301). Alexandria, VA: ASTD Press.

Carnes, B. (2010). *Making learning stick*. Alexandria, VA: ASTD Press.

Cercone, K. (2008). Characteristics of adult learners with implications for online learning design. *Association for the Advancement of Computing in Education Journal, 16*(2), 137–159.

Clark, R. C. (2010). *Evidence-based training methods: A guide for training professionals*. Alexandria, VA: ASTD Press.

Davis, D. & Davis, N. (2010). Selecting educational interventions for knowledge translation. *CMAJ, 182*(2), E89–E93.

Davis, D., O'Brien, M. A., Freemantle, N., Wolf, F. M., Mazmanian, P., & Taylor-Vaisey, A. (1999). Impact of formal continuing medical education: Do conferences, workshops, rounds, and other traditional continuing education activities change physician behavior or health care outcomes? *JAMA, 282*(9), 867–874.

Eraut, M. (2000). Non-formal learning and tacit knowledge in professional work. *British Journal of Educational Psychology, 70*(1), 113–136.

Flottorp, S. (2008). Do continuing education meetings and workshops improve professional practice and healthcare outcomes? A SUPPORT summary of a systematic review. Available from: http://epocoslo.cochrane.org/sites/epocoslo.cochrane.org/files/uploads/SURE%20Guides/Collected%20files/source/support%20summaries/forsetlund2009.pdf

Forsetlund, L., Bjørndal, A., Rashidian, A., Jamtvedt, G., O'Brien, M. A., Wolf, F., et al. (2009). Continuing education meetings and workshops: Effects on professional practice and health care outcomes. *Cochrane Database of Systematic Reviews,* (2), CD003030.

Grossman, R. & Salas, E. (2011). The transfer of training: What really matters. *International Journal of Training and Development, 15*(2), 103–120.

Guskey, T. R. (2003). Analyzing lists of the characteristics of effective professional development to promote visionary leadership. *NASSP Bulletin, 87*(637), 4–20.

Harden, R. M., Grant, J., Buckley, G., & Hart, I. R. (1999). BEME Guide No. 1: Best evidence medical education. *Medical Teacher, 21*(6), 553–562.

Mansvelder-Longayroux, D. D., Beijaard, D., Verloop, N., & Vermunt, J. D. (2007). Functions of the learning portfolio in student teachers' learning process. *Teachers College Record, 109*(1), 126–159.

O'Sullivan, P. S. & Irby, D. M. (2011). Reframing research on faculty development. *Academic Medicine, 86*(4), 421–428.

Pearce, J., Mann, M. K., Jones, C., Van Buschbach, S., Olff, M., & Bisson, J. I. (2012). The most effective way of delivering a Train-The-Trainers Program: A systematic review. *Journal of Continuing Education in the Health Professions, 32*(3), 215–226.

Schmitt, W. J. (2011). *Seminars, trainings and workshops: Effective preparation, creation, and implementation*. Trainplan Press (e-Book).

Sork, T. J. (1984). The workshop as a unique instructional format. In T. J. Sork (Ed.), *Designing and implementing effective workshops*. San Francisco, CA: Jossey-Bass. Published in: *New Directions for Continuing Education,* (22), 3–10.

Spruijt, A., Jaarsma, A. D. C., Wolfhagen, H. A. P., Van Beukelen, P., & Scherpbier, A. J. J. A. (2012). Students' perceptions of aspects affecting seminar learning. *Medical Teacher, 34*(2), e129–e135.

Steinert, Y. (1992). Twelve tips for conducting effective workshops. Medical Teacher, *14*(2–3), 127–131.

Steinert, Y. (2011). Commentary: Faculty development: The road less traveled. *Academic Medicine, 86*(4), 409–411.

Steinert, Y., Boillat, M., Meterissian, S., Liben, S., & McLeod, P. J. (2008). Developing successful workshops: A workshop for educators. *Medical Teacher, 30*(3), 328–330.

Steinert, Y., Mann, K., Centeno, A., Dolmans, D., Spencer, J., Gelula, M., et al. (2006). A systematic review of faculty development initiatives designed to improve teaching effectiveness in medical education: BEME Guide No. 8. *Medical Teacher, 28*(6), 497–526.

Stes, A., Min-Leliveld, M., Gijbels, D., & Van Petegem, P. (2010). The impact of instructional development in higher education: The state-of-the-art of the research. *Educational Research Review, 5*(1), 25–49.

Vermunt, J. D. & Endedijk, M. D. (2011). Patterns in teacher learning in different phases of the professional career. *Learning and Individual Differences, 21*(3), 294–302.

Vermunt, J. D. & Verloop, N. (1999). Congruence and friction between learning and teaching. *Learning and Instruction, 9*(3), 257–280.

Wilkerson, L. & Irby, D. M. (1998). Strategies for improving teaching practices: A comprehensive approach to faculty development. *Academic Medicine, 73*(4), 387–396.

Yardley, S. & Dornan, T. (2012). Kirkpatrick's levels and education 'evidence'. *Medical Education, 46*(1), 97–106.

Zanting, A., Verloop, N., & Vermunt, J. D. (2001). Student teachers' beliefs about mentoring and learning to teach during teaching practice. *The British Journal of Educational Psychology, 71*(1), 57–80.

Chapter 10
Intensive Longitudinal Faculty Development Programs

Larry D. Gruppen

10.1 Introduction

Many faculty developers recognize that, in order to have a major impact on such key faculty outcomes as educational leadership, scholarship, and skills, it is often necessary to make substantial investments in these faculty members. Although there are a variety of ways of making this investment, extending the duration and increasing the frequency of faculty development activities is a straightforward solution. Providing an intensive, longitudinal series of activities for a cohort of faculty also fits well with institutional goals to develop faculty members with more sophisticated levels of skill in particular domains, such as leadership, scholarship or educational development.

This chapter describes some of the characteristics of faculty development programs that are designed to provide faculty members with intensive training in a specific set of skills over an extended period of time. Although such programs go by many names, such as a 'Teaching Scholars Program' or 'Medical Education Fellowship' or 'Program for Physician Educators,' we will refer to them generically as intensive longitudinal faculty development programs. This chapter does not address degree-granting programs in health professions education or higher education (Tekian and Harris 2012), although there are a number of similarities.

L.D. Gruppen, Ph.D. (✉)
Department of Medical Education, University of Michigan Medical School,
Ann Arbor, MI, USA
e-mail: lgruppen@umich.edu

Y. Steinert (ed.), *Faculty Development in the Health Professions: A Focus on Research and Practice*, Innovation and Change in Professional Education 11, DOI 10.1007/978-94-007-7612-8_10, © Springer Science+Business Media Dordrecht 2014

10.2   What Are Intensive Longitudinal Programs?

Searle et al. (2006b) define this kind of faculty development program as 'a cohort of faculty members selected to participate in a longitudinal set of faculty development activities with the goals of improving the participants' teaching skills and of building a cadre of educational leaders for the institution' (p. 936). They trace the origins of this format back to the 1980s and the emergence of Family Medicine as a specialty. Indeed, in the United Kingdom, these origins go back to the 1960s. At that time, there was a significant need to develop a cadre of teachers to foster the development of the specialty, often by focusing on residents as future faculty members. As such, it was important to devote an intensive effort to faculty development and building the culture of the specialty through a cohort of learners. Since then, intensive longitudinal programs have proliferated and diversified in form and focus, both in the United Kingdom and North America.

A 2005–06 national survey of 127 United States medical schools sought to determine the scope and characteristics of this faculty development format (Thompson et al. 2011). Almost half of the responding schools had an intensive longitudinal program, most of which began in the 1990s or 2000s. In general, these are institutional investments, with a minority sponsored by individual departments. All of these programs are designed for working faculty members; that is, they are not 'sabbatical' activities but are intended to be manageable in the context of routine clinical and educational responsibilities. Although clinical faculty members tend to predominate as participants, most programs are open to basic science faculty and some to residents and allied health faculty as well. This survey identified almost 5,500 graduates of all the programs.

10.3   An Illustrative Program

The Medical Education Scholars Program (MESP) at the University of Michigan (Frohna et al. 2006; Gruppen et al. 2003) is representative of such intensive longitudinal faculty fellowship programs. Established in 1998 to promote educational scholarship, leadership and teaching skills among the faculty at the University of Michigan Medical School, it admits an annual cohort of approximately 12 faculty participants who apply to the program in a competitive admissions process. Admission priority is given to medical school faculty members, but faculty from other health professions schools and residents have also participated. Participants meet weekly from September through May for approximately 40 sessions. Each session is 3.5 h in length and emphasizes highly interactive instructional methods and activities. There are approximately 25 workshop facilitators in the MESP who come from numerous departments in the medical school and the university, as well as guest faculty from other institutions. Each participant identifies a curriculum development or educational research project to work on during the course of the program. The MESP is administered by a director (20 % effort) and an administrative coordinator (50 % effort) within the Department of Medical Education. The MESP charges each participant a modest fee to help defray these expenses, but the remainder of the program support comes from the Department of Medical Education budget.

A typical session of the MESP begins with an interactive workshop on a topic facilitated by a guest or local expert. A priority is placed on active participation and contribution, practical application, and shared thoughts and perspectives among the cohort of participants. The MESP Director is always present to ensure continuity among the various sessions by pointing out linkages to prior discussions and relevant implications to individual problems and projects. After the workshop, the facilitator leaves the room and the MESP cohort engages in what is termed an 'educational autopsy,' designed to not only evaluate the session but also to enter more deeply into an analysis of the structure and process that the facilitator used for the workshop. This autopsy provides feedback to the facilitator but also encourages the participants to think beyond the content of the workshop to its underlying process and the educational alternatives that might have been considered. The final hour of the session is devoted to a 'scholar's hour' in which a designated participant (in rotation) can use this time for their own goals. This might include getting feedback on an educational innovation, a journal club discussion, peer input on an educational project, or any number of other creative activities.

These activities are feasible only in the context of an intensive faculty development program in which participants have regularly scheduled, protected time to devote to acquiring and practicing specialized skills and competencies. Defining the MESP as a program for developing educational leaders and scholars reflects institutional priorities and explicitly echoes the scope of other specialized training programs, such as in biomedical research education or clinical administrative leadership development.

10.4 The Goals and Purposes of Intensive Longitudinal Programs

10.4.1 Enhancing Teaching Skills

During the first half of the twentieth century, teaching expertise had traditionally been assumed to be part of content expertise (Wilkerson and Irby 1998). In other words, anyone who mastered the discipline was competent to teach it. More recently, it has been recognized, both in education generally and in medical education specifically, that teaching skill and expertise is not an automatic consequence of disciplinary expertise (Harris et al. 2007; McLean et al. 2008; Shulman 1986). However, the development of educational skills in addition to disciplinary expertise has often been left to chance as individual faculty members learn to teach by observing their own teachers (Skeff et al. 1997a, b; Thompson et al. 2011). The lack of formal training in educational skills resulted in a haphazard learning process that produced faculty members who varied considerably in educational skill and sophistication. In their analysis of educational scholarship, Simpson and Fincher (1999) noted that medical schools need clearer criteria for evaluating the educational contributions of their faculty and need to provide an infrastructure to support the continuous development of faculty members as educational scholars and effective teachers. The intensive longitudinal faculty development program is one strategy for addressing these various institutional needs.

10.4.2   Supporting Educators

Faculty members must address many stressors in their roles as clinicians and educators, and burnout is an all too common hazard (McLean et al. 2008). Additional challenges in sustaining faculty productivity and vitality come from the growth of ambulatory and community-based teaching and the participation of faculty members hired primarily to provide patient care, who may not have planned a career that is primarily academic (Searle et al. 2006a). Although faculty development in general is intended to provide some protection against these risks by developing skills and support for teaching responsibilities, intensive longitudinal programs likely provide a greater degree of assistance by virtue of their intensity and community-building qualities. A cohort of a dozen faculty members who meet periodically over the course of a year invariably share their teaching frustrations and triumphs and come to recognize that they are not alone. The 'hidden curriculum' of many such programs includes the peer-mentoring and support of teachers who ordinarily work in isolation. The community-building potential of these programs is a major selling point and may contribute to the retention of valuable teaching faculty members (Moses et al. 2009).

Besides mutual support, participants in intensive longitudinal programs are motivated by many other goals. One that emerges repeatedly is the belief that participation in such a program will make them more competitive for educational leadership positions in medical schools, hospitals, and professional organizations. These positions carry with them greater expectations for being familiar and conversant with new methods of teaching and assessment (Searle et al. 2006a). Pursuing these positions and careers also requires evidence of productivity and quality that can be used by promotions committees; this is an explicit goal of a number of programs (Baldwin et al. 1995; Wilkerson et al. 2006).

10.4.3   Augmenting Education as a Scientific Discipline

Most programs strive to expand the participants' perspective on education beyond being just an area of practice to recognizing it as a scholarly discipline with a foundation of theory and empirical evidence (McLean et al. 2008). All such programs use this evidence base and relevant theoretical frameworks as critical resources and structures for the participants to use in their practical application, but many programs go further by seeking to enable participants to contribute to the scholarly foundation of medical education as a discipline (Harris et al. 2007; Sheets and Schwenk 1990). Many programs have sought to address this problem by including instruction in educational research principles and practices (Gruppen et al. 2006; Robins et al. 2006). This aspect recognizes the expanded definition of scholarship that includes teaching and educational innovation (Boyer 1990).

This emphasis seeks to promote teaching that is grounded in relevant theory and in best practices from the literature, thus improving the education of medical students and residents. It also seeks to foster a more thoughtful and informed use of the medical education literature by these faculty members. However, another explicit goal is to develop more and better educational researchers and to improve the quality of the empirical evidence in medical education. Although programs recognize that only a subset of participants are likely to devote much time to research, encouraging and empowering participants to do so is important not only to the individual programs and sponsoring institutions, but to the larger field of medical education as a whole. It is worth noting that an explicit focus on faculty development for building research capacity may require somewhat different considerations and structures than those typical of most intensive programs. (See Chap. 4 for further details.)

10.4.4   Developing Educational Leadership

As noted above, many participants in intensive longitudinal programs have personal goals to advance their own leadership roles, but many institutions have also recognized the need for developing educational leadership for their own local purposes (Hatem et al. 2006; Muller and Irby 2006). There is a growing need for and expectation of educational sophistication in many leadership positions, particularly those in graduate medical education, as program directors and coordinators adapt to the shifting focus on educational outcomes and performance instead of time on task (Gruppen et al. 2006; Wilkerson et al. 2006). Whereas informal learning on the job through years of experience might have been enough for success in these positions in the past, there is a growing recognition that more formal knowledge in a wide range of domains is becoming increasingly necessary. (See Chap. 3 for a discussion of leadership development.)

10.5   Evidence of Success

Given the goals and objectives of intensive longitudinal programs, what evidence exists that these goals are being achieved? Evaluating the impact of faculty development programs is often challenging. There is seldom a comparison group to whom to compare program graduates. In a rare example of a matched control group design, Hewson and Copeland (1999) were able to demonstrate that teaching evaluations from learners improved for faculty members in a relatively brief program focused on improving teaching skills as compared to the control group, which were comparable on teaching evaluation scores prior to the program. In addition, the outcomes and goals are difficult to measure and assessment methods with compelling evidence of validity are rare. As a consequence, many evaluations tend to rely on self-report measures and satisfaction ratings from participants, even while acknowledging that these data are among the less informative and useful for program evaluation (McLean et al. 2008). Other sources of evaluation data included participant activity levels (Elliot et al. 1999), analyses of professional networks (Morzinski and Fisher 2002; Moses et al. 2009), qualitative follow-up interviews (Burdick et al. 2010; Elliot et al. 1999; Gruppen et al. 2003), peer observation and evaluation of participants (Hatem et al. 2006), curriculum vitae content analysis (Gruppen et al. 2003; Morzinski and Simpson 2003; Morzinski and Schubot 2000), and learner evaluations (most programs). Some specific outcomes are also assessed through questionnaires and other means, such as attitudes towards learner-centered learning (Gordon et al. 1990). What follows are some evaluation methods and results that can be considered in judging the efficacy of this format of faculty development.

10.5.1   Satisfaction and Self-Efficacy

A repeated finding is that participants are highly satisfied with the experience and judge that they have learned a great deal from it (e.g. Burdick et al. 2010; Lown et al. 2009; Muller and Irby 2006). That this is so is perhaps unsurprising, given the self-selection inherent in these programs. Nonetheless, the unsolicited testimonials and the universal presence of high satisfaction indicate that these programs gratify some goals and objectives of the participants. There is also some supportive validity evidence available from interviews of secondary beneficiaries – individuals identified by program participants who might be affected by their participation in the program (Moses et al. 2006). The majority of these individuals acknowledged that the scholar they knew had improved as a teacher and education scholar and had enhanced their educational scholarship, educational programs, teaching, mentoring and leadership in the department.

10.5.2   Leadership and Career Development

Another frequently cited outcome of intensive longitudinal programs is the frequency with which graduates take on leadership positions, either within their institution or in national professional societies and organizations (Muller and Irby 2006; Steinert and McLeod 2006; Wilkerson et al. 2006). Up to 2/3 of these graduates attain such leadership positions after participation. At the Medical College of Wisconsin's program, one of the oldest, leadership positions more than tripled when comparing post-program rates with pre-program rates (Morzinski and Simpson 2003). This positive picture needs to be tempered, however, with the recognition that programs factor current or potential leadership into the admissions and selection process and identify it as a goal for the program, so the sample is predisposed for leadership.

There is also some evidence that the presence of intensive longitudinal programs increases the institution's ability to recruit educators and educationally oriented residents (Muller and Irby 2006). Other evidence points to a renewed interest in academic medicine and medical education as a career (Steinert and McLeod 2006) or increased faculty retention (Morzinski and Simpson 2003).

10.5.3 Developing a Community of Educators

As the development of a community of educators is a frequent objective of intensive longitudinal programs, there is great interest in being able to document this outcome. However, this is one for which there is no widely accepted or utilized measurement method. One analysis of 351 participants in 49 faculty fellowship programs in Family Medicine (Morzinski and Fisher 2002) indicated that participation was associated with a significant expansion of the participants' networks of collegial relationships. The relationships were most often with peers but also frequently with colleagues who could serve as mentors for various facets of career development. Other colleagues served as academic consultants.

An alternative technique that has been adopted for this purpose from the social sciences is network analysis. In a network analysis, program participants list the individuals with whom they interact in specified roles or for specified purposes. These identified individuals are combined for all the program participants and a social network is built (using computer software) to reflect the extent to which program participants interact as a community or in isolation from each other. The University of Arkansas program (which admits an interprofessional cohort) applied this methodology in a pre- and post-program design (Moses et al. 2009). Their analysis indicated a large expansion in network size and complexity for individuals and among the members of the program. This expansion was attributed, in part, to greater shared interests and better knowledge of resources and people. The members of the network were limited to those at the University, but others who have used network analysis note expansions from local into regional and national networks due to attending conferences that participants would not have attended before the program.

10.5.4 Scholarship and Productivity

For programs which seek to not only improve participant teaching skills but also their research and scholarship, the curriculum vitae (CV) is one source of outcomes that can be probed for evidence of the impact of participation. Several programs have developed methods for analyzing participant CVs to evaluate such program goals as promotions, new educational leadership roles, new curricular resources, scholarly publications, presentations and grants (Moses et al. 2009). When using a pre- and post-program comparison of participant productivity, such analyses frequently find statistically and practically significant increases in numbers of publications, presentations and educational grants (Gruppen et al. 2003; Morzinski and Simpson 2003; Rosenbaum et al. 2006; Simpson et al. 2006).

10.6 Characteristics of Intensive Longitudinal Programs

The preceding sections of this chapter have described the purposes of, and evidence for, intensive longitudinal faculty fellowship programs as one solution to a range of faculty development needs. For readers interested in pursuing this format further, it is important to note that, although these programs share some basic characteristics, there is a great deal of variation on how each one is designed and implemented. The present section highlights some of these characteristics with the goal of enabling readers to better frame their planning and decision-making.

10.6.1 Institutional Relevance

Most intensive longitudinal programs described in the literature begin with a careful study of institutional values and needs. Common issues include the need for accountability and effectiveness in the institution's educational mission, fostering and sustaining faculty in their educational roles, and adapting to the challenges and opportunities in the health care environment (Gruppen et al. 2006; McLean et al. 2008). Universally, these institutional goals appear in the program curriculum as segments devoted to the development of the individual participant's career, the instructional programs of the institution, institutional leadership, and the organization as a whole. Much of the variation among programs stems from the fact that each program is designed to meet the needs of its local faculty and institution (Searle et al. 2006b). A systematic review of faculty development programs (Steinert et al. 2006) highlighted the customization of most programs to a particular group of faculty members in a particular context. This customization increases the probability of successfully reaching program goals but it also makes generalizing across programs difficult. The importance of recognizing local contextual factors and the complexity of the faculty development process leads to the need to examine institutional and organizational factors, factors that have been largely ignored to date in many faculty development efforts.

The dynamic nature of aligning the goals of an intensive longitudinal program with the institution, and adapting to the inevitable changes in the institution (Gruppen et al. 2006), is well illustrated in the evolution of long-established programs. For example, the program at the Medical College of Wisconsin started in 1991 (Simpson et al. 2006). Its initial focus was on primary-care faculty and it emphasized a tight linkage between the educational needs of these faculty members with institutional priorities and academic reward structures. This linkage was challenged over the years as changes in institutional priorities, funding levels, new initiatives, competition for faculty time, and program vision required various alterations in program focus, structure, and logistics. Four tenets for adapting an intensive longitudinal faculty development program to the local environment emerged from this experience: (1) adaptability to changing environments and demands; (2) project-oriented faculty development as a powerful instructional strategy; (3) risk-taking role models in the program leadership; and (4) formative and summative program evaluation to provide data on program effectiveness (Simpson et al. 2006).

Similarly, changes in the institutional environment may be reflected in changing curricula, needs for improved or expanded assessment, and shifting philosophical emphasis on education as a mission of the school (e.g. Wilkerson et al. 2006). In other cases, particular institutional needs guide the focus and goals of the program at inception. The program at the University of Iowa illustrates this in its very specific program goal of training future faculty developers to do faculty development at the departmental level (Rosenbaum et al. 2005, 2006).

A special case of adapting an intensive longitudinal program to a particular audience is found in the Foundation for Advancement of International Medical Education and Research (FAIMER) regional institutes (Burdick et al. 2011). The five regional institutes, presently located in South Africa, Brazil, and India, share many of the same goals as programs at individual medical schools, such as enhanced leadership and management skills and improved teaching and assessment. However, the institutes are designed specifically as a model for focusing faculty development on community health outcomes. This model emphasizes the importance of social networks within a transnational perspective and emphasizes building a global community that is sensitive to resource-poor countries and institutions and addresses needs in the public sector. (See Chap. 15 for a more detailed description.)

10.6.2 Scope of the Targeted Participants

Each program is designed for a specifically targeted set of participants. The majority of programs are intended for faculty members at a single institution. However, there are a few exceptions to this rule. One is the Educational Scholars Fellowship program (Searle et al. 2006b), which is jointly sponsored by Baylor College of Medicine, the University of Texas Medical School at Houston, and the University of Texas Dental Branch at Houston. This collaboration is fostered by the close geographic proximity of the three institutions and rotates the directorship of the program among these institutions. In contrast, the Harvard Macy Program for Physician Educators is explicitly designed to accept participants from other institutions in North America and the world (Armstrong et al. 2003). The geographic dispersion of this program's cohort requires much more intensive periods of teaching on site – 2 weeks intensive followed by another week 6 months later – because these participants cannot readily gather for face-to-face sessions.

Most of the programs are open to both clinical and basic science faculty members, but the preponderance of participants come from the clinical departments; basic science faculty are greatly underrepresented (Rosenbaum et al. 2006; Steinert and McLeod 2006). The highest proportion of basic science faculty seems to be 10 % reported for the Baylor-UT program (Searle et al. 2006b). This disproportionate participation may reflect the emphasis of most programs on the training of physicians (medical students and residents) as contrasted with biomedical doctoral students. This emphasis may also limit the perceived value of participation by basic science faculty members. The imbalance may reflect differing perceptions between these groups of faculty of the importance of, and rewards associated with, improved teaching and educational scholarship. Similarly, most programs have originated in medical schools, so other health professions make up only a minority of participants.

10.6.3   Duration and Intensity

Of the programs surveyed in 2006 (Thompson et al. 2011), the median number of contact hours was 64, but there was a very large range (from 10 to 584). Overall program duration had a median of 10.5 months, ranging from less than 1 to 48 months. Most programs meet weekly or biweekly.

10.6.4   Curricular Elements

Virtually all of the programs are face-to-face and residential, although the program at UCLA combines a mix of face-to-face and online discussion (Wilkerson et al. 2006). The vast majority of programs provide the same curriculum to all participants in a given cohort, although the curriculum changes somewhat from year to year. The Teaching Scholars Program at McGill seems to be unique in its emphasis on an individualized program for each participant (Steinert et al. 2003; Steinert and McLeod 2006).

Teaching formats vary, but common methods are interactive presentations or workshops, observations and observed teaching activities, and reflective exercises (e.g. journals, written educational philosophies). Readings from the relevant literatures are an important element for grounding the participants in the theory and practices of education and related disciplines that are likely to be novel to them.

Projects are a major curricular element designed to provide participants with the opportunity to put into practice the educational principles they learn in the program (Beckman and Cook 2007). Many programs focus on curricular development projects, but research projects are also common. Individual project work typically requires consultation and input from program faculty and peers, but also from outside experts, to whom the program usually fosters access. Projects are often defined and implemented by individual participants, which enables them to express their personal interests. However, the individual project may not be very representative of the fact that most educational and research projects outside of the program are based on teams

Table 10.1 Primary foci, required products of fellows and program evaluation strategies of medical education fellowships across the USA (n = 55) (With permission from Thompson et al. 2011)

Primary focus[a]	No. (%)
Teaching skills	43 (78.2)
Scholarly dissemination	32 (58.2)
Curriculum design	29 (52.7)
Educational theory	26 (47.3)
Education research methods	26 (47.3)
Networking with other faculty	25 (45.5)
Educational leadership	24 (43.6)
Program evaluation	23 (41.8)
Use of educational literature	22 (40.0)
Evaluation of learners	21 (38.2)
Career advancement	21 (38.2)
Reflective practice	14 (25.5)

Required products of fellows[b]	No. (%)
Completion of scholarly project	44 (80.0)
Presentation./publication of scholarly project	36 (65.5)
Design of a curriculum	24 (43.6)
Entries into a journal (i.e. reflective writing)	14 (25.5)
Creation of a career development plan	13 (23.6)
Development of a learning contract	10 (18.2)
Implementation of a curriculum	10 (18.2)
Presentation of a grand rounds session	4 (7.3)

Evaluation methods[b]	No. (%)
Satisfaction questionnaires	48 (87.3)
Self-assessment questionnaires	32 (58.2)
Follow-up interviews	31 (56.4)
Number of educational activities begun or led by participant	24 (43.6)
Type of educational activity in which participant is involved	24 (43.6)
Direct peer observation/evaluation of participant	20 (36.4)
Curriculum vitae content analysis	20 (36.4)
Course/clerkship/seminar evaluations of participants	12 (21.8)
Portfolios	12 (21.8)

[a]Percentage of participants choosing 'primary focus'
[b]Totals equal more than 100 % because participants could select

and collaboration. There may also be value in considering projects that represent institutional needs and priorities rather than only individual preferences.

The most common curricular content include teaching skills, curricular design and various forms of scholarly dissemination, educational theory and research methods, networking, educational leadership, and program evaluation (Table 10.1, from Thompson et al. 2011). Some focus only on teaching skills (Hewson 2000) or faculty development (Rosenbaum et al. 2005), but most include a range of other skills and competencies.

10.6.5 Admissions Criteria

Most programs require applicants to document their interests in, and commitment to, education, often through evidence of past activities. Evidence of institutional (department or school) support (often in the form of a letter from the Chair or Division Chief) is also typical and used to indicate the potential the participant would have to make an impact after completing the program. Most programs require a personal statement describing their interest in the program and their goals. Cohort size is typically limited, with the size averaging around 10.

10.6.6 Communities of Practice

A characteristic common to virtually all of these programs is a focus on a community of practice (Wenger 1998). Program directors and developers recognize the importance of a supportive group of like-minded colleagues who can encourage and critique ideas in an environment that may not otherwise foster thoughtful and scholarly examination of critical educational problems. Developing such communities is important for a variety of reasons. Most of the fellowship programs consider learning to be a very social process that benefits from interchange and discussion among peers as well as with the program faculty (Salomon and Perkins 1998). Programs also recognize that medical education is inherently a 'team activity' that requires both the participation but also the cooperation of many members of the faculty. One might also predict that an expanded community of practice would result in greater impact or productivity of the individual participant or the community, but this link has not yet been demonstrated (Moses et al. 2009).

The nature of these communities varies among programs. Many programs bring together participants from various medical specialties; others focus on a single specialty. Some focus exclusively on physicians; others include multiple health professionals. Some are restricted to faculty members; others include residents and other levels of learners. All, however, explicitly foster the formation and health of a community of educational colleagues. Programs may vary in how much effort they devote to sustaining this community after participation in the program is completed and may vary in the number and types of activities used to develop these communities.

Participants benefit from the community of their peers but also need access to specialized expertise and similar resources. Thus, it is important that these communities bring together colleagues from different disciplines and specialties to promote a greater sense of connectedness within the institution, for building a community of educators, and sharing solutions to common problems. Although it is the local community of practice that is the most frequent focus, most programs seek to augment the larger national or international community of medical educators by encouraging participants to get involved in activities at those levels. Some examples include requiring attendance at a national or international medical education conference or course (Steinert et al. 2003; Steinert and McLeod 2006) and encouraging the submission and presentation of scholarly work at appropriate conference meetings (numerous programs).

10.6.7   Scholarship

The great majority of programs (Thompson et al. 2011) require a scholarly project as both a graduate requirement but also as an important vehicle for applying the principles taught in the program to a practical problem of relevance to the participant in their daily work responsibilities. Some programs also require the development of a curriculum whereas less common expected outcomes were reflective writing entries, or a career development or learning plan.

Getting participants to complete the projects is often a challenge. Some of the higher rates of completion approach 90 % (Simpson et al. 2006), but many programs attain much lower rates, nearer 60 % (e.g. Armstrong et al. 2003; Wilkerson et al. 2006). It is also common for the majority of these projects to focus on curricular or programmatic innovations rather than educational research. For example, the McGill Teaching Scholars Program found that 62 % of the participant projects focused on curriculum design or evaluation rather than educational research, as was the initial expectation (Steinert and McLeod 2006).

10.7   Future Directions for Intensive Longitudinal Faculty Development Programs

As these programs proliferate and mature, it is important to consider the issues and opportunities they may have to address in the future.

10.7.1   Reinvent the Wheel or Share It?

A major issue is that of sharing resources across programs. Given the similarities in curricula for most programs, it seems reasonable to consider the potential benefits of developing more portable curricular resources that reflect the best expertise available and make these a common, shared resource among programs (McLean et al. 2008; Steinert et al. 2006; Thompson et al. 2011). In addition to curricular resources, the need for content expertise as well as mentors for participants is a common need among programs. To date, most programs have sought to meet this need internally or by inviting visiting faculty from other institutions for a session. Whether there could be a more broadly shared, pooled resource of faculty expertise is worth exploring.

One vehicle for promoting such sharing is the recent development of a Directors of Medical Education Fellowship group, which meets during the annual meeting of the Association of American Medical Colleges. Similar sharing of ideas takes place among colleagues within other nations, and efforts to promote this sharing at an international level are growing through such events as the International Conferences on Faculty Development in the Health Professions in 2011 and 2013. Reasonable as this sharing might seem, it must overcome the resistance to curricula that are not locally developed and the considerable up-front costs of developing portable resources with little prospect of a concrete return on that investment.

10.7.2 Financial Challenges

These programs represent a variety of financial models, including central funding, reliance on departmental contributions, foundation support, and fee-based. Regardless of financial model, there are never enough resources to do everything that the program director, the institution, or the participants would like. It is also a common phenomenon for programs to start off with a sustainable level of funding, but, as time passes and novelty fades, to then see gradual reductions in their budget and begin to face cost-cutting requirements (Frohna et al. 2006; Gruppen et al. 2003; Robins et al. 2006). How programs address these constraints is not well documented in the literature but is a frequent topic at meetings of program directors.

Paying participants a stipend to protect their time for participation is fairly common, at least as programs start (e.g. Rosenbaum et al. 2006). However, it is often one of the first program expenses to get cut as funding becomes more constrained. Overall, it is not obvious that paying a stipend for participation is a necessity for program success. Most programs that have lost that funding have continued to have a good number of applicants. However, this change may have implications for a given institutional culture and, perhaps, for the participation of some members of the community.

Of course, these challenges pale in comparison to those faced in less resource-rich environments in which the needs for faculty development far outstrip the resources available. The Foundation for Advancement of International Medical Education and Research (FAIMER) is exploring ways to offer intensive faculty development in such countries (Burdick et al. 2010, 2011), but this is a challenge that needs to be embraced by other institutions as well.

10.7.3 Demonstrating Program Effectiveness

Longitudinal, intensive faculty development programs represent significant institutional investments in the growth and performance of its faculty members. Demonstrating the value of this investment is likely to become an increasingly important task for program directors. This requires both an assessment of program outcomes important to the institution and the individual participant and an accounting of the costs of these programs. As is true for most educational interventions and programs, accounting for the costs is a complex and often uncertain process. Direct salary and benefits costs for director and staff time are reasonably straightforward, as are other program expenses, such as food, materials, program travel, project costs, and, for some programs, stipends to participants for protected time to participate. However, there are numerous indirect costs that directors will need to consider: lost clinical revenue for participants, facilities costs, institutional resources, such as libraries and librarians, educational technologies, project consultants, guest faculty and speakers, and many more. Although difficult, efforts to document the costs of such programs, particularly on an individual participant basis, are important reference points for making decisions about the value of such investments (Bowen et al. 2006).

There also needs to be greater attention paid to institutional outcomes in addition to the more common individual participant outcomes (McLean et al. 2008). Relatively little is known about the impact of such programs on the institutional learning environment for students and residents or the professional environment for faculty members. Several programs document that their participants assume leadership positions in the institution, but what impact on the institution does their leadership provide? Do graduates of such programs have higher career satisfaction? Do they stay longer at their institution? Do they become better teachers who might foster better learning? (Griffith et al. 2000; Hewson and Copeland 1999) What are the institutional benefits of building a community of skilled educators and scholars?

A repeated lament in the literature on faculty development programs is the lack of outcomes evaluation and the limited scope of outcome data (McLean et al. 2008; Steinert et al. 2006; Wilkerson and Irby 1998). Although not focused exclusively on longitudinal intensive faculty development programs, Steinert et al.'s (2006) systematic review of 53 evaluation studies of the impact of faculty development programs on teaching effectiveness found that 74 % of the study outcomes were classified as 'reaction' outcomes, according to Kirkpatrick's framework (Kirkpatrick and Kirkpatrick 2006). Knowledge gains were assessed in 77 % of the studies, but virtually all of these were assessed through participant self-report, a notoriously biased method with questionable validity (Eva and Regehr 2005; Ward et al. 2002). Remarkably, 72 % of the studies assessed changes in teaching behaviors, but this outcome was specifically targeted by the review's search criteria. Behavioral changes were assessed through both self-report and learner or peer observations of teaching behaviors. A minority of the evaluation studies (19 %) examined the impact of faculty development programs on changes in organizational practice (3 studies) or changes in student or resident learning (1 study).

As in other domains of medical education, it is time to move beyond simple descriptions of programs and demonstrations that they 'work' to more sophisticated studies that compare alternative program formats or features. At present, such decisions are a matter of preference on the part of the program developer or facilitator rather than something guided by any empirical evidence of relative effectiveness. Improving the evidence base for intensive longitudinal programs will require both greater rigor in outcomes definition and measurement but, more importantly, the difficult step of actually comparing programs and their outcomes. At present, the evidence can be characterized as demonstrating quite clearly that an intensive longitudinal program is better than short programs or one-time workshops. What is needed is 'comparative effective studies' that directly compare programs with differing characteristics (duration, frequency, selection criteria, etc.) to determine whether these characteristics are critical to success. (See Chaps. 17 and 18 for further details.)

10.7.4   Evolution of the Model

As described earlier in this chapter, the intensive longitudinal faculty development model has many common features across various institutions. However, it is still a fairly new model and is likely to undergo divergent evolution as people use it for different purposes.

One branch of this evolution may be adapting the model to different outcomes and audiences. For example, the University of Michigan has applied the intensive longitudinal model to a program in health care administration for residents and is planning a patient safety and quality improvement program that utilizes the same model. One can speculate on other special domains or audiences that might fit the model: other health professionals and interprofessional cohorts, research mentoring, educational technology, biomedical PhD and postgraduate student educators, and others. The FAIMER Institutes have already been cited as an example of how the model can apply to a dispersed cohort of international participants (Burdick et al. 2010), but it is likely that other variants will be needed for programs that specifically target a participant cohort that includes international learners.

Another branch in the evolutionary tree may be the relationship of intensive longitudinal programs with other faculty development resources. Other chapters in this book describe a variety of formats for faculty development that have different goals, resource demands, and strengths and weaknesses. Ideally, these alternatives should fit together into a spectrum of resources for faculty at a given institution. One specific relationship that warrants more consideration is the link between intensive longitudinal programs and formal degree-granting programs, such as the expanding number of Masters' degree programs in health professions education (Tekian and Harris 2012). Some programs include graduate courses as part of the curriculum (Steinert et al. 2003), whereas others have arrangements by which participation in the program can count for credit towards a formal degree (Gruppen et al. 2006; Robins et al. 2006; Searle et al. 2006b). At the other end of the spectrum, creative links between intensive longitudinal programs and more traditional 'one-off' faculty development workshops might be considered as a feeder or recruitment mechanism for participation in an intensive longitudinal faculty development program.

10.8   Implications for Practice and Research

For those contemplating establishing an intensive longitudinal faculty development program, the characteristics of this model outlined above can serve as a framework for planning and discussion. The evaluation literature for these programs provides some guidance as to what outcomes can be expected and how success might be fostered. However, what is perhaps most important is to learn from the experience of these earlier programs. Hatem et al. (2009) summarized ten strategic steps in developing a program that merit our attention:

1. Defining an operating philosophy, values, and goals.
2. Establishing a curriculum that reflects the roles and responsibilities of fellows and faculty.
3. Employing a basic approach to adult learning.
4. Striving to achieve a balance between stated objectives and openness of discussion.
5. Creating optimum learning opportunities for the fellows to acquire and practice skills delineated in the curriculum.
6. Fostering interdisciplinary communication, team development, and the creation of a learning community.
7. Developing mindfulness and critical self-reflection.
8. Systematically reviewing each session.
9. Evaluating fellowship outcomes.
10. Planning for the future.

For those who already have such programs, it is important to recognize that they need to be periodically, if not continuously, evaluated for how well they fit the needs of the participants and the institutional environment. Not only does the program need to stay fresh and innovative, but the institution and its leaders need to be reminded about the contributions the program makes to individual participants and the institution itself. The argument for value of an intensive longitudinal faculty development program is necessarily a local one, but it can benefit from the collective experience, evidence, and purpose of the community of directors and facilitators of such programs. This sharing should extend beyond justifying these programs to sharing resources, assessment methods, and even comparisons among programs. Such mutual support and prompting will move the whole community forward.

10.9   Conclusion

Intensive longitudinal programs are an important format in the faculty development arsenal. This model allows for a greater depth of learning when compared with single-session workshops and enables a more comprehensive curriculum that addresses a range of integrated skills that can lead to a well-rounded health professional and leader. Intensive longitudinal programs are more than just an investment in the growth of individual faculty members; they are also investments in the health of the institution. The faculty members who graduate from these programs frequently give back to the institution in many ways, including higher-quality educational planning, better assessment methods, more informed decision-making, and educational leadership that is based on educational evidence and principles. The logistical details, curricular content, and primary goals of each program described in this chapter reflect the culture and context of the home institution. Although reasonable, this diversity highlights the need for further evaluation of the impact of these programs and studies to identify the key features that lead to success.

10.10 Key Messages

- Intensive longitudinal faculty development programs have proliferated over the past 15 years.
- These programs have reasonably good evidence for effectively achieving their goals for improving leadership, educational foundations, scholarly productivity, community building, and teaching.
- Although each program must adapt to the demands of its institutional home, there are considerable opportunities for programs to share ideas, curricular resources, and best practices.

References

Armstrong, E. G., Doyle, J., & Bennett, N. L. (2003). Transformative professional development of physicians as educators: Assessment of a model. *Academic Medicine, 78*(7), 702–708.

Baldwin, C. D., Levine, H. G., & McCormick, D. P. (1995). Meeting the faculty development needs of generalist physicians in academia. *Academic Medicine, 70*(1 Suppl.), S97–S103.

Beckman, T. J. & Cook, D. A. (2007). Developing scholarly projects in education: A primer for medical teachers. *Medical Teacher, 29*(2–3), 210–218.

Bowen, J. L., Clark, J. M., Houston, T. K., Levine, R., Branch, W., Clayton, C. P., et al. (2006). A national collaboration to disseminate skills for outpatient teaching in internal medicine: Program description and preliminary evaluation. *Academic Medicine, 81*(2), 193–202.

Boyer, E. L. (1990). *Scholarship reconsidered: Priorities of the professoriate.* Princeton, NJ: Carnegie Foundation for the Advancement of Teaching.

Burdick, W. P., Amaral, E., Campos, H., & Norcini, J. (2011). A model for linkage between health professions education and health: FAIMER international faculty development initiatives. *Medical Teacher, 33*(8), 632–637.

Burdick, W. P., Diserens, D., Friedman, S. R., Morahan, P. S., Kalishman, S., Eklund, M. A., et al. (2010). Measuring the effects of an international health professions faculty development fellowship: The FAIMER Institute. *Medical Teacher, 32*(5), 414–421.

Elliot, D. L., Skeff, K. M., & Stratos, G. A. (1999). How do you get to the improvement of teaching? A longitudinal faculty development program for medical educators. *Teaching and Learning in Medicine, 11*(1), 52–57.

Eva, K. W. & Regehr, G. (2005). Self-assessment in the health professions: A reformulation and research agenda. *Academic Medicine, 80*(10 Suppl.), S46–S54.

Frohna, A. Z., Hamstra, S. J., Mullan, P. B., & Gruppen, L. D. (2006). Teaching medical education principles and methods to faculty using an active learning approach: The University of Michigan Medical Education Scholars Program. *Academic Medicine, 81*(11), 975–978.

Gordon, G. H., Levinson, W., & Society for General Internal Medicine Task Force on Doctor and Patient. (1990). Attitudes toward learner-centered learning at a faculty development course. *Teaching and Learning in Medicine, 2*(2), 106–109.

Griffith III, C. H., Georgesen, J. C., & Wilson, J. F. (2000). Six-year documentation of the association between excellent clinical teaching and improved students' examination performances. *Academic Medicine, 75*(10 Suppl.), S62–S64.

Gruppen, L. D., Frohna, A. Z., Anderson, R. M., & Lowe, K. D. (2003). Faculty development for educational leadership and scholarship. *Academic Medicine, 78*(2), 137–141.

Gruppen, L. D., Simpson, D., Searle, N. S., Robins, L., Irby, D. M., & Mullan, P. B. (2006). Educational fellowship programs: Common themes and overarching issues. *Academic Medicine, 81*(11), 990–994.

Harris, D. L., Krause, K. C., Parish, D. C., & Smith, M. U. (2007). Academic competencies for medical faculty. *Family Medicine, 39*(5), 343–350.

Hatem, C. J., Lown, B. A., & Newman, L. R. (2006). The academic health center coming of age: Helping faculty become better teachers and agents of educational change. *Academic Medicine, 81*(11), 941–944.

Hatem, C. J., Lown, B. A., & Newman, L. R. (2009). Strategies for creating a faculty fellowship in medical education: Report of a 10-year experience. *Academic Medicine, 84*(8), 1098–1103.

Hewson, M. G. (2000). A theory-based faculty development program for clinician-educators. *Academic Medicine, 75*(5), 498–501.

Hewson, M. G. & Copeland, H. L. (1999). Outcomes assessment of a faculty development program in medicine and pediatrics. *Academic Medicine, 74*(10 Suppl.), S68–S71.

Kirkpatrick, D. L. & Kirkpatrick, J. D. (2006). *Evaluating training programs: The four levels. (3rd Ed.).* San Francisco, CA: Berrett-Koehler Publishers.

Lown, B. A., Newman, L. R., & Hatem, C. J. (2009). The personal and professional impact of a fellowship in medical education. *Academic Medicine, 84*(8), 1089–1097.

McLean, M., Cilliers, F., & Van Wyk, J. M. (2008). AMEE Guide No. 36: Faculty development: Yesterday, today and tomorrow. *Medical Teacher, 30*(6), 555–584.

Morzinski, J. A. & Fisher, J. C. (2002). A nationwide study of the influence of faculty development programs on colleague relationships. *Academic Medicine, 77*(5), 402–406.

Morzinski, J. A. & Schubot, D. B. (2000). Evaluating faculty development outcomes by using curriculum vitae analysis. *Family Medicine, 32*(3), 185–189.

Morzinski, J. A. & Simpson, D. E. (2003). Outcomes of a comprehensive faculty development program for local, full-time faculty. *Family Medicine, 35*(6), 434–439.

Moses, A. S., Heestand, D. E., Doyle, L. L., & O'Sullivan, P. S. (2006). Impact of a teaching scholars program. *Academic Medicine, 81*(10 Suppl.), S87–S90.

Moses, A. S., Skinner, D. H., Hicks, E., & O'Sullivan, P. S. (2009). Developing an educator network: The effect of a teaching scholars program in the health professions on networking and productivity. *Teaching and Learning in Medicine, 21*(3), 175–179.

Muller, J. H. & Irby, D. M. (2006). Developing educational leaders: The Teaching Scholars Program at the University of California, San Francisco, School of Medicine. *Academic Medicine, 81*(11), 959–964.

Robins, L., Ambrozy, D., & Pinsky, L. E. (2006). Promoting academic excellence through leadership development at the University of Washington: The Teaching Scholars Program. *Academic Medicine, 81*(11), 979–983.

Rosenbaum, M. E., Lenoch, S., & Ferguson, K. J. (2005). Outcomes of a Teaching Scholars Program to promote leadership in faculty development. *Teaching and Learning in Medicine, 17*(3), 247–253.

Rosenbaum, M. E., Lenoch, S., & Ferguson, K. J. (2006). Increasing departmental and college-wide faculty development opportunities through a teaching scholars program. *Academic Medicine, 81*(11), 965–968.

Salomon, G. & Perkins, D. N. (1998). Individual and social aspects of learning. *Review of Research in Education, 23*(1), 1–24.

Searle, N. S., Hatem, C. J., Perkowski, L., & Wilkerson, L. (2006a). Why invest in an educational fellowship program? *Academic Medicine, 81*(11), 936–940.

Searle, N. S., Thompson, B. M., & Perkowski, L. C. (2006b). Making it work: The evolution of a medical educational fellowship program. *Academic Medicine, 81*(11), 984–989.

Sheets, K. J. & Schwenk, T. L. (1990). Faculty development for family medicine educators: An agenda for future activities. *Teaching & Learning in Medicine, 2*(3), 141–148.

Shulman, L. S. (1986). Those who understand: Knowledge growth in teaching. *Educational Researcher, 15*(2), 4–14.

Simpson, D. E. & Fincher, R.M. (1999). Making a case for the teaching scholar. *Academic Medicine, 74*(12), 1296–1299.

Simpson, D. E., Marcdante, K., Morzinski, J., Meurer, L., McLaughlin, C., Lamb, G., et al. (2006). Fifteen years of aligning faculty development with primary care clinician-educator roles and academic advancement at the Medical College of Wisconsin. *Academic Medicine, 81*(11), 945–953.

Skeff, K. M., Stratos, G. A., Mygdal, W., DeWitt, T. A., Manfred, L. M., Quirk, M. E., et al. (1997a). Faculty development. A resource for clinical teachers. *Journal of General Internal Medicine, 12*(Suppl. 2), S56–S63.

Skeff, K. M., Stratos, G. A., Mygdal, W. K., DeWitt, T. G., Manfred, L. M., Quirk, M. E., et al. (1997b). Clinical teaching improvement: Past and future for faculty development. *Family Medicine, 29*(4), 252–257.

Steinert, Y., Mann, K., Centeno, A., Dolmans, D., Spencer, J., Gelula, M., et al. (2006). A systematic review of faculty development initiatives designed to improve teaching effectiveness in medical education: BEME Guide No. 8. *Medical Teacher, 28*(6), 497–526.

Steinert, Y. & McLeod, P. J. (2006). From novice to informed educator: The Teaching Scholars Program for Educators in the Health Sciences. *Academic Medicine, 81*(11), 969–974.

Steinert, Y., Nasmith, L., McLeod, P. J., & Conochie, L. (2003). A Teaching Scholars Program to develop leaders in medical education. *Academic Medicine, 78*(2), 142–149.

Tekian, A. & Harris, I. (2012). Preparing health professions education leaders worldwide: A description of masters-level programs. *Medical Teacher, 34*(1), 52–58.

Thompson, B. M., Searle, N. S., Gruppen, L. D., Hatem, C. J., & Nelson, E. A. (2011). A national survey of medical education fellowships. *Medical Education Online, 16*, Art. 5642. Available from: http://www.ncbi.nlm.nih.gov/pmc/articles/PMC3071874/pdf/MEO-16-5642.pdf

Ward, M., Gruppen, L., & Regehr, G. (2002). Measuring self-assessment: Current state of the art. *Advances in Health Sciences Education, 7*(1), 63–80.

Wenger, E. (1998). *Communities of practice: Learning, meaning, and identity.* New York, NY: Cambridge University Press.

Wilkerson, L. & Irby, D. M. (1998). Strategies for improving teaching practices: A comprehensive approach to faculty development. *Academic Medicine, 73*(4), 387–396.

Wilkerson, L., Uijtdehaage, S., & Relan, A. (2006). Increasing the pool of educational leaders for UCLA. *Academic Medicine, 81*(11), 954–958.

Chapter 11
Faculty Development Online

David A. Cook

11.1 Introduction

With the growing presence of computers and Internet technologies in our personal and professional lives, it is no surprise that computer-assisted learning has shown dramatic growth over the past decade. These technologies act as prostheses – enabling activities that would otherwise not be possible (Amin et al. 2011). Interest in the field of computer-assisted instruction (as measured by research publications) continues to grow rapidly (Adler and Johnson 2000; Cook et al. 2008b). One study suggests that online continuing medical education (CME) may dominate over half of all CME activities by 2017 (Harris et al. 2010). Since Google, Facebook, YouTube and smartphones are increasingly used by faculty and students, it seems timely to consider how these and other electronic tools might be harnessed to promote faculty development.

The broad field of e-learning encompasses all educational interventions that use electronic technologies, including instruction using computers, Internet, mobile devices, audio tapes or CDs, video tapes or DVDs, and satellite TV. Online learning (also called Web-based learning) is e-learning that uses the Internet. This chapter will first offer a brief introduction to online learning in general, followed by an argument for online learning in faculty development, a review of what has already been done, an overview of options and key principles for instructional design, and next steps for current practice and future research. Although this chapter focuses on online learning, many of the principles apply to other e-learning activities.

D.A. Cook, MD, MHPE (✉)
Division of General Internal Medicine and Office of Education Research,
College of Medicine, Mayo Clinic, Rochester, MN, USA
e-mail: cook.david33@mayo.edu

Y. Steinert (ed.), *Faculty Development in the Health Professions: A Focus on Research and Practice*, Innovation and Change in Professional Education 11, DOI 10.1007/978-94-007-7612-8_11, © Springer Science+Business Media Dordrecht 2014

11.2 Online Learning: A Brief Introduction

11.2.1 What Is Online Learning?

Online learning is, simply put, the process of learning with support from the Internet or a local intranet. Virtually any use of the Internet could be construed as a learning activity (for example, we learn something each time we read the news). However, as commonly used and for the purposes of this chapter, online learning refers more specifically to *learning while engaged in online activities deliberately designed and sequenced to achieve defined learning objectives*. This can be accomplished in several different ways, including the presentation of instructional materials (e.g. online tutorials), communication systems that facilitate learning-focused discussions (computer-supported collaborative learning), and activities that permit practice with authentic scenarios (computer simulations). The Glossary (in Appendix A) contains definitions for these and other terms.

It is also important to recognize what online learning is *not*. The Internet has many applications in medical education in which the primary intent is not to directly facilitate the achievement of defined learning objectives. These include online postings of course information (syllabi or handouts), archives of face-to-face lectures (e.g. PowerPoint slides or videotaped lectures), online administration of tests and course evaluations, and administrative communications. Likewise, the Internet is increasingly used for social (e.g. Facebook) and information-seeking activities that do not constitute online learning as defined above. However, while these activities do not constitute online learning by themselves, each could comprise an element *within* an online learning course. For example, posting online the slides (or an archived video) from a faculty development workshop would not constitute online learning; however, these slides (or video) could be an integral part of a structured learning program with defined enrollment, objectives, and post-course assessment.

11.2.2 Is Online Learning Better than Face-to-Face?

Since the origin of the computer, investigators have attempted to determine whether computer-assisted learning – and more recently the subgroup of online learning – is more or less effective in comparison with traditional approaches to learning (Clark 1983). The conclusion of this research is that there is, on average, no significant difference between computer and non-computer approaches. One systematic review of 76 studies comparing online learning with traditional approaches found negligible differences (Cook et al. 2008b). A website dedicated to this phenomenon – www.nosignificantdifference.org – has catalogued hundreds of studies with the same bottom line. Yet although the average difference approaches zero, for a given study the differences vary widely, sometimes favoring online, and at other times favoring traditional learning. The key factor appears to be not the medium (computer or traditional) but the appropriateness of that medium for the instructional objectives, and the effectiveness of the instructional methods.

The implication for educators is that there is nothing magical about online learning that makes it inherently better than other forms of instruction (such as face-to-face lectures or small groups) (Cook and McDonald 2008). Online learning may solve some problems but not others, and will typically create new problems as well. Traditional methods frequently remain the better choice. In reality, the ideal option often involves a blending of both approaches as discussed in Sect. 11.7.

The appropriateness of online learning for a given situation requires the alignment of multiple factors including the instructional objectives, intended instructional content, learners, and learning context. Making these decisions requires an understanding of the potential advantages and disadvantages of using these technologies (Cook 2007), as discussed below and in the Glossary. The other key factor, the instructional methods, will be discussed in Sect. 11.4.

11.2.3 Advantages and Disadvantages of Online Learning

11.2.3.1 Advantages

The advantages and disadvantages discussed below pertain to online learning generally (Cook 2007), although some are particularly salient to online faculty development. Perhaps the most obvious advantage of online learning is that physical distances become irrelevant. Faculty development courses have reached learners across the state (Langlois and Thach 2003), country (Anshu et al. 2008; Wearne et al. 2011), and world (Ladhani et al. 2011; McKimm and Swanwick 2010). Distance learning also enables economies of scale for many courses: once an online learning tutorial has been developed, class size is limited only by server capacity and bandwidth. Moreover, an online tutorial or other individual course component (such as an animation, video clip, or simulation) could subsequently be used again in another course (e.g. 'reusable learning objects').

Online learning also allows flexibility in the timing of participation. Learners can access an online learning tutorial or simulation at any time, day or night. Asynchronous online discussions also offer flexibility, although participants need to respond to communications from other group members in a timely manner and adhere to agreed-upon schedules. For example, one group used an online approach to encourage clinical assessment skills among busy surgical faculty (Pernar et al. 2012).

Since online course materials are housed at a central location, updates can be implemented quickly and easily. Learning resources such as tutorials also persist long after the course ends. Faculty members may thus return to a useful tutorial when planning a course or conducting a research study, or reference the text of a relevant online discussion when trying to solve a difficult leadership challenge.

Online learning offers the capability to individualize learning through self-adjustment or automated adaptation. For example, most online courses permit learners to take control of the learning environment by slowing down when material is new or difficult, and moving quickly if material is familiar (self-pacing). Some courses also allow learners to select among different learning opportunities within a given course (self-selection). In computer-adaptive instruction, the computer uses information about the learner (baseline knowledge, learning style, or motivation to learn) to alter, and thus optimize, the learning experience.

Online learning also offers the opportunity to try creative new instructional methods for engaging learners and encouraging deep and durable learning. For example, an asynchronous online discussion might allow learners time to reflect on a question and craft a thoughtful response. Online simulations could give faculty members the opportunity to rehearse new skills in a simulated teaching or research experience, as virtual patients do for clinical medicine. Other innovative approaches include games, interactive models, computer animations, and incorporation of audio and video clips. Creative methods in online faculty development include computer simulations of organizational change (Richman et al. 2001) and interviewing standardized patients using a videoconference feed (Kobak et al. 2006).

Finally, online learning facilitates learner assessment, tailored feedback based on these assessments, and documentation that educational objectives were achieved (Cook 2007).

11.2.3.2 Disadvantages

However, online learning is not without its disadvantages. Offsetting the potential economies of scale are the large up-front costs associated with developing online learning. Crafting an effective online course requires a substantial investment in planning, testing, technical expertise, and computer infrastructure. At least one faculty development program underestimated this investment, leading to delays and frustration in program implementation (Lewis and Baker 2005). Also, economies of scale are less apparent in online discussions, in which demands on instructor time usually increase with each additional learner.

Technical difficulties are nearly inevitable in all teaching activities, but they may be more important in an online course. An instructor could improvise in a face-to-face course in which the DVD player malfunctioned. By contrast, even a minor technical problem can have a substantial influence on the appearance, content, and functionality of an online course, with resultant negative effects on satisfaction and learning (Dyrbye et al. 2009). Moreover, problem recognition may be delayed, and troubleshooting may require substantial time from both learners and instructors.

Online learning unmasks inferior instructional design in the same way that it magnifies technical problems. In contrast to a face-to-face course in which a talented instructor can get by with minimal preparation, instruction in online learning must be explicitly planned and implemented, as will be discussed below. While poor instructional design is certainly not unique to online learning, online learning appears to be much more sensitive to this problem.

The full potential of individualized instruction has only rarely been realized. Computer-adaptive instruction is not as easy as it sounds (Cook et al. 2008a), and when it has been accomplished, the benefits in comparison with non-adaptive instruction are fairly minimal to-date (Landsberg et al. 2012). Self-driven adaptations are simpler, but still require the development of alternate learning materials and pathways, ideally with proven benefit for certain learner subtypes. Thus, in most current online courses, the individualization consists only of the variation in the timing and pace of instruction.

Flexibility in time and location means that the learner using online learning tutorials and simulations is often studying alone, which can create a sense of isolation. Even courses that require learners to collaborate, such as an online discussion group, may be less engaging and less socially fulfilling than a face-to-face equivalent. This is not a trivial issue, particularly when it comes to engagement and satisfaction with faculty members as learners (Dyrbye et al. 2009; Steinert et al. 2002; Wearne et al. 2011). This problem may be more acute for faculty who are less comfortable using computers (although this concern is largely hypothetical, and in one study of continuing medical education no correlation was found between age and online participation (Schoen et al. 2009)). Also, for some topics (e.g. 'how to lead a small group') instructor modeling of behavior is an important element that would be lost in an online course.

Finally, a transition to online faculty development could create political tensions among faculty if, for example, online learning were perceived as yet another unfunded mandate that consumes personal time for professional activities.

11.3 Innovations: Creative Approaches to Online Faculty Development

Online learning addresses many of the barriers frequently encountered in faculty development initiatives. Online learning can be designed to allow involvement according to each participant's schedule, which can be a significant impediment for faculty members with busy clinical calendars, teaching schedules, administrative responsibilities, and travel commitments. Similarly, the capability to involve learners regardless of physical location addresses another significant obstacle when reaching out to faculty members at rural and community sites and at other institutions. Online learning also permits access to 'just-in-time' education. Documentation of completion is often helpful, especially for those requiring continuing education credits.

The topics and key modalities of 20 online faculty development initiatives are summarized in Table 11.1. A more detailed analysis of this evidence has been presented elsewhere (Cook and Steinert 2013). Online learning has been most often described for faculty development in clinical teaching and assessment. However, it has also been used to train in business administration (Dean et al. 2001; Fox et al. 2001), financial planning (Richman et al. 2001), critical appraisal of the literature (Macrae et al. 2004), and research skills (Kobak et al. 2006; Kotzer and Milton 2007). These studies employed a wide variety of online modalities and instructional designs, including tutorials, online discussions via discussion board, chat, and email

Table 11.1 Articles describing computer-assisted faculty development activities

Author (Year)	Scope	Topic	Description
Dean et al. (2001)	Distance learning program in the USA	Business administration	Virtual (online) classroom, online homework assignments, face-to-face sessions
Fox et al. (2001)	Distance learning program in the UK	Leadership (change management)	Online tutorial with discussion board
Richman et al. (2001)	Distance learning program in the USA	Financial planning (part of larger leadership course)	Computer simulation of budgeting and strategic planning
Janicik et al. (2002)	1 school in the USA	Assessment and feedback	Web module: video clip, survey, tutorial
Steinert et al. (2002)	1 school in Canada	Small group teaching	Discussion board and e-mail listserv following face-to-face workshop
Langlois and Thach (2003)	16 counties in 1 state in the USA	Clinical teaching	8 Web modules; also videotape, paper handouts, and face-to-face workshops
Macrae et al. (2004)	Surgeons scattered across Canada (academic and community sites)	Critical appraisal of literature	Internet-based journal club (e-mailed articles and discussion)
Lewis and Baker (2005)	Distance learning program in the USA	Master degree in education for health professionals	Various online courses in the graduate degree program
Coma del Corral et al. (2006)	Distance learning program in Spain	Research methods	Online chat (synchronous discussion), Web-based resources
Kobak et al. (2006)	Distance learning program in the USA	Rater training (for clinical research)	Online tutorial, practice interview with 'patient' via Internet videoconference
Bramson et al. (2007)	Clinical preceptors (site not specified)	Clinical teaching	Face-to-face workshop, e-mail listserv, discussion board, video, CD-ROM
Kotzer and Milton (2007)	1 hospital in the USA	Research (review board policies)	12 brief e-mails
Anshu et al. (2008)	Multiple medical schools spread across India	Teaching and assessment (part of FAIMER fellowship in medical education)	E-mail listserv discussion

Dyrbye et al. (2009)	Distance learning program in the USA, learners from multiple countries	Master degree in health professions education	Various online courses in the graduate degree program
Anshu et al. (2010)	Multiple medical schools spread across India	Teaching and assessment (part of FAIMER fellowship in medical education)	E-mail listserv discussion
McKimm and Swanwick (2010)	155 countries	Clinical teaching	16 online modules
Paulus et al. (2010)	1 school in the USA	Online teaching	Face-to-face and virtual (online) workshops; online discussion board
Ladhani et al. (2011)	30 countries	Community-based medical education (part of FAIMER fellowship in medical education)	Online discussion board role play (part of larger online course)
Wearne et al. (2011)	Multiple rural and urban sites across Australia	Clinical teaching	Not defined
Pernar et al. (2012)	1 school in the USA	Clinical teaching and feedback	27 very brief e-mailed 'bullets' on effective strategies

listserv, computer simulations, video clips, role playing, and live assessments of a training subject at a distance.

The most common problem encountered with online faculty development is lack of participation. Several reports note low faculty engagement (Bramson et al. 2007; Langlois and Thach 2003; Steinert et al. 2002), leading one group to describe their initiative with online discussion as 'an experiment that failed' (Steinert et al. 2002). Some courses, however, have had great success (Macrae et al. 2004; Ladhani et al. 2011). The reasons for these differences remain uncertain, but several solutions have been proposed. Some authors suggest that only when courses successfully meet a need perceived by faculty will they invest the necessary time and energy to participate in an online course (Paulus et al. 2010; Steinert et al. 2002; Wearne et al. 2011). Others reported that careful organization, clear communication, and assistance with technical problems were key (Dyrbye et al. 2009; Janicik et al. 2002; Langlois and Thach 2003; Ladhani et al. 2011; Lewis and Baker 2005; Wearne et al. 2011). Yet others suggested that time to complete course activities, clear expectations, and relevance to near-future teaching activities were essential (Ladhani et al. 2011; Langlois and Thach 2003; Paulus et al. 2010; Pernar et al. 2012). Given the absence of clear evidence to support one solution over another, perhaps the most important lesson is that those responsible for faculty development must be aware of the potential for low participation, anticipate this, and plan in advance to address this challenge.

A related but distinct problem regards online communication and the development of a sense of community. Several studies found that online communities can enhance interactions among faculty (Anshu et al. 2008, 2010; Bramson et al. 2007; Wearne et al. 2011), while others found the opposite (i.e. that faculty members met the online initiative with opposition, disinterest, and lack of engagement (Fox et al. 2001; Ladhani et al. 2011; Steinert et al. 2002)). The key difference appears to be the motivation behind the online community. Online communities seem to prosper when they meet an otherwise unfulfilled need, such as bridging the distance among rural physicians (Wearne et al. 2011). Less successful initiatives attempted to replace existing face-to-face interactions, or lacked a cohesive structure (Bramson et al. 2007; Langlois and Thach 2003; Steinert et al. 2002). Online communication has also been noted to be a challenge, with at least one study noting that the absence of voice inflection or body language can breed misunderstanding (Dyrbye et al. 2009), although at least one group overcame these barriers by using a conversational communication style and encouraging contributions from all participants (Anshu et al. 2008).

In summary, educators have used online learning for faculty development on multiple topics in diverse locations using a variety of creative approaches. However, these initiatives have not been equally effective, and the reasons for this variation are only partially understood. Going forward, health professionals engaged in online faculty development should: (1) learn from what others have done (see Table 11.1); (2) anticipate and plan to address low participation, which might include providing adequate time and emphasizing educational needs; (3) optimize communication; (4) implement current best practices (see Sects. 11.4 and 11.5); and (5) consider conducting new investigations to advance our understanding of best practices (see Sect. 11.8).

11.4 Instructional Design Part 1: Options

Online learning comes in many flavors or configurations, including tutorials, online communities, simulations, and performance support. While these classifications are neither mutually exclusive nor collectively comprehensive, they provide a useful framework to discuss this technology and its educational applications. Each of these will be discussed in turn. (These and other key terms are defined in the Glossary in Appendix A.)

11.4.1 Online Tutorials

Just as a face-to-face lecturer might use a chalkboard, PowerPoint slides, a video clip, and a brief case scenario, an online instructor might design a tutorial incorporating a variety of technologies and instructional approaches such as multimedia, interactive games, practice cases, and self-assessment tools. Online tutorials possess all of the advantages and disadvantages listed above, most notably the advantages of flexibility in time, location, and pace of instruction, but with the disadvantage of large up-front development costs. A simple online faculty development tutorial on the topic of learner assessment might consist of learning objectives, PowerPoint slides (designed for this purpose – not borrowed from a face-to-face course!), and a self-assessment with feedback. A more advanced module might additionally ask faculty members to rate several video clips, and then compare their scores with those of an expert.

When to use online tutorials? Computer-based tutorials will be most useful when learners are separated in time or space (such as conflicting schedules or working at physically distinct sites).

An effective online tutorial requires more than simply taking the slides or video of an existing face-to-face course and posting them on the Web. As noted below, the science of online tutorials is fairly well-developed, and applying this science requires considerable planning and attention to implementation. Remember that the goal of instruction is mental activity on the part of the learner; information processing and construction of new knowledge. Since physical activity (such as clicking the mouse) does not guarantee mental activity, effective instructional designs focus on facilitating mental activity. Opportunities for self-assessment and feedback, reflection, and interaction with other learners can facilitate this. The development cost and other disadvantages should be balanced against potential advantages. Technical support is essential. Learning management systems such as Blackboard or free, open-source Moodle can be helpful in organizing the course.

11.4.2 Online Collaboration: Blogs, Wikis and Discussion Boards

Internet-mediated communication has facilitated the development of so-called online collaborative learning communities (Sandars et al. 2012). This approach is common in faculty development, with half of the courses shown in Table 11.1 incorporating online collaboration. Online collaboration can use a variety of tools including wikis, blogs, discussion boards, instant messaging, social networks and virtual worlds. In the virtual equivalent of a face-to-face small group, learners can interact to share experiences and information and learn together. As with face-to-face small groups, online learner interaction serves both a social function and as a stimulus to active learning. In both online and face-to-face discussions the teacher may offer some didactic teaching (e.g. a brief tutorial), but most of the learning occurs in the group conversation. Teachers assume the role of facilitators – defining the scope of the discussion, monitoring the discussion and providing guidance as needed, and steering learners to useful resources.

When to use online collaboration? Collaborative learning is particularly effective during the integration phase of instruction (reflection and debate), when opinions and practices vary, and when deliberately developing relationships among learners. Some learners feel more comfortable contributing to a conversation online rather than face-to-face, and asynchronous discussion allows time to reflect and pursue further study before responding. Many online communication tools create a permanent archive of the conversation.

Face-to-face groups can meet with the instructor for a small group discussion, or the instructor can simply give an assignment and let the learners decide the timing, location, and frequency of group meetings required to complete the final product. Similarly, there are a variety of approaches to online collaboration. As noted above, online collaborative faculty development activities have not always been successful. While the evidence base is inconclusive, it would seem that key ingredients include faculty buy-in (best achieved by focusing on a perceived need), clear objectives, and explicit expectations in terms of participation and final product (Lewis and Baker 2005; Paulus et al. 2010; Steinert et al. 2002; Wearne et al. 2011).

Most online communication is asynchronous, with a delay between sending a message and receiving the response. Tools for asynchronous communication include e-mail, discussion boards, blogs, and wikis. Synchronous communication is real-time, and is mediated through live audio or audio-video communication (e.g. Skype) and instant text messaging. The degree of instructor involvement and observation varies greatly among these options; that is, the instructor can easily monitor all activity on a school-sponsored discussion board, whereas if learners use a social network discussion board the instructor may have no information about the group activity. This isn't necessarily bad, but it does change course operations and limit the information available to the instructor for assessment.

11.4.3 Online Simulations

Online simulations attempt to emulate real-life events on a computer screen. Evidence suggests that efficient application of knowledge requires experience with a large number of similar problems. Rather than wait for such problems to occur in real life, supplementing the mental 'case library' with simulated experiences may encourage knowledge application to new settings. Online simulations provide an efficient way to provide such experiences. Online simulations for faculty development could replicate a faculty-on-learner clinical assessment, the analysis of research data, or a sticky administrative problem.

When to use online simulations? Face-to-face and online lectures, tutorials, and discussions are probably more efficient for the development of core knowledge. The role for online simulations, then, is to allow learners to consolidate this knowledge and practice applying it in a variety of situations.

The key consideration in teaching with online simulations involves the selection, sequencing, and implementation of cases. Ideally, cases on a given topic would start off relatively simple (and perhaps with some guidance in decision-making) and progress to more challenging cases with greater complexity and less guidance. Technological sophistication does not equate with better learning. Much attention is paid to the fidelity or realism of the online simulation, but these concerns are likely ill-founded. Not only is high fidelity expensive, but there is some evidence to suggest that it can paradoxically impede rather than enhance learning. Written case studies have been used for decades in law, medicine, and business administration, and in many situations a simple text narrative may yet be sufficient. Some educators have found that working through a virtual case as a group is more effective than working alone, or that online simulations are most effective as part of a blended learning activity (e.g. having a face-to-face group discussion once everyone has completed the case).

11.4.4   Performance Support (Just-in-Time Learning)

Performance support (just-in-time learning) involves delivering educational information just when the learner needs that information. A faculty member might need support, for example, when planning a course, teaching or assessing learners, conducting research, or writing a manuscript. Information delivery can be triggered by some observed or planned event ('pushed' to the provider during or just prior to the moment of need) or requested by the faculty member ('pulled' from online searchable resources). The educational advantages of just-in-time delivery are at least two-fold. First, this is a moment when learners will be receptive to the material, since it (hopefully) will enable them to complete the required activity more effectively. Second, because a knowledge gap has been identified and prior knowledge activated, learners are primed to integrate this new information into their existing knowledge structure.

As useful as this sounds, it has limitations. It takes time to read, digest, and assimilate this information, and if 'pushed' information arrives at an inconvenient time (e.g. during a pressing manuscript deadline or on a busy clinical workday), faculty members may ignore or even resent the information. Also, just-in-time learning may not substitute for other instructional approaches because the ad hoc, unstructured information may be improperly integrated with what the learner already knows. Thus, performance support – at least at present – is just that: support. It should not replace other instructional methods.

11.4.5 Emerging Technologies: Online Games, Immersive Environments, Social Networks and Mobile Devices

Technologies continually evolve and change, and with each evolution come challenges in determining the new technology's role and redefining roles for older technologies (Sandars 2012). Three new technologies are emerging within the field of online learning with potential to permanently alter the landscape. Online games (Graafland et al. 2012) and immersive environments (Wiecha et al. 2010) can engage learners intensely, and to the degree that this promotes learning they may be a highly effective learning tool. Social networks have revolutionized how relationships are formed and maintained, and show great promise in facilitating online learning communities (Sandars 2010; Sandars et al. 2012). Mobile devices have transformed our use of computers, and for many people have become part of their moment-to-moment existence; yet it remains unknown how the small screen and typically brief interactions will impact learning.

These technologies, and others that will undoubtedly arise in the future, will make instructional design a continuously moving target. Fortunately, teachers can be successful using both old and new technologies if they focus on the fundamentals – as discussed in the next section.

11.5 Instructional Design Part 2: Evidence-Based Principles

11.5.1 Fundamental Principles

The fundamental principles of effective learning are the same for online approaches as for face-to-face. However, while these principles are often instinctively or extemporaneously applied in face-to-face instruction, online instructional designs must be explicitly planned and implemented. The pages that follow will first provide a brief review of general principles of instruction, followed by some principles specifically developed for multimedia instruction (i.e. online learning).

The ultimate goal in faculty development is the same as in instruction for other learners – namely, to help learners develop new knowledge, and then recall and apply this knowledge in real-life settings (i.e. so-called 'transfer'). This involves more than just effectively transmitting information. Learning is more than accumulation of information, but rather involves organizing, reorganizing, and linking new information and experiences with prior knowledge and past experience. This process, known as *elaboration*, constitutes the core of all learning (Bransford et al. 2000) and plays a critical role in faculty development.

Current models of the learning process postulate three distinct regions of cognitive activity: sensory input (primarily visual and auditory), working memory, and long-term memory (van Merriënboer and Sweller 2005). Elaboration takes place in the working memory, where it merges new information (from the senses) and old knowledge (from long-term memory). Online learning will be most effective to the extent that it encourages learners to elaborate robust, meaningful knowledge structures.

11.5.2 First Principles of Instructional Design

Countless theories attempt to explain how learning occurs, but although these theories differ in fundamental ways, they actually share many common elements in their implications for the design of instruction. Merrill (2002) reviewed dozens of educational theories and models in search of such common themes, reasoning that themes present in multiple theories are likely to be true. In so doing, he identified five 'first principles of instruction,' namely:

1. Problem-based: Instruction should be situated in the context of real life problems. Such problems should reflect the range of tasks the learners might encounter in practice. The level of difficulty should be commensurate with the learners' level of training, and ideally would progress (i.e. become more challenging) over the course of instruction.
2. Activation of prior knowledge: 'learning is promoted when relevant previous experience is activated' (Merrill 2002, p. 46). Activation brings knowledge and experiences from long-term memory back into working memory, where these can be integrated with new information and experiences. Knowledge can be activated by analyzing or trying to solve problems, responding to questions, generating questions on the topic, or engaging in hands-on experience.
3. Demonstration: 'learning is promoted when the instruction demonstrates what is to be learned, rather than merely telling information about what is to be learned' (p. 47). Demonstrations might involve providing a verbal or written example of a concept, a picture or video of a procedure, or a diagram of a process. Multiple examples (and contrasting counter-examples) illustrating different perspectives are often helpful. Demonstrations are intended to build accurate mental models of how to apply knowledge in practice.
4. Application of learning: 'learning is promoted when learners are required to use their new knowledge or skill to solve problems' (p. 49). Evidence suggests that novice learners benefit from guidance and coaching during early stages. However, guidance should be gradually withdrawn as they progress, such that in the end they solve problems independently.
5. Integration: 'learning is promoted when learners are encouraged to integrate (transfer) the new knowledge or skill into their everyday life' (p. 50). This occurs most directly when they apply it in real practice, but integration can also be encouraged when learners actively reflect on what they have learned, teach a principle to others, or defend or debate their newfound knowledge.

For example, in an online course on research design, a junior faculty member might first be asked to read a journal article and identity strengths and weaknesses of study design (activation of prior knowledge). Later, the instructor might provide examples of several different designs, contrasting their strengths and weaknesses and showing examples from recent literature (demonstration). Next, the faculty member might complete a series of practice exercises requiring the selection and justification of an ideal study design for a given situation (application in the context of real-life examples). As a final step, the faculty member could apply this new knowledge to his or her own research project, or engage in a mock debate with another course participant on the ideal study design for a given scenario.

Or, in an online course on learner assessment, a faculty member might start by rating a videotaped clinical encounter between a medical student and a patient. Identifying areas of disagreement in comparison with an experienced rater and using these to generate a personal list of learning objectives would activate prior knowledge. Next, the faculty member could view a series of short clips extracted from other clinical encounters that illustrate both good and inferior performance (demonstration). Later, he or she might rate additional clips of unknown skill level (application) and discuss and defend ratings with other course participants (integration).

11.5.3 Designing Effective Multimedia

Once an overall instructional plan has been developed using Merrill's first principles or an alternative model, the online instructor must create a website that encourages learning. To guide such decisions, Mayer (2005) has developed a theory of multimedia learning based on decades of empiric research. These evidence-based principles are relevant to computer-assisted instruction, PowerPoint presentations, and other uses of audio and video in instruction. A very brief summary of selected principles is offered below; for a more complete discussion of the underlying evidence and how to implement these principles, readers are encouraged to consult Mayer's original works (Clark and Mayer 2008; Mayer 2005).

11.5.3.1 Multimedia Principle: People Learn More from Graphics and Words than from Words Alone

A picture is worth a thousand words, and it comes as no surprise that graphics, photographs, animations, and short video clips can greatly enhance learning. Images and videos can be used to provide examples (and non-examples) of an object, to offer a topic overview or organization scheme, to demonstrate steps in a procedure or process, or to illuminate complex relationships among content, concepts, or time or space. However, not all graphics are created equal: as noted below, poorly designed or irrelevant graphics add nothing or may actually impede learning.

11.5.3.2   Modality Principle: When There Are Graphics, Present Words as Speech Rather than Onscreen Text

Working memory receives new information through separate visual and auditory pathways. Just as traffic moves more efficiently on a four-lane highway, learning improves when both input pathways are optimally used – i.e. both graphical (visual) and spoken (verbal) communication. Thus, it would be more effective to show a picture, chart, or diagram, and use narration to explain the salient teaching points, rather than using text alone.

However, it is usually counterproductive to narrate on-screen (akin to when a live lecturer reads their slides verbatim). Such redundancies actually impede learning because the working memory must reconcile differences between these two input streams (including, for example, if the learner is reading faster than the narrator). Exceptions to this rule include when learning in a non-native language, if the learner has a learning disability, or if the information is particularly complex. Otherwise, avoid narrating on-screen text.

11.5.3.3   Contiguity Principle: Related Information Should Be Located Together

It is common to include an explanatory legend at the bottom of a figure. However, this separation of information consumes cognitive capacity that could be directed towards elaboration (identifying relationships within the new information and linking these with prior knowledge). To lower cognitive load, the contiguity principle suggests locating words adjacent to or embedded within relevant parts of the figure. The same principle applies to non-graphical elements, such as carefully synchronizing spoken words with graphics (especially animations), putting the directions for an exercise on the same page as the exercise itself, or presenting the question and the answer/feedback together when providing formative feedback on an online test.

11.5.3.4   Coherence Principle: Avoid the Extraneous (Less Is More)

Teachers in both face-to-face and online settings often add cartoons or photos to presentations for aesthetic value (to 'spice up' a lecture), but such decorative graphics can actually impede learning rather than enhance it. The same applies to extraneous sounds, interesting but irrelevant stories, unnecessarily detailed descriptions, and most animations. Interesting but irrelevant details detract from learning.

Why is it wrong to show a photo of my last Caribbean vacation? First, it probably doesn't really help to motivate learners. As John Dewey once stated, 'When things have to be made more interesting it is because interest itself is wanting. The thing, the object is no more interesting than it was before' (Dewey 1913, pp. 11–12). More importantly, extraneous information taxes cognitive capacities, distracts learners from more relevant material, and disrupts the elaboration of appropriate mental links.

The learner might also (subconsciously, in working memory) attempt to make the extraneous information part of the permanent knowledge structure, or activate and then incorporate inappropriate prior knowledge. The end result is weak or flawed knowledge structures. The instructional purpose of words, graphics, and multimedia is to help learners construct mental representations. Anything extraneous to this purpose should probably be removed. If it doesn't facilitate learning, leave it out.

11.5.3.5 Personalization Principle: A Conversational Tone and Relationship with the Instructor Improves Learning

Of course, the coherence principle doesn't mean the teacher shouldn't share personal information and stories; feeling connected with the instructor improves learning. A conversational (rather than formal) tone also helps promote learning. In addition, it helps for the instructor to share appropriate background information about him or herself.

11.6 Implementation

Developing an online course requires the coordination of content expertise, technical expertise, financial support, and technological infrastructure. However, successful implementation requires more than just successful development. Encouraging and enabling learner participation, ensuring appropriate instructor and technical support, and course evaluation all require additional planning and resources. A full consideration of these issues is beyond the scope of this text, but a list of ten tips is provided in Table 11.2.

Table 11.2 Ten tips for successful online learning

Recommended strategies
Perform a needs analysis and specify goals and objectives
Determine technical resources and needs
Evaluate commercial or open-source software and use it if it fully meets local needs
Secure commitment from all participants and identify and address potential barriers to implementation
Develop content in close coordination with website design and encourage active learning (adhere to fundamental principles of instructional design described in text)
Follow a timeline
Facilitate and plan to encourage use by the learner (make website accessible and user-friendly, provide time for learning, and motivate learners)
Evaluate learners and course
Pilot the website before full implementation
Plan to monitor online communication and maintain the site by resolving technical problems, periodically verifying hyperlinks, and regularly updating content

Adapted from Cook and Dupras (2004)

Three points are sufficiently important and frequently forgotten as to warrant specific mention. First, given the flexibility in time and location, online learning activities are often simply added to existing schedules. This should be avoided whenever possible. Not only will time barriers reduce participation rates, but failure to commit appropriate resources sends a message to learners that the course goals are unimportant.

Second, health professionals should not underestimate the time required to develop and maintain an online course (Cook and Dupras 2004). Whenever possible, it is helpful to borrow or purchase previously-developed content ('reusable learning objects' or entire courses) rather than develop these from scratch (respecting, of course, copyright and other legal rights).

Third, those involved in the development and delivery of online instruction will likely require faculty development themselves. Training needs include both technical skills and instructional design skills. Technical skill development should address how to use specific devices (e.g. desktops, tablets, smartphones, etc.) and software applications (e.g. course development applications such as Articulate, learning management systems such as Blackboard and Moodle, social networking tools such as Facebook, and other online tools such as YouTube and Google). Even when an institution has a strong team of technical experts, those engaged in online teaching must possess at least a basic understanding of the tools they intend to use. Yet perhaps more important than technical expertise are skills in instructional design – understanding when to use an online vs. traditional approach, when to use one online modality over another, and how to design the online experience to effectively promote learning (as discussed in detail above). Consider implementing an online component to the faculty development activity, as this facilitates learning not only through didactic instruction, but also through the experience itself (Paulus et al. 2010). Nothing will acquaint a teacher with how to facilitate an online learning discussion quite like engaging in an online discussion as a student!

11.7 Integrating Online and Other Learning Activities

The central decision in the development of online learning is not whether or not educators should use it – they should. Rather, the germane questions are when to use it, and how to use it effectively once that choice has been made. Merrill's (2002) and Mayer's (2005) principles address the 'how' question. There is less empiric evidence to answer the 'when' question. However, I believe this is primarily a decision of convenience and need (Cook 2006). As noted above, both face-to-face and online approaches can be effective, and both have advantages and disadvantages. The choice to use one or another should consider instructional objectives, logistic constraints (e.g. time, learner location), and available resources (e.g. technical support and infrastructure).

However, this is rarely an either-or decision. This chapter might have given the impression that instructors must choose between online and face-to-face learning activities. On the contrary, so-called blended learning – combining multiple modalities such as face-to-face, computer, video, and simulation – has been historically used in at least one-fourth of online courses (Cook et al. 2010). Many of the faculty development initiatives listed in Table 11.1 included both online and face-to-face elements. In the future, blended learning will become even more common and the boundaries differentiating online from other modalities will be increasingly blurred. Soon, we will no longer distinguish online and face-to-face approaches any more than we currently distinguish lectures that use slides or chalkboards.

In developing blended learning, instructors should carefully consider the selection, sequence, and relative proportion of online vs. other activities (Hull et al. 2009). Ideally, activities will target the strengths of each modality. For example, a blended course on assessment might include a face-to-face baseline test, online tutorials with core information, online discussion to define and recognize key rating criteria, online practice with video clips, face-to-face role play with other faculty members, and a face-to-face final test.

11.8 Evaluation and Research

A detailed exposition on evaluation is beyond the scope of this chapter. More detailed discussion can be found elsewhere in this book (see Chaps. 17 and 18) and in other sources (Cook 2010; Cook and Dupras 2004). However, all online courses should be evaluated for at least two purposes: to identify areas for improvement the next time the course is offered (formative evaluation), and to determine if course objectives were achieved (summative evaluation).

Many educators wonder if their online course could be the subject of formal research. Of course, the answer is yes – but it is important to consider the research question. The majority of studies (well over 100) have asked 'Does online learning work [in comparison with no intervention]?' The answer is, almost without exception, 'Yes.' (Cook et al. 2008b) Numerous studies have also asked, 'Is online learning better/worse than traditional instruction?' Here the answer varies widely, but as noted above the answer is that, on average, there is no significant difference. Unfortunately, both of these questions do little to inform the development of future online learning activities. The key questions proposed above are 'When should we use online learning?' and 'How can we use it effectively when we do?' These questions should constitute the focus of future research in the field. Answering these questions will require comparison, not with a placebo arm or traditional instruction, but with alternate online instructional approaches. Useful information will also derive from rigorously conducted qualitative research (Lingard 2007), and from so-called 'realist' approaches (Wong et al. 2012). Of course, there may be room for descriptions of innovations such as those in Table 11.1. But as online learning for faculty development becomes less of a novelty, such reports will less often meet the bar required for peer-reviewed publication. Those contemplating formal research in online learning are encouraged to consult previously published research agendas (Cook 2005; Cook et al. 2010) and experts in the field as they plan their study.

11.9   Conclusion

The future looks promising for online faculty development. Although the studies reporting such experiences are few, and not all were successful, the number of successes appears to be improving in recent years. Online tutorials, collaborative communities, simulations, and even games could help to overcome existing barriers and thereby add substantial value to faculty development initiatives. Those charged with developing such initiatives should not feel obliged to use online learning if it does not address a perceived need. Yet when needs do exist, online learning can resolve many barriers, particularly those of distance, scheduling, and self-pacing. In many cases, the ideal approach will blend activities from both online and other learning approaches to capitalize on the strengths of each. Blurred boundaries between online and 'traditional' approaches will increasingly be the norm.

Much remains to be learned about how to effectively implement online faculty development activities. For the moment, educators can rely on evidence from other fields. Going forward, it would be highly desirable for educators to collect evidence to inform when to use online learning for faculty development and how to use it effectively.

11.10   Key Messages

- Online learning is neither better nor worse than face-to-face instruction. Health professionals should use the approach most appropriate to local needs.
- The success of online faculty development initiatives varies widely. Keys to success include focusing on a perceived need, careful planning, facilitating clear communication, and developing a sense of community.
- Evidence from other fields can inform effective instructional design.
- Blending online and face-to-face instruction is increasingly common, and boundaries between these two options are increasingly blurred. Blended learning, properly done, capitalizes on the strengths of both approaches and is often more effective than either approach alone.

Appendix A: Glossary of Terms

Computer Tutorials

The online equivalent of a lecture; typically comprised of varying combinations of multimedia (see below). Online tutorials might also include activities to encourage engagement and deep learning such as computer simulations, interactive games and models, self-assessment tools, and hyperlinks to full-text journal articles or other online resources.

Online Discussion Boards

Discussion boards facilitate online group activities by providing a place to post messages and documents as part of an ongoing discussion. The group could alternatively do this using email, of course, but the key with a discussion board is that conversations are threaded; meaning that a response message (post) is linked with the post that prompted the response. It winds up looking like the branches of a tree – the first question is the main trunk, each response is a branch from that trunk, subsequent posts are branches from that branch, and so forth. Nearly always, teachers monitor the discussion board to observe the direction and depth of the discussion, keep people on track, and mediate the occasional online 'disagreement.'

Online Simulations

Online simulations are case-based computer programs that simulate real-life clinical scenarios. In clinical education, the most common computer simulations are virtual patients (Cook and Triola 2009). Simulations for faculty development might include virtual students (for practicing assessment or teaching), virtual research studies, or virtual leadership case scenarios.

Online Games

Online educational games are 'voluntary [online] activit[ies] structured by rules, with a defined outcome (winning, losing) or other quantifiable feedback (e.g. points) that facilitates reliable comparisons of in-player performances' (Thai et al. 2009, p. 11). Games typically have explicit goals and a compelling storyline (Tobias et al. 2011), and thus have the potential to engage learners and encourage their continued practice with the objective of improved knowledge and skill acquisition and application. However, the benefits of online educational games in medical education are still largely hypothetical, with only a few descriptions and even fewer comparative studies (Graafland et al. 2012).

Learning Management Systems

Learning Management Systems (LMS) are web-based software packages that facilitate the management and delivery of learning content and resources to learners. They provide important features such as secure log on, administration and tracking of tests and surveys, submission of assignments, monitoring of course participation, and content reuse and sharing across modules. Many also offer tools to facilitate learning such as discussion boards, wikis, and blogs. Examples include Blackboard, Sakai, and Moodle (an open-source [free] LMS).

Multimedia

Multimedia refers to the use of text, narration, other sounds, videos (with or without sound), slideshows, images, animations, and more. Appropriate use of multimedia can dramatically enhance learning over text alone. However, inappropriate use of multimedia can actually detract from learning.

Web 2.0

Web 2.0 represents a collection of web-based technologies that enable and encourage a collaborative, user-focused approach to design, maintain, and evaluate material. Blogs, wikis, social networks, and virtual worlds (discussed below) are Web 2.0 technologies. The content of these sites is determined by the collective efforts of its users and is in a constant state of change. Most Web 2.0 technologies were initially developed for entertainment and social functions (YouTube, Wikipedia, Facebook), but educators have begun to explore their potential for interactive instruction and assessment.

Social Media: Wikis, Blogs, Whiteboards, Instant Messaging, Social Networks and Virtual Worlds

Social media software refers to a variety of tools that allow individuals to easily produce content and/or communicate with others through online virtual networks. In education, these methods can promote and facilitate online collaboration for groups separated by distance and, except for whiteboards, time. In addition to discussion boards (above), options include:

- Wikis: Web sites or documents that groups create together. Everyone can edit the same document, making it a true group effort. Wikis can be created synchronously (everyone working at the same time) or asynchronously (individuals each contribute at a time convenient for them).
- Blogs: dated message postings organized chronologically (in contrast to discussion boards, which are threaded). Blogs are often individual (similar to a diary) but they can easily be used for group activities. Group blogs are usually asynchronous.
- Whiteboards: essentially the same as whiteboards in face-to-face classrooms – namely, participants can write or draw whatever they want. As participants view online, the image of the whiteboard is constantly updated. Whiteboards are, of necessity, synchronous – everyone must be participating 'live.'

- Instant messaging: real-time text communication between one or more individuals. The conversation is usually archived. Many online tools, educational and otherwise, offer instant messaging.
- Online social networks: an online service or site designed to promote communication and networking. Facebook is currently the leading example, and incorporates elements of blog and instant messaging along with media sharing (photos, audio, and video clips).
- Virtual Worlds: simulated environments in which users 'live' and interact via graphical representations of a real person called avatars. Some educators have used virtual worlds such as Second Life for presenting educational materials.

Reusable Learning Objects

Digital reusable learning objects are collections of instructional materials – text and multimedia – designed to meet a specific instructional objective, with little dependence on the surrounding educational context. This permits them to be repurposed for multiple learning applications. For example, a reusable learning object on how to perform a t-test could supplement a first-year medical school epidemiology course, be made available to residents as a resource for their scholarly projects, and comprise a core part of an online faculty development course.

Authoring Software: Technology for Rapid Multimedia Development

In recent years, a number of user-friendly software applications have been developed to assist non-programmers to easily develop professional-appearing online learning courses. Such 'authoring software' assembles digital media files into polished, interactive presentations, and makes online course development accessible to do-it-yourself teachers.

References

Adler, M. D. & Johnson, K. B. (2000). Quantifying the literature of computer-aided instruction in medical education. *Academic Medicine, 75*(10), 1025–1028.

Amin, Z., Boulet, J. R., Cook, D. A., Ellaway, R., Fahal, A., Kneebone, R., et al. (2011). Technology-enabled assessment of health professions education: Consensus statement and recommendations from the Ottawa 2010 Conference. *Medical Teacher, 33*(5), 364–369.

Anshu, Bansal, P., Mennin, S. G., Burdick, W. P., & Singh, T. (2008). Online faculty development for medical educators: Experience of a South Asian program. *Education for Health, 21*(3), 175.

Anshu, Sharma, M., Burdick, W. P., & Singh, T. (2010). Group dynamics and social interaction in a South Asian online learning forum for faculty development of medical teachers. *Education for Health, 23*(1), 311.

Bramson, R., Vanlandingham, A., Heads, A., Paulman, P., & Mygdal W. (2007). Reaching and teaching preceptors: Limited success from a multifaceted faculty development program. *Family Medicine, 39*(6), 386–388.

Bransford, J. D., Brown, A. L., & Cocking, R. R. (Eds.). (2000). *How people learn: Brain, mind, experience, and school.* Washington, DC: National Academy Press.

Clark, R. C. & Mayer, R. E. (2008). *E-learning and the science of instruction: Proven guidelines for consumers and designers of multimedia learning.* San Francisco, CA: Pfeiffer.

Clark, R. E. (1983). Reconsidering research on learning from media. *Review of Educational Research, 53*(4), 445–459.

Coma del Corral, M. J., Guevara, J. C., Luquin, P. A., Peña, H. J., & Mateos Otero, J. J. (2006). Usefulness of an internet-based thematic learning network: Comparison of effectiveness with traditional teaching. *Medical Informatics & the Internet in Medicine, 31*(1), 59–66.

Cook, D. A. (2005). The research we still are not doing: An agenda for the study of computer-based learning. *Academic Medicine, 80*(6), 541–548.

Cook, D. A. (2006). Where are we with web-based learning in medical education? *Medical Teacher, 28*(7), 594–598.

Cook, D. A. (2007). Web-based learning: Pros, cons and controversies. *Clinical Medicine, 7*(1), 37–42.

Cook, D. A. (2010). Twelve tips for evaluating educational programs. *Medical Teacher, 32*(4), 296–301.

Cook, D. A., Beckman, T. J., Thomas, K. G., & Thompson, W. G. (2008a). Adapting web-based instruction to residents' knowledge improves learning efficiency: A randomized controlled trial. *Journal of General Internal Medicine, 23*(7), 985–990.

Cook, D. A. & Dupras, D. M. (2004). A practical guide to developing effective Web-Based Learning. *Journal of General Internal Medicine, 19*(6), 698–707.

Cook, D. A., Garside, S., Levinson, A. J., Dupras, D. M., & Montori, V. M. (2010). What do we mean by web-based learning? A systematic review of the variability of interventions. *Medical Education, 44*(8), 765–774.

Cook, D. A., Levinson, A. J., Garside, S., Dupras, D. M., Erwin, P. J., & Montori, V. M. (2008b). Internet-based learning in the health professions: A meta-analysis. *JAMA, 300*(10), 1181–1196.

Cook, D. A. & McDonald, F. S. (2008). E-learning: Is there anything special about the E? *Perspectives in Biology and Medicine, 51*(1), 5–21.

Cook, D. A. & Steinert, Y. (2013). Online learning for faculty development: A review of the literature. *Medical Teacher, 35*(11), 930–937.

Cook, D. A. & Triola, M. M. (2009). Virtual patients: A critical literature review and proposed next steps. *Medical Education, 43*(4), 303–311.

Dean, P. J., Stahl, M. J., Sylwester, D. L., & Peat, J. A. (2001). Effectiveness of combined delivery modalities for distance learning and resident learning. *Quarterly Review of Distance Education, 2*(3), 247–254.

Dewey, J. (1913). *Interest and effort in education.* Boston, MA: Houghton Mifflin Co.

Dyrbye, L., Cumyn, A., Day, H., & Heflin, M. (2009). A qualitative study of physicians' experiences with online learning in a masters degree program: Benefits, challenges, and proposed solutions. *Medical Teacher, 31*(2), e40–e46.

Fox, N., O'Rourke, A., Roberts, C., & Walker, J. (2001). Change management in primary care: Design and evaluation of an internet-delivered course. *Medical Education, 35*(8), 803–805.

Graafland, M., Schraagen, J. M., & Schijven, M. P. (2012). Systematic review of serious games for medical education and surgical skills training. *British Journal of Surgery, 99*(10), 1322–1330.

Harris, J. M. Jr., Sklar, B. M., Amend, R. W., & Novalis-Marine, C. (2010). The growth, characteristics, and future of online CME. *Journal of Continuing Education in the Health Professions, 30*(1), 3–10.

Hull, P., Chaudry, A., Prasthofer, A., & Pattison, G. (2009). Optimal sequencing of bedside teaching and computer-based learning: A randomised trial. *Medical Education, 43*(2), 108–112.

Janicik, R., Kalet, A., & Zabar, S. (2002). Faculty development online: An observation and feedback module. *Academic Medicine, 77*(5), 460–461.

Kobak, K. A., Engelhardt, N., & Lipsitz, J. D. (2006). Enriched rater training using internet based technologies: A comparison to traditional rater training in a multi-site depression trial. *Journal of Psychiatric Research, 40*(3), 192–199.

Kotzer, A. M. & Milton, J. (2007). An education initiative to increase staff knowledge of Institutional Review Board guidelines in the USA. *Nursing & Health Sciences, 9*(2), 103–106.

Ladhani, Z., Chhatwal, J., Vyas, R., Iqbal, M., Tan, C., & Diserens, D. (2011). Online role-playing for faculty development. *Clinical Teacher, 8*(1), 31–36.

Landsberg, C. R., Astwood, R. S. Jr., Van Buskirk, W. L., Townsend, L. N., Steinhauser, N. B., & Mercado, A. D. (2012). Review of adaptive training system techniques. *Military Psychology, 24*(2), 96–113.

Langlois, J. P. & Thach, S. B. (2003). Bringing faculty development to community-based preceptors. *Academic Medicine, 78*(2), 150–155.

Lewis, K. O. & Baker, R. C. (2005). Development and implementation of an online master's degree in education program for health care professionals. *Academic Medicine, 80*(2), 141–146.

Lingard, L. (2007). Qualitative research in the RIME community: Critical reflections and future directions. *Academic Medicine, 82*(10 suppl), S129–S130.

Macrae, H. M., Regehr, G., McKenzie, M., Henteleff, H., Taylor, M., Barkun, J., et al. (2004). Teaching practicing surgeons critical appraisal skills with an Internet-based journal club: A randomized, controlled trial. *Surgery, 136*(3), 641–646.

Mayer, R. E. (2005). Cognitive theory of multimedia learning. In R. E. Mayer (Ed.), *The Cambridge handbook of multimedia learning,* (pp. 31–48). New York, NY: Cambridge University Press.

McKimm, J. & Swanwick, T. (2010). Web-based faculty development: e-learning for clinical teachers in the London Deanery. *Clinical Teacher, 7*(1), 58–62.

Merrill, M. D. (2002). First principles of instruction. *Educational Technology Research and Development, 50*(3), 43–59.

Paulus, T. M., Myers, C. R., Mixer, S. J., Wyatt, T. H., Lee, D. S., & Lee, J. L. (2010). For faculty, by faculty: A case study of learning to teach online. *International Journal of Nursing Education Scholarship, 7*(1), Article 13.

Pernar, L. I., Beleniski, F., Rosen, H., Lipsitz, S., Hafler, J., & Breen, E. (2012). Spaced education faculty development may not improve faculty teaching performance ratings in a surgery department. *Journal of Surgical Education, 69*(1), 52–57.

Richman, R. C., Morahan, P. S., Cohen, D. W., & McDade, S. A. (2001). Advancing women and closing the leadership gap: The Executive Leadership in Academic Medicine (ELAM) program experience. *Journal of Women's Health & Gender-Based Medicine, 10*(3), 271–277.

Sandars, J. (2010). Social software and digital competences. *InnovAiT, 3*(5), 306–309.

Sandars, J. (2012). Technology and the delivery of the curriculum of the future: Opportunities and challenges. *Medical Teacher, 34*(7), 534–538.

Sandars, J., Kokotailo, P., & Singh, G. (2012). The importance of social and collaborative learning for online continuing medical education (OCME): Directions for future development and research. *Medical Teacher, 34*(8), 649–652.

Schoen, M. J., Tipton, E. F., Houston, T. K., Funkhouser, E., Levine, D. A., Estrada, C. A., et al. (2009). Characteristics that predict physician participation in a Web-based CME activity: The MI-Plus study. *Journal of Continuing Education in the Health Professions, 29*(4), 246–253.

Steinert, Y., McLeod, P. J., Conochie, L., & Nasmith, L. (2002). An online discussion for medical faculty: An experiment that failed. *Academic Medicine, 77*(9), 939–940.

Thai, A. M., Lowenstein, D., Ching, D., & Rejeski, D. (2009). *Game changer: Investing in digital play to advance children's learning and health.* New York, NY: Joan Ganz Cooney Center.

Tobias, S., Fletcher, J. D., Dai, D. Y., & Wind, A. P. (2011). Review of research on computer games. In S. Tobias & J. D. Fletcher (Eds.), *Computer games and instruction,* (pp. 127–222). Charlotte, NC: Information Age Publishing Inc.

van Merriënboer, J. J. G. & Sweller, J. (2005). Cognitive load theory and complex learning: Recent developments and future directions. *Educational Psychology Review, 17*(2), 147–177.

Wearne, S., Greenhill, J., Berryman, C., Sweet, L., & Tietz, L.. (2011). An online course in clinical education - Experiences of Australian clinicians. *Australian Family Physician, 40*(12), 1000–1003.

Wiecha, J., Heyden, R., Sternthal, E., & Merialdi, M. (2010). Learning in a virtual world: Experience with using Second Life for medical education. *Journal of Medical Internet Research, 12*(1), e1.

Wong, G., Greenhalgh, T., Westhorp, G., & Pawson, R. (2012). Realist methods in medical education research: What are they and what can they contribute? *Medical Education, 46*(1), 89–96.

Part IV
Practical Applications

Chapter 12
Faculty Development to Promote Role-Modeling and Reflective Practice

Karen V. Mann

12.1 Introduction

Role-modeling and reflective practice are increasingly recognized as important elements in teaching and learning in the health professions. As our understanding of these areas of practice grows, we appreciate that faculty members need preparation and support to use them effectively. In this chapter, role-modeling and reflection will be addressed, and the underpinning literature and theory will be summarized. Each will be addressed individually; however, as we explore these two important areas, their integral relationship to each other will become apparent. Implications for faculty development practice will conclude the chapter.

Reflection and role-modeling are important in all faculty roles; however, this chapter will focus on the teaching role of faculty members as the vast majority of literature about faculty development for these topics addresses their effective use in teaching and learning. The principles, however, may be applied in the context of other faculty roles and practices.

12.1.1 Why Is Faculty Development for Role-Modeling and Reflective Practice Important?

Role-modeling remains an extremely influential method of teaching and learning. Yet, Kenny et al. (2003) noted that 'conceptually, role-modeling is a 'black box' for

K.V. Mann, BN, M.Sc., Ph.D. (✉)
Division of Medical Education, Faculty of Medicine, Dalhousie University,
Halifax, NS, Canada
e-mail: karen.mann@dal.ca

Y. Steinert (ed.), *Faculty Development in the Health Professions: A Focus on Research and Practice*, Innovation and Change in Professional Education 11, DOI 10.1007/978-94-007-7612-8_12, © Springer Science+Business Media Dordrecht 2014

both teachers and learners. Educators lack an adequate understanding of the process through which learners respond to models and of how practitioners of varying quality and commitment exert their influence' (p. 1205).

Traditionally, role-modeling has been accepted as a naturally occurring teaching process, one that 'happens' spontaneously rather than being planned. Learners can learn implicitly from role models through observations of their behavior and its consequences (Bandura 1986); however, learners also have an active role in learning from role models, ultimately creating for themselves a configuration of attitudes, behaviors and orientations, gleaned from the multiple and varied examples they have encountered. Faculty members are often unaware that role-modeling can be a deliberate activity and that we are always role-modeling even when not intending to do so (Hafferty and Franks 1994). The concept of role-modeling is important, as professionals are not acting a role; they are embodying it (Bleakley et al. 2011).

Faculty development for reflection and reflective practice is important at more than one level. First, it is important for faculty to be able to help learners to reflect, to enhance their learning, and to prepare for the self-regulation required in practice. Reflection and self-awareness are critical to developing professional identity. Second, learning about and experiencing reflection is important for faculty members themselves, as it allows them to explore their teaching practices, understand their underlying values, and learn from their practice. This can in turn effect change in teaching practice and also in role-modeling.

12.2 Role-Modeling

12.2.1 Why Is Role-Modeling Important?

Role-modeling is identified by faculty members as integral to their teaching and cited by students as a major influence on their learning all aspects of their professional role. Indeed, it is suggested that role models are central to the moral enculturation of developing professionals who take on the attitudes, values and attributes of their chosen profession (Hafferty and Franks 1994). The influence of role models is generally viewed to be at the individual level, in helping the learner to develop desired skills and attributes. However, role-modeling is also important at the collective level, as models play an important role in helping learners enter the community of practice of their profession. Learners gradually become more involved in the community while developing their professional identity and competence (Cooke et al. 2010). Activities, roles and relationships are modeled by more senior peers, other health professionals and other learners. The literature also supports that professional caring and patient-centeredness can be modeled effectively in the learner-teacher relationship, and that such modeling can have long-lasting effects (Cavanaugh 2002; Haidet and Stein 2006). Novice teachers report that role models were important in their non-formal learning at work and their professional development (Cook 2009). Lastly, Weissmann et al. (2006) suggest that role models may counter the negative effects of the hidden curriculum.

12.2.2   Conceptual Approaches to Understanding Role-Modeling

Role-modeling is a fundamental process, and our understanding of it draws from several fields. The goal of this section is to summarize some relevant understandings of role-modeling to provide a foundation for designing effective faculty development programs and activities.

The idea of 'role' originates in sociology and the roles that individuals perform in their everyday lives in society. Generally, people have and manage multiple roles in the various aspects of their lives. Roles carry with them ways of behaving, rights and obligations. The concept of role-modeling addresses how roles are enacted, and how others learn to enact those roles through observation. In contemporary medical education, the concept has been operationalized by the Royal College of Physicians and Surgeons of Canada as a group of roles the individual physician enacts as part of the overall role of 'physician' (Royal College of Physicians and Surgeons of Canada 2012).

Role-modeling is also an important concept in psychology and learning. Bandura (1986) described the powerful learning that occurs from observing the actions of others and the consequences of their behavior. Learning in this way is referred to as 'observational' or 'vicarious'. Examples of this abound in our lives.

Role-modeling also contributes to building self-efficacy, or people's expectations that they can successfully execute a particular task or set of tasks in a domain (Bandura 1997). Bandura asserts that self-efficacy can be learned through observing the performance of others.

Lastly, social anthropology has evolved the theory of Communities of Practice to broaden our understanding of apprenticeship (Lave and Wenger 1991). In this conception, learners develop not only skills and knowledge; they also develop their professional identity. Learning is a process of joining a community and learning occurs by participating in the authentic activities of the community. Along their journey toward full membership in the community, learners participate through doing, but also through watching and listening. They learn *from* talk, through listening to community members talk about their practice and their world; they also learn *to* talk, as this is key to their participation in the community (Lave and Wenger 1991).

These varying conceptual perspectives illuminate the complexity of learning from role models. Certain assumptions underpin the belief that role-modeling is an effective means of learning. First, especially regarding professional behavior and development of professional identity, we may assume that the values of the teacher and the learner are similar. However, historical events, culture and societal influences result in changes in societal values; these are sometimes most evident across generations. Second, we may assume that those observing will understand the intent of the role model's behavior. However, observing a role model cannot be equated with understanding exactly what the model intended. To ensure understanding, the model must be capable of and willing to reflect with learners to clarify what was intended, especially since not all observed situations have the desired outcome.

Particularly where values and professional behavior are modeled, reflecting openly allows the model to make explicit the values and standards guiding his/her behavior. Learners, in turn, can consider these against their own developing values (Kenny et al. 2003). Importantly, modeling does not require *one* way of doing things; it requires adaptability and recognition that what needs to be modeled is the approach that has the most explanatory value in the current context (Bleakley et al. 2011).

Cruess et al. (2008) classified the characteristics of effective role models, including clinical competence, teaching skills and personal qualities. Others have identified similar characteristics (Jochemson-van der Leeuw et al. 2013; Wright and Carrese 2002). Cruess et al. (2008) propose an iterative process of learning from role-modeling which involves: active observation of a role model; making the unconscious conscious; reflection and abstraction; translating insights into principles and actions; and generalization of learning and behavior change. This model draws on the cycle of experiential learning described by Kolb (1984); it also explicitly recognizes the process of unconscious incorporation of values by observers. Eraut (2004) has also described 'learning without being aware that we have learned' as part of the informal and non-formal learning that occurs at work. Bleakley et al. (2011) argue that our traditional approaches to role-modeling are no longer adequate; for the transformation of medical education to occur, we must move from role-modeling based on charisma to role-modeling based on capability.

Through the many experiences encountered throughout their education, learners construct a professional identity. Identity is shaped by the interactions with the entire culture of medical education, both specifically and generally. Through modeling, members of the practice community enact the community's values. This includes not only the particular aspects of the physician's knowledge and skills, but also the quality of team interactions, teaching, coaching and assessment. In Bleakley et al.'s (2011) view, moral commitment to the highest levels of patient care and commitment to high standards of role-modeling within the community are required. For faculty, this also involves an understanding of the cultural history of our actions and the hidden curriculum – how it shapes professional identity for both teachers and learners.

The research literature consistently supports role-modeling as an integral form of learning, highlighting the potential benefits of faculty development to help faculty to be more mindful and deliberate in their teaching through modeling. Three examples illustrate this. Riley and Kumar (2012) asked doctors and medical students to first define and then indicate how they had learned professionalism and how they thought it best taught. Role models were the second most often reported source of teaching and learning about professionalism, second only to experience; learning from role models was not always through positive examples. Goldie et al. (2007) identified role models as important in the socialization process, allowing medical students to enter the community of practice of the medical profession.

Faculty members and residents in surgery reflected on how they had learned professionalism (Park et al. 2010). Both role-modeling and reflection were included. Learners in surgery described that effective learning from role models involved three elements of observation, reflection and reinforcement. They noted the importance of being able to observe faculty members, to reflect on what they had seen or experienced followed by an opportunity to practice these behaviors, and most importantly, to have them reinforced by faculty. Understanding role-modeling as a process rather than an event could help faculty members to maximize its learning potential.

12.3 Reflection and Reflective Practice

This section of the chapter focuses on reflection and reflective practice. The goal in so doing is to highlight its importance, illuminate our understanding of its conceptual underpinnings, and identify important issues for faculty development.

12.3.1 Why Are Reflection and Reflective Practice Important?

Reflection and reflective practice are deemed by many to be integral to professional practice. Epstein and Hundert (2002) define competence as 'the habitual and judicious use of communication, knowledge, technical skills, clinical reasoning, emotions, values, and reflection in daily practice for the benefit of the individual and community being served' (p. 226). In their definition, reflection becomes a 'habit of mind'.

The literature regarding the role of reflection in teaching, learning and practice has been developed in several fields (Boud et al. 1985; Moon 2004; Schön 1983, 1987). Reflection has been proposed as a critical means of learning from experience, both in the moment, following an event, and in anticipation of events. Reflection has been associated with enhanced learning, deep learning, making meaning of events, and understanding one's practice in a larger context (Mann et al. 2009). It has also been associated with improved diagnostic accuracy in complex problems (Mamede et al. 2008). Reflection is intimately related to self-assessment, as effective self-assessment and self-regulation rely on the capability to reflect on one's practice. Lastly, reflection plays an important role in facilitating the acceptance of feedback and its incorporation into practice (Sargeant et al. 2009).

Reflection on both successes and failures can be used by teachers to improve their practice (Pinsky and Irby 1997; Pinsky et al. 1998). Reflection is also a means of uncovering one's expertise and building upon it by exploring beneath the everyday activities and experience of practice, thus learning to understand its underlying values and foundations. Although the literature suggests that some individuals may inherently be more oriented toward reflection than others, there is evidence that these capabilities can be learned and that they can impact practice (Mann et al. 2009). Reflection can be both an individual and a collective activity. Reflection at a group, or collective, level allows for sharing of norms and reflecting on values; it can also lead to transformation at an institutional level (Frankford et al. 2000).

Preparing faculty for reflection and reflective practice in their teaching addresses three goals. The first goal is to assist faculty members to develop skills to reflect on their own teaching experience and practice, both to identify future goals, and to understand and uncover the expertise, attitudes and values which underlie it. The second goal is to enable faculty to support and guide learners to acquire these capabilities, to prepare learners effectively for a lifetime of maintaining and improving professional competence. The third goal (related to the first) may be to enable the faculty members to situate their teaching as a social process, in the context of the society within which it occurs.

Bleakley et al. (2011), writing in medical education, have described the need for medical educators to experience and understand the dynamic process of which they are a part. They suggest that reflection in and on practice is essential to teachers in developing themselves and becoming involved in the scholarship of teaching.

12.3.2 Conceptual Approaches to Understanding Reflection

The definition of reflection has been complicated by its origin in different fields of study. In 1995, Brookfield, in his book, *Becoming a Critically Reflective Teacher,* suggested:

> Reflective practice has its roots in the Enlightenment idea that we can stand outside of ourselves and come to a clearer understanding of what we do and who we are, by freeing ourselves of distorted ways of reasoning and acting (Brookfield 1995, pp. 214–215).

Two assumptions are present in this definition: the first is that reflective practitioners can examine their own practice to understand it better, and uncover the values, assumptions and experience that drive it, and second, that a plurality of models of good teaching exist. Brookfield cautioned that reflection had become a catch-all term, overused and in danger of becoming ritualized and trivialized. Boud and Walker (1998) also identified the challenges of teaching reflection in a professional context, and identified ritualization as a potential risk.

Models of reflection have their origin in education (Boud et al. 1985; Dewey 1933; Schön 1983) and more recently have been linked to cognition and cognitive psychology (Moon 2004). Models which have been most influential share certain characteristics which include: an *iterative* dimension within which there is a return to experience to critically analyze and learn from it; and a *vertical* dimension incorporating different levels and depths of reflection, from a superficial description of events to a more profound and deeper analysis (Mann et al. 2009).

Schön (1987) described reflection as a means by which teachers might understand their relation to their learners, thus potentially altering the traditional power relations in apprenticeship. By helping the learner to acquire different approaches to reflection, the teacher can facilitate the learner becoming more self-directed, more able to account for the work they are doing, and therefore more equal in the relationship.

However, Bleakley et al. (2011) cautioned that reflection is really 'appreciation' of a situation. Critical reflexivity, which can bring about change in our educational practice and systems, involves looking at what values inform our practice. These authors further underlined that developing skills of reflection and reflexivity is a learning process.

Schön's (1987) model of reflection is probably the best known in professional education. This model includes an iterative process of *reflection-on-action* after an event and *reflection-in-action* during an event or experience. Although predominantly associated with reflection 'on' events, Schön also emphasized reflection 'in the moment', a moment-to-moment awareness of our actions in the context and of the responses we make to those conditions. This aspect of reflection, or self-monitoring, has been further explored by several authors (Moulton et al. 2007).

Further, although his work was mainly associated with individual reflection, Schön (1987) also described 'reflection in community', or collective reflection, where professionals can learn together through sharing good practices and offering peer support in democratic structures. Collective reflection also offers the opportunity for learning vicariously, improving group members' self-efficacy and sharing and constructing group norms and values.

An essential aspect of teaching practice is 'phronesis' or *practical knowing*. Practical knowing and 'the way we do things', have been described as contributing to our personal 'theory in action' which underlies our actions (Argyris and Schön 1974). Reflection and critical reflexivity allow us to uncover what those theories are. Sfard (1998) reminds us that learning theories are not value free, and that understanding our values and what drives our practice are essential to bringing about change in our learners, ourselves and our institutions. Sfard (1998) identified two predominant metaphors for learning which underlie our practical knowledge: acquisition and participation. These two models are particularly relevant to faculty developers. Our programs must balance acquisition – or the building up of skills and knowledge which are the property of the individual alone – with participation, where the faculty member participates in the collective work of building a shared construction of knowledge.

12.4   Faculty Development for Role-Modeling and Reflective Practice

The literature describing approaches to faculty development can be clustered into three areas. These are: approaches to enhance humanistic teaching through personal and professional growth; approaches to improve role modeling; and approaches to enhance reflection. This section will address each in turn.

12.4.1   Approaches to Enhance Humanistic Teaching

There are several examples of faculty development to enable faculty to better teach attributes of humanistic care. Role-modeling is but one; however, it is a critical aspect of that teaching (Haidet et al. 2008).

Programs that address role-modeling and reflection share certain characteristics: they are longitudinal, extending over a period of time; they involve a stable group of faculty so that an atmosphere of safety and trust may be built; and they alternate or combine sessions on particular aspects of humanistic care with those that focus on individual and shared reflection. These approaches have been replicated across several schools, and have been evaluated carefully and regarded as successful.

Enhancing the human dimensions of care. Branch et al. (2009) describe such a program which may serve as an illustrative example. Although drawn from medical education, its structure and outcomes seem applicable across the health professions.

This longitudinal faculty development program was offered in five US medical schools and involved promising teachers chosen from volunteers. The facilitators together developed and implemented a faculty development curriculum to enhance humanistic teaching. The program content and structure reflected both the literature and an analysis of teaching encounters of highly regarded role models.

The program occurred over 18 months to support group process that would foster reflection; it included an experiential learning component to allow for practice of new skills relevant to role-modeling and alternating sessions for reflecting on values and attitudes. Reflective activities included narrative writing, Balint groups, and opportunities to discuss renewal and meaning. Participants discussed critical incidents, appreciative narrative enquiries and personal goals.

A variety of outcomes and measures were reported. Branch et al. (2009) developed and utilized a previously validated 10-item questionnaire, the Humanistic Teaching Practice Effectiveness Questionnaire, which included questions about listening skills, personal inspiration, stimulating reflection and illustrating humanistic care. They found that, when rated by students, participants outperformed a group of peer controls who had not participated in the program, scoring significantly higher on all ten items ($p < .05$). Importantly, the authors found a difference of 8–13 %, which they considered sufficiently robust to make the results of practical significance as well.

In programs using reflective activities such as those described above, reflections have been triggered by individual experience and group events, and have taken the form of appreciative inquiry (e.g. Quaintance et al. 2010) Appreciative inquiry chooses not to focus on things that are not going well and need improvement; instead, it focuses on successful processes and outcomes, and analyzes them critically with a view to creating more of them (Kowalski 2008).

Learning about professionalism. Quaintance et al. (2010) described a method for teaching professionalism that helped faculty to consider not only what they teach, but how they teach, through introducing such constructs as situated learning, explicit role-modeling and appreciative inquiry. In their approach, students interviewed faculty members about their experiences of professionalism, following which the students reflected upon and then wrote about the teachers' stories. Rich and generally positive stories resulted that conveyed the major principles of professionalism, including humanism, accountability, altruism and excellence; similarly, the students' reflections demonstrated awareness of the same principles. The authors concluded that narrative reflective storytelling could both assist faculty to reflect on their experience and deepen students' understanding of professionalism.

Reflective learning for junior faculty. Faculty development of this nature may also be effective when offered to junior faculty. Higgins et al. (2011) demonstrated benefits from such a program and described a phased model of development over 4 years of a group's work. The three phases included: becoming caring, humanistic doctors; becoming humanistic role models while teaching; and becoming empathetic leaders.

Group norms also developed, moving through empathy, compassion, fairness and courage. Courage related to the participants' ability to articulate their values and to live by them in their professional work. The authors suggest that group support, cohesion and validation encouraged adoption of common values among the participants that informed their professional development over the 4 years, and subsequently influenced them as their careers progressed.

The literature on excellence in clinical teaching demonstrates the relationship of role-modeling and reflection. Weissmann et al. (2006) found that awareness of oneself as a role model is an attribute of excellent clinical teachers. These authors described a wide range of behaviors modeled by faculty members, which they classified as nonverbal behaviors; demonstrations of respect; building a personal connection; eliciting and addressing patients' emotional responses to illness; and faculty self-awareness. Teachers reported reflecting on their own behavior as well as reflecting with learners. Self-awareness as a role model was underpinned by reflection, which allowed faculty members to act more deliberately to make changes to the clinical environment to facilitate compassionate care. The authors suggest that role models may counter the effects of the hidden curriculum.

It appears that faculty development for role-modeling and reflection positively impacts faculty behavior in these areas. Although several reports are iterations of the same program and principles, it is notable that positive outcomes were seen at all five sites, suggesting a broader applicability. The significance of these results is that benefits may accrue not only to learners, but to faculty members who experience professional development and renewal.

Two studies described reflection in clinical teaching in medicine (Pinsky and Irby 1997; Pinsky et al. 1998). Distinguished clinical teachers were surveyed regarding the role of reflecting on both instructional success and failure in their professional development as teachers. They identified using both reflection-in-action and reflection-on-action. However, they most frequently described 'anticipatory reflection' or learning from and incorporating previous experience into teaching. Reflecting on failures was seen as equally important to reflecting on successes. Both studies support the role of reflection in the ongoing professional development of teachers.

12.4.2 Approaches to Support and Improve Role-Modeling

Cruess et al. (2008) describe strategies to improve role-modeling at both the individual and the institutional level. Strategies to improve individual performance include: awareness of being a role model; making and protecting time to teach; awareness of reflection; the need to make the implicit explicit; and participating in staff/faculty development.

Kenny et al. (2003) recommended faculty development which clarified the meaning of roles and role-modeling, discussed standards, assisted faculty to reflect, and provided safe spaces for reflection and debriefing.

Steinert et al. (2005) developed a systematic, integrated faculty development program to support the teaching and evaluation of professionalism. The program's main messages were making the implicit explicit and the importance of role-modeling. Program evaluation, using participants' intended changes to their teaching, indicated that role-modeling would be the teaching strategy of choice for many participants.

Boerebach et al. (2012) studied the relationship between teaching performance and residents' perceptions of a teacher as a role model. Of the many factors which might influence how the physician was viewed, the largest predictor was the faculty member's teaching performance. There were some specific relationships between particular teaching skills and effects on role-modeling. The authors suggested that one effective approach in improving role-modeling was to invest effort in improving faculty's teaching performance.

Importantly, improving role-modeling cannot be accomplished at the individual level alone. The institution plays a key role. Efforts have been made to understand the learning environment on the premise that the context of student learning interacts with their experience and affects not only the student's development as a professional but also the ways in which faculty members can and do act. Haidet et al. (2005) report the development of the 'C3', an instrument to characterize the patient-centeredness of clinical learning environments. At the institutional level, Cruess et al. (2008) suggest that faculty work together to improve the institutional culture, particularly to affect the structure so that teaching is valued and time is available to teach. The goal is to create an environment which supports positive role-modeling.

Faculty development efforts can support initiatives such as those described and can assist faculty to reflect on the information to improve both their own individual practice and the larger institutional environment.

12.4.3 Approaches to Improve Reflection

Faculty development approaches to improve reflection have been developed in two broad directions. In the first, the goal is to improve faculty's ability to use reflection with their learners. In the second, the focus is on enhancing faculty's ability to develop reflective practice in their own work, arguing that by learning and using these approaches, faculty members will be more able to deliberately modify their own approaches and to facilitate learners' use of the same reflective activities.

12.4.3.1   Helping Faculty to Use Reflection with Learners

Defining and assessing reflection in learners. Acquisition of reflective skills has become increasingly emphasized in nursing education. Yet little has been written about preparing teachers to promote development of those skills in learners and novice teachers report feeling unprepared (Braine 2009). Dekker-Groen et al. (2011) used a Delphi process to define reflection and to identify a framework of required teaching competencies. The resulting framework identified six domains, the most important of which were coaching students and stimulating student thinking.

Aronson et al. (2009) recognized that a wide variety of activities may be labeled as 'reflection'; further, although the literature on reflection identifies analytic, evidence-based and temporal or behavioral change components, the authors found many reflective activities in their faculty to be unstructured and poorly evaluated. In response, they designed a 3 h faculty development session to: define reflection; describe the five applications of reflection in medical education; evaluate written reflections for reflective ability; and discuss a rubric for the evaluation of reflective ability. Despite a small number of participants, the authors found evidence that a single session resulted in educators being able to design exercises to develop reflective ability in their learners. These authors subsequently developed resources which are available to assist both teaching and evaluating reflection (Aronson et al. 2012; O'Sullivan et al. 2010).

Wald et al. (2012) have also developed and evaluated a rubric entitled the Reflection Evaluation for Learners' Enhanced Competencies Tool (REFLECT) to both assess learners' reflection, but also to assist faculty in providing feedback that will promote reflective capacity.

Using Reflection to Foster the Acceptance of Feedback. Another important role of reflection is as a vehicle allowing exploration of feedback and enhancing the ability to accept and incorporate feedback to improve practice. This is important both for faculty members' practice and for their ability to help learners use feedback effectively. A recent model to assist learners to utilize reflection is the ECO model (Sargeant et al. 2011). This model outlines three steps to help the facilitator improve the learner's ability to accept and use feedback: emotion, content and outcome. By processing and acknowledging the emotion, the learner/recipient can be assisted to reflect on the feedback and to make a plan for how it might be used. This model can be useful for both faculty and students. Faculty can use such an approach to help learners accept feedback and incorporate it. Understanding this model may also assist faculty to be better able to reflect on feedback they receive.

Modeling Reflection and Reflective Practice. Weissmann et al. (2006) studied excellent clinical teachers from four US medical schools. These teachers taught mainly through modeling a variety of humanistic behaviors in their interactions with students and patients, and by modeling self-awareness and reflection. The faculty members identified self-reflection as the primary method by which they developed and refined their teaching strategies; they also noted the importance of modeling reflection for learners.

12.4.3.2   Becoming a More Critically Reflective Teacher

A rich literature exists in general education about faculty development to promote reflection, which helps to situate faculty development in the health professions within a larger context. This literature focuses on assisting faculty members to develop as reflective practitioners, believing this to be fundamental to any sustained change in teaching practice, and that focusing only on skills or methods is insufficient.

Amundsen and Wilson (2012) published a conceptual review of the educational development literature in higher education. There were 29 papers identified where the goal was to engage faculty in a process of reflection, both individual and collaborative, with the purpose of changing or clarifying their conceptions of teaching and learning and linking this to change in their teaching practices.

Faculty participants in these initiatives engaged in reflection and discussion in a variety of ways, sometimes prompted by reflecting on their own practices in relationship to a personal goal, to a colleague's practice, to literature, or to newly developed knowledge. The review raised the question of individual improvement of teaching practice versus engaging teachers in the improvement of teaching as a socially situated process. Initiatives promoting reflection are among those that focus not only on the individual's teaching but on changing teaching at a more transformative level.

An example may be informative. Hubball et al. (2005) explored how faculty members used reflection and incorporated it into their 'real life' work. This study, which involved faculty from several higher education disciplines, both mirrors reported experience in health professions education and exemplifies the outcomes that we wish to achieve: improved teaching and learning. The authors defined reflection as 'thoughtful consideration and questioning of what we do, what works and what doesn't work, and what premises and rationales underlie our own teaching and that of others' (Hubball et al. 2005, p. 60). Expected outcomes included that faculty members would develop a critically reflective teaching practice; think critically about curriculum and pedagogical issues; and articulate their own values about teaching and learning. Over 8 months, participants engaged in activities such as journal reflections on readings, developing a personal teaching philosophy, and developing a teaching dossier. The authors used an instrument, the Teaching Perspectives Inventory (Collins and Pratt 2011; Pratt and Collins 2013), to help participants to look more deeply at the underlying values and assumptions which guided their teaching practice. The Teaching Perspectives Inventory (TPI) identifies five perspectives or lenses through which educators view their work. Each perspective brings a blend of beliefs, intentions and actions, framing views of teaching, learners, learning, content and context. The authors found that the TPI stimulated greater reflection on teaching practices, which in turn contributed to changes in participants' (self-reported) TPI scores. The TPI emphasizes the plurality of ways in which good teaching can occur. This is particularly relevant when we think of role-modeling; many different approaches to a problem may be modeled.

Barriers to reflection were also identified and included inadequate time for reflection and unclear expectations and goals for reflection activities. Participants identified the importance of 'habitualizing' reflection and the lack of cultural norms supporting reflection in academe. The messages of the wider literature resonate strongly with our experiences as teachers and learners in the health professions.

Studies in general education provide many parallels to the studies reported earlier, in which teachers in medicine and the health professions have engaged in critical reflection on their practice. Readers may find it helpful to consult the summary of all studies presented in Table 12.1.

12.5 Guidelines for Faculty Development Practice

Promoting faculty development for role-modeling and reflection is a rich area for faculty development. Taken together, the conceptual underpinnings for each offer us several implications for practice. These implications, drawn from the literature, are presented below as principles which may guide the design of faculty development initiatives.

1. **Raising awareness of the impact of role-modeling can improve faculty members' awareness of themselves as models.** Encourage faculty members to discuss and share experiences with role-modeling, both as a learner and as a teacher. This can be accomplished informally, but also in seminars or in interactive discussions. Faculty can benefit from reflecting on how they themselves have learned from role models, both in the past and currently. Further, helping faculty members to realize that they are modeling ways of being even when they are unaware of it can help them to be more deliberate about the behaviors they wish to model.
2. **Attention to improving teaching performance can lead to changes in role-modeling behavior.** Teaching performance is closely related to role-modeling and to how teachers are viewed as role models. This is especially true of teachers in the health professions where teaching is inseparable from communication and interactions with patients and other team members. Concentrating on improving teaching, and awareness of one's own teaching, can lead to improvements in role-modeling as well.
3. **The institution's role is critically important in creating an environment in which the best attributes of professional practice can be modeled.** Encourage faculty members to explore the setting and climate of their workplace, and to reflect on how it supports or hinders their ability to model the kind of practice they would like. This may also include exploration of the hidden curriculum and how they may model some of its values unknowingly. Learners and staff can also contribute to this discussion and to developing shared approaches.
4. **Short, one-time interventions are unlikely to provide the opportunity for lasting change**. Like the learners they work with, faculty members need time and support to make changes and grow professionally. The most successful approaches involve stable groups who meet regularly to discuss and share

Table 12.1 A summary of selected reports of interventions to improve reflection and role-modeling in faculty members

Authors	Year	Intervention/Program	Length of program	Strategy	Outcomes
Hubball, Collins & Pratt	2005	Certificate Program on Teaching and Learning in Higher Education	8 months	Individual learning plans were developed consisting of various reflective activities based on a prior learning assessment	Depth of reflection on teaching increased following the program
Aronson, Chittenden & O'Sullivan	2009	Faculty Development Workshop in Teaching Reflection	3 h	Small group seminar consisting of a presentation, an evaluation of reflective ability of students and residents, a critique of current reflective exercises, and a discussion around educational approaches to promote critical reflection	Faculty members developed a better understanding of reflection as demonstrated by their ability to create appropriate exercises focused on the development of reflective abilities of learners
Branch, Frankel, Gracey, Haidet, Weissmann, Cantey, Mitchell & Inui	2009	Longitudinal Faculty Development Program	18 months	Combination of experiential learning of skills and reflective learning to explore attitudes and values	Positive impact was demonstrated on humanistic teaching skills and personal and professional attributes of participants in the program
Quaintance, Arnold & Thompson	2010	Teaching and Modeling of Professionalism	Dependent on participation	Narrative storytelling and reflection through writing	Students were able to identify and internalize concepts of professionalism
Higgins, Bernstein, Manning, Schneider, Kho, Brownfield & Branch	2011	Longitudinal Faculty Development	18 months	Combination of small group facilitated experiential learning of skills and role modeling with reflective learning	Participants developed as teachers and leaders and increased awareness through appreciative inquiry and critical reflection

Suchman, Williamson, Litzelman, Frankel, Mossbarger & Inui, Relationship-Centered Care Initiative Discovery Team	2004	Development of an Informal Curriculum and Promotion of Mindfulness	Individual interviews occurred over 3 months	Appreciative narrative approach and open forum to elicit and disseminate inspiring narratives about the informal curriculum at its best	Initial assessment showed an organizational identity shift towards reinforcing values of the formal curriculum
Steinert, Cruess, Cruess & Snell	2005	Faculty Development Program for Teaching and Evaluation of Professionalism	Varied by participation	Used think tanks, workshops, and evaluation	Self-reported changes in teaching and practice, new educational initiatives, and more effective use of role modeling

experience and to engage with new learning. This continuity provides the opportunity to build an atmosphere of trust among members.

5. **Faculty members need time and opportunity to practice new skills and to receive feedback on their experience**. In addition to providing regular meetings, interventions with faculty members should allow time for participants to test new learning in their practice. This may involve trying a new teaching approach on one's own or working with a colleague to observe and provide feedback to each other. Once there has been an opportunity to practice, reflection with the group can maximize learning for both the individual and the group.

6. **Teaching practices are improved by reflecting on one's own teaching and the values that underlie it**. This notion links reflection to improving teaching and role-modeling. Skills in reflection can be learned. Faculty members need support and structure to understand what reflection involves, and to understand how they can learn from their own practice, not just to improve it but to uncover their own expertise. They also need support in learning and acquiring these skills.

7. **Reflecting on both teaching successes and failures can help faculty members to improve their teaching**. Teachers can learn from both successes and failures, and incorporate what they learn into their teaching. The importance of trusted colleagues and an environment that supports learning are paramount for the development of critical reflexivity.

8. **Learning to use reflection in their own practices allows faculty members to model this for learners and peers.** As faculty members become familiar with, and more confident in, using reflection to enhance their own learning, they can use these skills with the learners they teach.

9. **Various resources are available to support faculty members in involving learners in reflection.** These include models for reflecting and rubrics for evaluation. Structured models may provide a scaffold for both teachers and learners. They also provide a framework for structured feedback to learners.

10. **Feedback models can be helpful to support faculty members in assisting learners to reflect**. The ECO model (Sargeant et al. 2011) can be used by faculty members both to reflect and enhance their own use of feedback and also when they are working with learners. Similarly, the rubric developed by Wald et al. (2012) may be helpful.

11. **Involving more junior faculty members may lead to long-term benefits**. By having the opportunity to participate in a community of faculty colleagues, it seems that over time, junior faculty members experience both personal growth and an increase in the ability to collaboratively create a shared value system. These values can sustain faculty members and they can support each other in enacting them.

12. **It is important to help faculty members build their self-efficacy in this area.** Self-efficacy is important to faculty both in their own use of reflection in their teaching and in their work with learners. Experience, practice and feedback, as well as observing others, can build self-efficacy.

13. **A variety of reflective activities should be used.** Faculty members will find that some activities will suit them better than others. No one activity will work for all. As they are exposed to a variety of approaches, faculty members will also have more options to use in their teaching.
14. **Reflection will be most effective when it is situated in the faculty member's own experience and practice**. Reflection should be ongoing, linked to other activities and always be authentically related to the individual's teaching, the context of their work, the setting and the learners they teach.
15. **It is critically important to provide a safe place for faculty to reflect, debrief and discuss their experiences.** The importance of safety for faculty members to develop the skills in reflection and role-modeling cannot be overestimated. Communities and groups of faculty who have the opportunity to develop as a group can share experience and develop common values. The development of shared norms and values can, in turn, support both individual and institutional transformation.

12.6 Conclusion

The goal of this chapter was to present current thinking about role-modeling and reflection and to stimulate our collective thinking about how these strategies might be incorporated into our faculty development practices to assist both teachers and learners.

Skills in role-modeling and reflection are important for effective teaching and learning. However, they are not easily acquired in short or one-time exposures alone, although these activities may be helpful in raising awareness. The literature suggests instead that such faculty development may be most effective when longitudinal opportunities for faculty members are also provided to enable them to acquire skills and to use those skills to reflect on their own teaching practice and experience. Further, this process can be enhanced when these activities occur in the context of groups which form communities that are supportive and share common values. The role of the institution in supporting such development emerges clearly.

Although the focus of the chapter has been on role-modeling and reflection in the context of teaching, the potential importance of these skills crosses all the aspects of faculty members' practices, including research and administration. Some suggested implications for practice have also been presented as principles which may guide the development of programs which are suited to the needs of our faculty members and the contexts of our institutions.

Preparing faculty members for role- modeling and reflective practice offers rich possibilities: for faculty members, it can provide an enhanced awareness of themselves as teachers and opportunities for personal and professional development; learners can benefit from their interactions with faculty members who encourage them to be reflective in their learning and development, and who use the power and process of role-modeling effectively; and institutions derive the benefits of the vitality that results from learning and growth among their members.

12.7   Key Messages

- Role modeling remains a significant influence on learners as they develop their professional identity.
- Faculty members can be helped to be more effective as role models through increased awareness of themselves as role models, an understanding of the standards and values they wish to transmit, and learning to use role modeling deliberately in their teaching.
- The influence of the institution is of critical importance in supporting and promoting effective role modeling. The goal is to create an environment that promotes optimal role modeling and student learning.
- Reflection and reflective practice are essential capabilities of competent professionals. Faculty members need support to develop these skills.
- Ability to reflect critically on one's experience as a teacher can result in changed teaching practices. It can also help faculty members to assist learners to use reflection for learning, and to learn from their experience throughout their practice.

Acknowledgements Grateful appreciation and thanks are extended to Dr. Anna Macleod for her feedback on an earlier version of this chapter, and to Dr. Yvonne Steinert, both for the invitation to write this chapter, and secondly, for her patience and thoughtful feedback as the ideas were developed.

References

Amundsen, C. & Wilson, M. (2012). Are we asking the right questions? A conceptual review of the educational development literature in higher education. *Review of Educational Research, 82*(1), 90–126.

Argyris, C. & Schön, D. A. (1974). *Theory in practice: Increasing professional effectiveness.* San Francisco, CA: Jossey Bass.

Aronson, L., Chittenden, E., & O'Sullivan, P. (2009). A faculty development workshop in teaching reflection. *Medical Education, 43*(5), 499.

Aronson, L., Kruidering, M., & O'Sullivan, P. S. (2012). The UCSF faculty development workshop on critical reflection in medical education: Training educators to teach and provide feedback on learners' reflections. MedEdPORTAL. Available from: www.mededportal.org/publication/9086

Bandura, A. (1986). *Social foundations of thought and action: A social cognitive theory.* Englewood Cliffs, NJ: Prentice Hall.

Bandura, A. (1997). *Self-efficacy: The exercise of control.* New York, NY: W. H. Freeman.

Bleakley, A., Bligh, J., & Browne, J. (2011). *Medical education for the future: Identity, power and location.* New York, NY: Springer.

Boerebach, B. C. M., Lombarts, K. M. J. M. H., Keijzer, C., Heineman, M. J., & Arah, O. A. (2012). The teacher, the physician and the person: How faculty's teaching performance influences their role modelling. *PLoS One, 7*(3), Art. e32089.

Boud, D., Keogh, R., & Walker, D. (1985). *Reflection: Turning experience into learning.* New York, NY: Nichols Publishing Company.

Boud, D. & Walker, D. (1998). Promoting reflection in professional courses: The challenge of context. *Studies in Higher Education, 23*(2), 191–206.

Braine, M. E. (2009). Exploring new nurse teachers' perception and understanding of reflection: An exploratory study. *Nurse Education in Practice*, *9*(4), 262–270.

Branch, W. T. Jr., Frankel, R., Gracey, C. F., Haidet, P. M., Weissmann, P. F., Cantey, P., et al. (2009). A good clinician and a caring person: Longitudinal faculty development and the enhancement of the human dimensions of care. *Academic Medicine*, *84*(1), 117–125.

Brookfield, S. (1995). *Becoming a critically reflective teacher*. San Francisco, CA: Jossey-Bass.

Cavanaugh, S. H. (2002). Professional caring in the curriculum. In G. Norman, C. P. van der Vleuten, and D. Newble. (Eds.), *International handbook of research in medical education*, (pp. 981–996). Dordrecht, NL: Kluwer Academic Publishers.

Collins, J. B. & Pratt, D. D. (2011). The teaching perspectives inventory at 10 years and 100,000 respondents: Reliability and validity of a teacher self-report inventory. *Adult Education Quarterly, 61*(4), 358–375.

Cook, V. (2009). Mapping the work-based learning of novice teachers: Charting some rich terrain. *Medical Teacher*, *31*(12), e608–e614.

Cooke, M., Irby, D. M., & O'Brien, B. C. (2010). *Educating physicians: A call for reform of medical school and residency*. San Francisco, CA: Jossey-Bass.

Cruess, S. R., Cruess, R. L., & Steinert, Y. (2008). Role-modelling: Making the most of a powerful teaching strategy. *BMJ, 336*(7646), 718–721.

Dekker-Groen, A. M., van der Schaaf, M. F., & Stokking, K. M. (2011). Teacher competences required for developing reflection skills of nursing students. *Journal of Advanced Nursing*, *67*(7), 1568–1579.

Dewey, J. (1933). *How we think*. Boston, MA: Heath.

Epstein, R. M. & Hundert, E. M. (2002). Defining and assessing professional competence. *JAMA*, *287*(2), 226–235.

Eraut, M. (2004). Informal learning in the workplace. *Studies in Continuing Education*, *26*(2), 247–273.

Frankford, D. M., Patterson, M. A., & Konrad, T. R. (2000). Transforming practice organizations to foster lifelong learning and commitment to medical professionalism. *Academic Medicine*, *75*(7), 708–717.

Goldie, J., Dowie, A., Cotton, P., & Morrison, J. (2007). Teaching professionalism in the early years of a medical curriculum: A qualitative study. *Medical Education*, *41*(6), 610–617.

Hafferty, F. W. & Franks, R. (1994). The hidden curriculum, ethics teaching, and the structure of medical education. *Academic Medicine*, *69*(11), 861–871.

Haidet, P., Hatem, D. S., Fecile, M. L., Stein, H. F., Haley, H. L., Kimmel, B., et al. (2008). The role of relationships in the professional formation of physicians: Case report and illustration of an elicitation technique. *Patient Education and Counseling*, *72*(3), 382–387.

Haidet, P., Kelly, P. A., & Chou, C.; Communication, Curriculum, and Culture Study Group. (2005). Characterizing the patient-centeredness of hidden curricula in medical schools: Development and validation of a new measure. *Academic Medicine*, *80*(1), 44–50.

Haidet, P. & Stein, H. F. (2006). The role of the student teacher relationship in the formation of physicians: The hidden curriculum as process. *Journal of General Internal Medicine*, *21*(Suppl. 1), S16–S20.

Higgins, S., Bernstein, L., Manning, K., Schneider, J., Kho, A., Brownfield, E., et al. (2011). Through the looking glass: How reflective learning influences the development of young faculty members. *Teaching and Learning in Medicine*, *23*(3), 238–243.

Hubball, H., Collins, J., & Pratt, D. (2005). Enhancing reflective teaching practices: Implications for faculty development programs. *The Canadian Journal of Higher Education*, *35*(3), 57–81.

Jochemson-van der Leeuw, H. G., van Dijk, N., van Etten-Jamaludin, F. S. & Wieringa-deWaard, M. (2013). The attributes of the clinical trainer as a role model: A systematic review. *Academic Medicine*, *88*(1), 26–34.

Kenny, N. P., Mann, K. V., & MacLeod, H. (2003). Role-modeling in physicians' professional formation: Reconsidering an essential but untapped educational strategy. *Academic Medicine*, *78*(12), 1203–1210.

Kolb, D. A. (1984). *Experiential learning: Experience as the source of learning and development*. Englewood Cliffs, NJ: Prentice-Hall.

Kowalski, K. (2008). Appreciative inquiry. *The Journal of Continuing Education in Nursing, 39*(3), 104.

Lave, J. & Wenger, E. (1991). *Situated learning: Legitimate peripheral participation.* Cambridge, UK: Cambridge University Press.

Mamede, S., Schmidt, H. D., & Penaforte, J. C. (2008). Effects of reflective practice on the accuracy of medical diagnoses. *Medical Education, 42*(5), 468–475.

Mann, K., Gordon, J., & MacLeod, A. (2009). Reflection and reflective practice in health professions education: A systematic review. *Advances in Health Sciences Education, 14*(4), 595–621.

Moon, J. A. (2004). *A handbook of reflective and experiential learning: Theory and practice.* London, UK: Routledge.

Moulton, C. A., Regehr, G., Mylopoulos, M., & MacRae, H. M. (2007). Slowing down when you should: A new model of expert judgment. *Academic Medicine, 82*(10 Suppl.), S109–S116.

O'Sullivan, P., Aronson, L., Chittenden, E., Niehaus, B., & Learman, L. (2010). Reflective ability rubric and user guide. MedEdPORTAL. Available from: www.mededportal.org/publication/8133

Park, J., Woodrow, S. I., Reznick, R. K., Beals, J., & MacRae, H. M. (2010). Observation, reflection, and reinforcement: Surgery faculty members' and residents' perceptions of how they learned professionalism. *Academic Medicine, 85*(1), 134–139.

Pinsky, L. E., & Irby, D. M. (1997). 'If at first you don't succeed': Using failure to improve teaching. *Academic Medicine, 72*(11), 973–976.

Pinsky, L. E., Monson, D., & Irby, D. M. (1998). How excellent teachers are made: Reflecting on success to improve teaching. *Advances in Health Sciences Education, 3*(3), 207–215.

Pratt, D. D. & Collins, J. B. (2013). *Teaching perspectives inventory.* Available from: http://www.teachingperspectives.com

Quaintance, J. L., Arnold, L., & Thompson, G. S. (2010). What students learn about professionalism from faculty stories: An 'appreciative inquiry' approach. *Academic Medicine, 85*(1), 118–123.

Riley, S. & Kumar, N. (2012). Teaching medical professionalism. *Clinical Medicine, 12*(1), 9–11.

Royal College of Physicians and Surgeons of Canada. (2012). CanMEDS. Retrieved July, 2012, from http://www.royalcollege.ca/portal/page/portal/rc/canmeds

Sargeant, J. M., Mann, K. V., van der Vleuten, C. P., & Metsemakers, J. F. (2009). Reflection: A link between receiving and using assessment feedback. *Advances in Health Sciences Education, 14*(3), 399–410.

Sargeant, J., McNaughton, E., Mercer, S., Murphy, D., Sullivan, P., Bruce, D.A. (2011). Providing feedback: Exploring a model (emotion, content, outcomes) for facilitating multisource feedback. *Medical Teacher, 33*(9), 744–749.

Schön, D. A. (1983). *The reflective practitioner: How professionals think in action.* New York, NY: Basic Books.

Schön, D. A. (1987). *Educating the reflective practitioner.* San Francisco, CA: Jossey-Bass.

Sfard, A. (1998). On two metaphors for learning and the dangers of choosing just one. *Educational Researcher, 27*(2), 4–13.

Steinert, Y., Cruess, S., Cruess R., & Snell, L. (2005). Faculty development for teaching and evaluating professionalism: From programme design to curriculum change. *Medical Education, 39*(2), 127–136.

Suchman, A. L., Williamson, P. R., Litzelman, D. K., Frankel, R. M., Mossbarger, D. L., & Inui, T. S. (2004). Toward an informal curriculum that teaches professionalism: Transforming the social environment of a medical school. *Journal of General Internal Medicine, 19*(5 Pt. 2), 501–504.

Wald, H. S., Borkan, J. M., Taylor, J. S., Anthony, D., & Reis, S. P. (2012). Fostering and evaluating reflective capacity in medical education: Developing the REFLECT rubric for assessing reflective writing. *Academic Medicine, 87*(1), 41–50.

Weissmann, P. F., Branch, W. T., Gracey, C. F., Haidet, P., & Frankel, R. M. (2006). Role-modeling humanistic behavior: Learning bedside manner from the experts. *Academic Medicine, 81*(7), 661–667.

Wright, S. M. & Carrese, J. A. (2002). Excellence in role-modelling: Insight and perspectives from the pros. *CMAJ, 167*(6), 638–643.

Chapter 13
Faculty Development for Curriculum Change: Towards Competency-Based Teaching and Assessment

Linda Snell

13.1 Introduction

As health care advances and knowledge of effective educational strategies evolves, curriculum renewal in health professions education is a given. Ensuring that faculty members can effectively function within a new curriculum implies that faculty development has a key role to play in curriculum change, at the individual, organizational and systems level. This chapter discusses the relationship between faculty development and curriculum change, and then uses the example of a move to a competency-based curriculum to illustrate how faculty development can help to bring about change at multiple levels.

There is a reciprocal relationship between new curricula and faculty development. Preparing faculty is a necessary adjunct to facilitate the design, implementation and evaluation of new curricula. As well, faculty development may drive change to a new curriculum, through creating a need or fostering a change in attitudes, increasing 'buy-in', or building capacity by improving knowledge or enhancing skills in a content area such that it can be taught better.

13.1.1 What Does Curriculum Change Include?

The term 'curriculum change' in this chapter is used to encompass curriculum renewal as well as the development or implementation of new curricula. Curriculum change can include the implementation of new curriculum models, the integration

L. Snell, MD, MHPE, FRCPC, FACP (✉)
Centre for Medical Education and Department of Medicine,
Faculty of Medicine, McGill University, Montreal, QC, Canada

Royal College of Physicians and Surgeons of Canada, Ottawa, ON, Canada
e-mail: linda.snell@mcgill.ca

Y. Steinert (ed.), *Faculty Development in the Health Professions: A Focus on Research and Practice*, Innovation and Change in Professional Education 11, DOI 10.1007/978-94-007-7612-8_13, © Springer Science+Business Media Dordrecht 2014

of new content areas, or explicitly teaching areas that were previously learned implicitly, situating learning in new contexts or including new faculty members in teaching. Examples of new curriculum models are competency- or outcomes-based approaches (Frank et al. 2010b) or technology-enhanced learning. New content areas might include explicit teaching about patient safety, professionalism, health advocacy or humanistic values. Examples of new contexts include moving learning to ambulatory settings, using simulation or developing a distributed education model. New faculty may include adding community-based supervisors or an inter-professional team as teachers. To add even more complexity, many of these changes may be undertaken as concurrent initiatives (Jolly 2002), so that identifying a specific faculty development need may be complicated.

13.1.2   What Are Faculty Members' Needs When New Curricula Are Implemented?

Faculty development activities can assist leaders, curriculum planners and health professions teachers prepare for change or respond to it effectively. Teachers might have to learn about new content areas, different roles for teachers or novel strategies for teaching, learning or assessment. Curriculum planners and leaders must become familiar with new curriculum models, educational planning and strategies to lead change (Jolly 2002; Steinert 2011b). They may also have to facilitate a change in faculty attitudes, such as supporting buy-in to a new system, or trying to encourage the 'unlearning' of entrenched teaching methods. Finally, faculty development can enhance educators' skills so that the impact of a new curriculum can be evaluated appropriately.

13.2   The Relationship Between Faculty Development and Curriculum Change

The published literature describing the relationship between faculty development and curriculum renewal in the health professions is scant. Most articles describe faculty development programs that support curriculum implementation; only a few address the use of faculty development to drive curriculum change. In addition, most of the articles outline activities to assist individual faculty members improve skills; a minority also discuss the issues relating to changes at the institutional or systems level (Dath and Iobst 2010; Farmer 2004; Jolly 2002).

13.2.1   New Curriculum Models and Faculty Development

In the past few decades, a number of new curriculum approaches have been introduced into health professions education. These have included problem-based methods, integrated models, outcomes-based education, spiral curricula, and longitudinal, community- or ambulatory-care-based and disseminated programs. These have been described briefly by Kusurkar et al. (2012) and Jolly (2002). Two models, problem-based learning and competency-based education, will be discussed in this section to illustrate how faculty development can be used to bring about curriculum change. The former, PBL, is now well established and lessons can be learned from the process of curriculum change. The latter, CBE, is gaining acceptance and provides a model for future application.

13.2.1.1   Faculty Development for Problem-Based Curricula

In the late twentieth century, many medical schools followed the recommendations of the GPEP Report (Physicians for the Twenty-First Century 1984) and other national reports, and developed new curricula that were more student-centered and focused on problems. The GPEP report recommended that faculty development be an integral part of curriculum renewal, and a few papers have reviewed the role of faculty development in these changes.

Grand'Maison and Des Marchais (1991) described a comprehensive faculty development approach to support the change to a problem-based learning (PBL) curriculum in Sherbrooke, Canada. Their faculty development program, which utilized a variety of formats and strategies, included a '2-day introductory workshop to initiate teachers into educational principles and their application in the new program, a 1-year basic training program in medical pedagogy requiring 100 h of participation, a 1-day workshop on PBL and a 3-day training program in PBL tutoring' (p. 557), followed by an annual 'refresher' course. The formats in the shorter programs included discussions, readings, individual work and assignments and experiential practice activities. The 1-year program included self-instructional modules with 'homework', regular small group discussions, and the opportunity to apply what had been learned. The major goals were to change faculty attitudes with an increased emphasis on the process of learning (as opposed to teaching), to encourage faculty members to learn the scientific basis of medical education and the knowledge and skills of teaching and learning, and to apply these to their daily teaching activities. Because of limited resources and local expertise at the onset, a systematic approach to development was taken. Outside experts trained a small group of locally-involved educators, then observed these faculty members as they provided faculty development activities and gave them constructive feedback. The local educators eventually implemented the programs independently. Faculty members who had a stronger background in education were encouraged to become 'mentors in the art of faculty development' and to be responsible for maintaining the quality of the programs. Those involved in implementing the new curriculum were invited to become instructors, with the strategic aim of increasing their expertise in education. There was a high attendance rate and a low attrition rate, perhaps in part attributable to the mandatory nature of the two introductory activities; that is, all faculty members wishing to teach were required to attend. The authors concluded that their faculty development programs, particularly the activities aimed at changing attitudes, 'had a significant impact on the successful shift from a traditional to a problem-based, small-group tutorial curriculum' (p. 561). They also commented that faculty activities must be continuous and tightly based on needs, and that activities to change attitudes must be initiated a long time before curriculum change is started. Developing a cadre of faculty members with broad expertise in education to act as faculty development instructors and as mentors contributed to the change. The lessons learned led them to believe 'that faculty development was… a prerequisite of curriculum change in medical schools' (p. 561).

Nayer (1995) reviewed faculty development initiatives in a change to problem-based learning curricula in seven medical schools. In each school, she found that the teacher (tutor) role in a PBL curriculum was more student-centered, and that this required a change in the orientation of faculty members. In this context, faculty development needed to do more than just develop the required skills; rather, it had to focus on the role of the teacher as well. Nayer also noted that, in the few faculty development programs that have been evaluated, faculty members changed attitudes and improved knowledge and gained teaching skills.

Farmer (2004) described a sequence for designing and implementing comprehensive faculty development programs for a change to a PBL curriculum. She outlined three stages of change: curriculum transition, curriculum implementation and curriculum advancement. In the first phase, programs presented the new curriculum approach and developed basic abilities such as PBL tutor skills and skills in case writing and assessment. Programs for the second phase enhanced teaching and assessment abilities. The final phase provided advanced training for teaching excellence. Within this three- stage sequence she outlines a number of strategies specifically addressing change in attitudes or culture. In the first phase, faculty members were given opportunities to understand the new curriculum approach. In the second, they were given opportunities for reflection and personal development. This was facilitated by allowing faculty members access to their teaching evaluations. In the final phase, teaching excellence was recognized, and as also mentioned by Licari (2007), appropriate rewards systems were developed. This included institutional recognition of leadership and scholarship activities associated with curriculum change. Farmer also points out that faculty development programs can have a positive effect on organizational culture as well as on individual faculty values.

The papers in this section describe in detail the systematic approaches to faculty development needed to implement PBL curricula. Overall, factors leading to faculty improvement in many of these studies included: (1) a multifaceted approach with varied faculty development strategies including longitudinal or modular programs starting early in the proposed curriculum change; (2) a mix of theoretical presentations, group work, practice sessions (microteaching), and experiential sessions such as role playing; and (3) a phased approach from novice to advanced content.

13.2.1.2 Faculty Development for Competency-Based Curricula

A more recent change in curriculum models has been the adoption of a competency-based approach. Competency-based education (CBE) has been defined as:

…an approach to preparing physicians for practice that is fundamentally oriented to graduate outcome abilities and organized around competencies derived from an analysis of societal and patient needs. It deemphasizes time-based training and promises greater
accountability, flexibility and learner-centeredness (Frank et al. 2010a, p. 636).

In a competency-based curriculum, fundamental competencies, often organized
in a framework, are taught, observed and assessed according to explicit criteria. In
CBE, the outcomes (competencies) are not isolated elements of knowledge or a skill
but rather integrate:

…multiple components … [of] knowledge, skills, values [or] attitudes that are applied in
practice. In CBE, learners assume greater responsibility for their own learning and assessment than in traditional approaches. Since competencies are observable, they can be measured and assessed and compared to a standard to ensure their acquisition and application.
Competencies can be assembled like building blocks to facilitate progressive development
(Frank et al. 2010b, p. 641).

Moreover, learners are expected to demonstrate their competence along a developmental continuum of milestones, and assessment focuses on criterion-referenced
direct observation.

Dath and Iobst (2010) have commented on the importance of faculty development in the transition to competency-based education. At the level of the individual,
teachers working within a CBE paradigm need faculty development to improve
their knowledge of CBE and the competencies being acquired, their facility in
teaching within this model and their ability to use new ways to assess learners. The
authors also noted the need for front-line teachers 'to understand, accept, teach, and
evaluate domains of practice [i.e. content areas, competencies] beyond medical
expertise' (p. 685). Medical teachers who were not explicitly taught according to
these competencies during their own training need to learn to teach them to their
learners. At the level of the institution, Dath and Iobst (2010) noted the utility of
faculty development to address resistance to change. At the systems level, faculty
development activities can improve understanding of, and confidence in, CBE
principles, to 'pave the way' for new credentialing and accreditation processes. The
authors described an example of system-level engagement, concurrent with the
introduction of the CanMEDS framework in Canada in 1996 (Frank and Danoff
2007), where faculty development was included as one of the requirements of
implementation. Dath and Iobst (2010) also described university-based and national
faculty-oriented initiatives, including workshops and presentations-on-demand,
each supported by a group of specifically trained national clinician educators and
extensive online and print resources. A more formal national 'train-the-trainer'
workshop series served to educate and promote local 'champions' for the various
competencies at each medical school in Canada. As well as providing content about
a specific competency, the series included practice in educational design to help
local champions understand how best to provide faculty development at their own
institutions. The authors conclude that the transition to a CBE approach may be
slow; however, they suggest that an approach to faculty development aimed at institutions and systems, as well as at individuals, may facilitate the adoption of a
competency-based curriculum. This approach should include a number of methods,

using multiple formats and enlisting 'early adopters', demonstrating how faculty members can identify fundamental competencies in their own practice and then explaining how to teach and assess them.

13.2.2   Addressing Attitudes, Buy-In, Resistance and Organizational Culture Change

When implementing curriculum change, faculty members may need to become more enthusiastic about the change or be more motivated to move away from what may be firmly entrenched teaching or assessment approaches or curriculum models. They may also fear a 'loss of control' or become antagonistic to change (Farmer 2004). Faculty development activities must therefore not only address skills acquisition needed for new curricula, but also tackle a change in attitudes and organizational culture (Carraccio et al. 2002).

Lanphear and Cardiff (1987) noted that curriculum renewal can be threatening to faculty members, who may resist the change or simply refuse to adopt it. They described a multistep program to facilitate the change to a longitudinal pathology curriculum that emphasized problem-solving and independent learning. The program included organizational development, instructional development and faculty development. They suggest that one of the first steps in curriculum change is to bring faculty members into active participation early in the change process. In their case, this involved including all stakeholders and constituencies in the decision-making process about the new curriculum, soliciting objectives from all teachers, and requiring regular performance reports. These activities gave faculty members a sense of involvement in decision-making and in the direction and amount of progress towards the curriculum change. The second step was the institution of training in the teaching methods required by the new curriculum. In this step, faculty members also contributed their own ideas into the curriculum goals and process. The final step gave faculty members the opportunity to clarify their priorities for teaching and professional roles, and included activities that addressed, for example, personal growth, conflict resolution and career planning. The institution of these steps led to a curriculum change solidly anchored in the attitudes and philosophy of the department, and allowed the faculty to 'make a success of a new curriculum because they could claim it as their own' (p. 491).

Based on these studies, it would appear that one of the early stages of curriculum change should be to focus on addressing the organizational culture and ensuring that there is faculty understanding of the need for change. In this context, Zaidi et al. (2010) found that a facilitator training workshop associated with a move to a problem-based learning curriculum did not just improve faculty members' teaching skills but also stimulated their interest in the curriculum and in a student-centered approach; it also increased their desire to be facilitators.

Curriculum change and the associated faculty development process must also 'become a core value of the school's culture' (Licari 2007). In addition to the standard instructional development activities, Licari suggested that the development of a reward system for faculty members to encourage new curriculum development and innovation be considered. For example, providing faculty with 'incentives, time to plan, credit for development of learning experiences, rewards and recognition for innovative teaching' (p. 1510), and even recognition of these activities for promotion and tenure, may serve to foster culture change. As Licari eloquently stated 'programs need to help faculty members navigate from the current steady state of a traditional curriculum through the unknown white-water rapids inevitably created by curriculum change' (p. 1509).

In this section, we have underscored the role of faculty development programs in focusing on changing attitudes and organizational values to facilitate the smooth implementation of new curricula. Effective programs have involved faculty members at the onset, initiated faculty development activities early in the change process, used multiple strategies to recognize faculty contributions to change, and addressed culture change at an individual and at an institutional level.

13.2.3   Leading a Curriculum Change

Curriculum renewal implies the need for individuals to lead the change, and faculty development programs have the potential to prepare current or future leaders to implement new curricula. A number of authors have noted the need to address leadership skills with specific faculty development activities (Farmer 2004; Jolly 2002; Steinert 2011a; Swanwick 2008).

In 2002, Jolly, in reviewing the literature on faculty development for curriculum implementation, identified the need for developing a strong leadership to sustain and support new curriculum strategies. In the third phase of her faculty development program, Farmer (2004) also highlights the need to nurture leadership skills. She suggests that teaching curriculum leaders about Complex Adaptive Systems (CAS) theory may facilitate change.

Swanwick (2008) notes that the institution of faculty development activities requires 'effective and sympathetic leadership from postgraduate training institutions, hospitals and health authorities' (p. 339). He also comments on the need for the development of management and leadership skills for those leading educational change. In Chap. 3, Swanwick and McKimm describe a number of faculty development content areas and strategies to enhance leadership skills, many of which are highly relevant to leading curriculum change.

These concepts are underscored by Steinert (2011b) who has noted that faculty development can serve to promote organizational change in a number of ways. In addition to achieving more 'traditional' faculty development goals such as implementing the change and enhancing organizational capacities, it can help to build consensus and generate support and enthusiasm, Similarly, Lanphear and Cardiff (1987) described specific features and actions of leaders that facilitated a curriculum change. These included explicit support of the change by departmental chairs, engagement of faculty members in the change process, effective communication skills, focused appointment of education experts, and effective management of conflict and change. Many of the factors and skills described by Lanphear and Cardiff (1987) and Steinert (2011b) are 'learnable' and could be addressed in a faculty development program for those leading change.

13.2.4 Enhancing Research Skills Related to Curriculum Change

In order to fully understand curriculum change, it should be evaluated. Faculty development activities can also be used to enhance faculty scholars' education research skills so that they can evaluate the impact of a new curriculum. Examples of these skills include applying an educational research design or methodology, using a valid program evaluation model such as that described by Musick (2006), or developing needs assessment tools or program evaluation measures to assess process or outcomes. Research on curriculum change can enhance our knowledge about curriculum in general, defining needs, teaching and learning strategies, and assessment methods. As well, the resulting evaluations of new curricula can guide decisions about further curriculum change.

13.3 Twenty-First Century Curricula, Competencies and the Need for Faculty Development

Health professions education curricula have evolved over the past few decades, with the adoption of outcomes-based approaches to curricula and an increased emphasis on the use of competency frameworks at all levels of medical education. Competency-based curriculum approaches have been implemented at both undergraduate and graduate levels in a number of health professions. This curriculum approach builds on the evolution of our understanding of competence. In pure CBE, fundamental competencies are learned outside of a time-based framework. Assessment focuses on direct observation, using explicit criteria over developmental stages (Holmboe et al. 2010).

Faculty development is essential to fostering this curriculum change. It can enhance the acquisition of content for teaching fundamental competencies (e.g. leadership, health advocacy, professionalism) that may previously have been learned implicitly by faculty teachers. As well, it can foster the development of potentially unfamiliar teaching and assessment skills (e.g. explicit role modeling, fostering reflection, using portfolios, using simulation methods for intrinsic roles).

In the rest of this chapter, the implementation of a competency-based model and the teaching and assessment of fundamental competencies will be used to illustrate the importance of faculty development for curriculum change. However, many of the principles described above apply equally well to other curriculum initiatives.

13.3.1 Contemporary Competency Frameworks and Content Areas

Examples of contemporary competency frameworks that have been adopted in a number of constituencies include *The Scottish Doctor* (Simpson et al. 2002), the US *ACGME Competencies* (Swing 2007), the National Undergraduate Framework in the Netherlands (Laan et al. 2010) and the *CanMEDS 2005 Physician Competency Framework* (Frank and Danoff 2007). Other similar frameworks have also been implemented in nursing, physiotherapy and occupational therapy (Verma et al. 2006). Although each framework is slightly different, the metacompetencies or 'roles' in most frameworks include some variation of (clinical) expertise, problem solving, health advocacy/prevention, communication skills, teamwork/collaboration, leadership and management, teaching skills, life-long learning, critical appraisal and professionalism (Verma et al. 2009). The competencies other than clinical expertise have been called the 'intrinsic roles' in that they are 'inherent, fundamental or essential to the practice of medicine, integrated with each other and the Medical Expert Role' (Sherbino et al. 2011, p. 697).

These competency frameworks comprise complex 'metacompetencies' that are divided into component parts, which are learned over time with milestones or markers along the way. Competencies have been described as multi-dimensional, dynamic, developmental, and contextual in nature, integrating knowledge, skills and behaviors in practice (Frank et al. 2010b; Snell and Frank 2010).

One of the most frequently-used approaches is the CanMEDS (Canadian Medical Education Directions for Specialists) framework, now adopted in over two dozen jurisdictions worldwide, in medicine at the medical school and residency level, as well as in nursing, occupational therapy, physical therapy, medical radiation technology, social work, psychology, midwifery and other health professions (Royal College of Physicians and Surgeons of Canada, Ottawa: unpublished data, 2013). Some of these programs have adopted pure competency-based models, such as the University of Toronto Orthopedics residency (Wadey et al. 2009) and the Cleveland Clinic undergraduate medical program (Dannefer and Henson 2007). The CanMEDS framework is perhaps successful because it has educational utility and was derived from a systematic needs assessment that included the perspectives of the public on what they hoped their physicians would model (Frank and Danoff 2007).

13.3.2 Innovative Approaches for Teaching and Assessing Fundamental Competencies

Although these fundamental competencies have been recognized for years as essential areas for learners in all health professions education contexts, they have usually been acquired tacitly through work-based learning and have not been assessed specifically. In fact, only recently have they started to be taught explicitly and assessed formally. With a move to competency-based education, this will become even more formalized, with the content better defined and a need for objective assessment of actual performance, milestones and outcomes.

CBE provides a clear description of intended outcomes rather than suggesting particular learning strategies or formats. However, many of the competencies, particularly the intrinsic ones beyond medical expertise (e.g. communication skills, teamwork, leadership skills, health advocacy, professionalism, as described in Sherbino et al. 2011), place an emphasis on skills, behaviors and attitude change rather than solely on knowledge acquisition. These competencies are often not effectively acquired using traditional teaching strategies such as didactic methods alone. As well, work-based learning alone is not considered to be adequate for the acquisition of these abilities. A change in approach to learning is implicit in a change to a competency-based curriculum. There will need to be increased attention to student-centeredness and flexibility, for example by providing outcomes (either milestones or abilities of graduates), and then allowing the learner to select from a number of routes (learning strategies) to acquire a competency. As well, there should be alignment of learning activities with assessment and a more active engagement of teachers in assessment by direct observation. Finally, there is a spiral development of concepts, knowledge, and skills, delineated by milestones along the way to full acquisition of competence (Harris et al. 2010). As can be imagined, this philosophical approach may not be familiar to most faculty members, who will need to understand, accept and be comfortable with this new paradigm.

To address this change, a number of emerging or innovative educational approaches have evolved, each thought to be effective for learning or assessing one or more of the fundamental competencies. These include, for example, teaching techniques to promote reflection, explicit role modeling (Cruess et al. 2008), simulation methods, team-based learning, and OSTEs (objective structured teaching exercises) (Boillat et al. 2012). Newer formative and summative assessment methods include the mini-CEX, work-based assessment methods such as direct observation and formative feedback, multisource feedback and the use of portfolios (Holmboe et al. 2010; Iobst et al. 2010). As well, many faculty members or clinical supervisors may not be familiar with some of the content of these competencies, which they may have learned implicitly, and as a result they may not have a 'vocabulary' or framework to teach them. They may also not be comfortable with using the range of teaching or assessment approaches described here. More importantly, some faculty members may not 'buy-in' to either the competency framework or even to the need to teach the competencies explicitly (Snell and Frank 2010).

13.3.3   Strategies for Faculty Development in CBE

For those moving towards a CBE approach, or implementing explicit teaching of fundamental competencies beyond that of medical expertise, it has been proposed that many of the challenges to meeting expectations of a competency-based

Table 13.1 Effective faculty development formats and strategies for a move to competency-based education

Formats
Workshops and other small group activities
Short courses
Longitudinal programs
Self-instructional modules, including on-line formats
Lectures and other didactic activities
Strategies
Simulation methods, such as OSTEs
Peer mentoring
Experiential learning
Role-play
Practical sessions, such as microteaching (practice with observation and immediate feedback)
Reflective exercises

curriculum can be addressed with faculty development (Holmboe and Snell 2011). Faculty development may serve a number of roles. It facilitates the design of novel curricula in which to learn desired competencies. As well, faculty development programs can teach teachers and supervisors about the content of the competencies and how to use teaching and assessment approaches effectively. At an institution or systems level, faculty development activities can encourage buy-in, develop faculty development leaders, evaluate the success of new curricula, and promote further curriculum change.

Faculty development can address both the competency (the content) and the educational methods (the process) (Dath and Iobst 2010; Scheele et al. 2008). For instance, commonly-used faculty development strategies such as workshops, short courses and experiential activities like OSTEs (Objective Structured Teaching Activities; Boillat et al. 2012) can combine teaching of both. This has some advantages, as many teachers may not attend a pure 'content'-based faculty development session (saying, for example, 'I already know about teamwork'), yet they will attend a combined session (such as one on 'faculty development for teaching and assessing collaborator skills'). An example is the CanMEDS Train-the-Trainer series (e.g. Cruess et al. 2009; Snell et al. 2010), 2- to 3-day workshops which teach advanced content about a single CanMEDS competency (such as Health Advocate). At the same time, these workshops provide skills in faculty development, such as using the education cycle, workshop planning and implementation, and program evaluation. Other faculty development strategies and formats discussed elsewhere in this volume include on-line learning, role modeling, mentoring, and peer coaching. These have not been discussed much in the literature as it pertains to faculty development for CBE, but many strategies could reasonably be used to teach faculty members, as listed in Table 13.1.

Given that most competencies are not acquired by learners at a single moment but developed over time, it makes sense to consider a progressive/longitudinal and integrated faculty development approach for teachers (Steinert 2011b). This has systems and policy implications, as a change to a competency-based curriculum, with new roles for teachers and students and greater involvement of faculty, implies a significant investment in faculty development (Taber et al. 2010).

13.4   A Proposed Model

Throughout this chapter, three elements of faculty development for curriculum change have been discussed: the 'content' (i.e. what the learner – and sometimes the teacher – has to learn; the 'process' (i.e. how the student learns and is assessed on the content); and the faculty development formats and strategies (i.e. how to teach the teachers the content and process). One could think of these three elements on three axes, each in a different direction, forming a cube, as in Fig. 13.1.

Two examples of this model are given. In the first example, shown in Fig. 13.2, a student is learning competencies within the CanMEDS competency framework, so the 'content' includes the seven CanMEDS Roles. The clinical student can learn these competencies in a number of ways (i.e. the 'process'), through observing role models, reflection or discussion of case vignettes; he or she can also learn these competencies both in the workplace and using simulation approaches. For the specific competency of communication skills, the student can attend mandatory activities in a simulation-based environment, with practice communicating in varied simulation scenarios. The student is debriefed following the scenario and reflects on the skills learned. Faculty members design the scenarios and act as debriefers. For teachers new to simulation scenario design, an effective form of faculty development would be peer mentoring. In this case, an experienced designer would assist a new teacher to develop communication scenarios at the appropriate level.

In the second example, pictured in Fig. 13.3, residents are being assessed on the ACGME competencies (the 'content'). A number of new or evolving potential

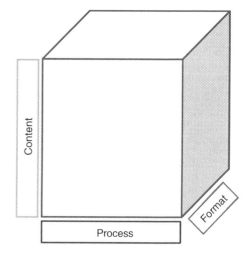

Fig. 13.1 Three-dimensional model relating the *Content* (WHAT trainees learn or are assessed on), *Process* (HOW trainees learn/are assessed), and faculty development *Format* or strategy (HOW faculty members learn Content or Process)

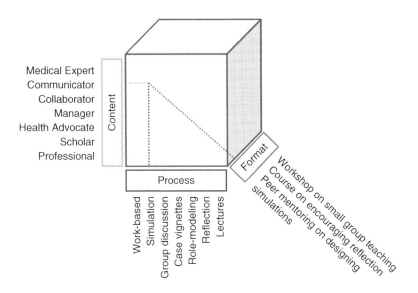

Fig. 13.2 Example of model using the CanMEDS competency framework and common learning strategies at the student level

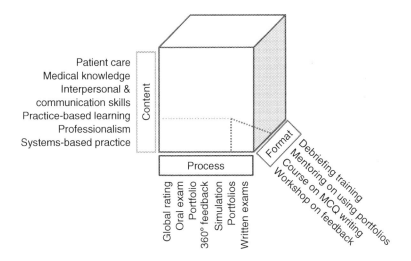

Fig. 13.3 Example of model using the ACGME competency framework and common assessment strategies at the resident level

assessment methods (i.e. the 'process') are used. The resident may be required to keep a portfolio to demonstrate achievement of competence in Practice-Based Learning. Faculty members may need instruction in the use of portfolios as an assessment tool. This might be done through mentoring or through a workshop on encouraging reflection using portfolios.

This model should not be thought of as static. Competencies are learned and assessed within an institution or system, where new teaching strategies and assessment tools are implemented and the curricula in which these competencies are learned evolve. There are also a number of other factors or variables that are too complex to depict in a static diagram. For example the 'size' of the small cubes within the big cube may vary depending on the emphasis of the content within the curriculum, the frequency with which the teaching or assessment method is used, or the acceptability of the faculty development method.. Another variable is the 'level' of the faculty development initiatives, and whether they are aimed at novice or advanced teachers.

From a practical perspective, this model can be used as a 'blueprint' by a faculty developer who wants to ensure that their faculty can teach and assess each competency. The specific competency and the desired teaching or assessment processes are identified. A faculty development strategy is chosen to match these. On the other hand, a new teaching or assessment strategy which might be applicable to more than one competency can be taught. During the faculty development activity, examples can be drawn from relevant 'matching' competencies.

13.5   A Case Study

In this section, the fundamental competency of professionalism is examined as a case study. The goal is to illustrate best practices for providing faculty development both to enhance teaching and assessment and to promote curriculum change. In the essential area of professionalism, a learner must acquire core knowledge, apply this knowledge in progressively more realistic contexts, and develop and express behaviors that reflect professional practice (Steinert et al. 2007). Faculty members who teach professionalism must be able to explicitly 'articulate its core concepts and demonstrate appropriate behaviors. This requires that faculty development should start with [learning] a cognitive base that includes the definition of professionalism, its historical roots, its relationship to the ever-changing social contract between medicine and society, and the obligations necessary to sustain professional status. 'New' teaching strategies for professionalism may include activities that will promote self-reflection, awareness and change in the learner. Finally, professionalism must be evaluated in a valid and reliable fashion' (Steinert et al. 2005, p. 128), and faculty members must learn new assessment methods.

13.5.1   *Teaching and Assessing Professionalism*
at McGill University

The increasing emphasis on professionalism in medicine motivated the Faculty of Medicine at McGill University to introduce formal teaching about the competency of professionalism at both the undergraduate and residency level. This teaching starts on the first day of medical school and is built sequentially through the undergraduate and postgraduate program, reinforcing the same concepts and allowing application to the appropriate level and context of the learner as their professional identity is formed.

Although the teaching strategies include didactic methods to transmit core knowledge, most of the learning occurs in small groups or in the clinical context and workplace, and much of it is longitudinal in nature as professional identity is formed over time. Learning occurs in multiple settings: in classrooms, using simulation, integrated within various preclinical and clinical experiences, and during resident workplace learning. A flagship course in the undergraduate medical program is the 'Physician Apprenticeship' where groups of six students meet regularly with the same faculty member, a practicing physician, over the entire 4 years of the undergraduate curriculum (Steinert et al. 2010). All individuals who come into contact with students need to use the same definitions and vocabulary and be aware that they are role models. The 'importance of residents in the learning experience of medical students led to the recognition that further education of residents as role models was required' (Steinert et al. 2007, p. 1063). A faculty-wide half day on professionalism is held annually for all 2nd-year residents, to reinforce the concepts of professionalism and to emphasize their role as models of professional behavior. In all these learning activities, the same cognitive base is taught and the same 'vocabulary' is built.

The assessment of professionalism is equally important. As a result, the principles and attributes of professionalism that are taught are also assessed, both in the learners and in the faculty and resident teachers (Todhunter et al. 2011). More recently, the MMI (multiple-mini-interview) method used for student selection has included assessing for professional attributes and behaviors in entering students.

The goal overall is to lead to a 'culture change', with faculty members not just teaching and assessing professionalism, but also demonstrating exemplary professionalism.

13.5.2   Faculty Development for Professionalism at the Teacher Level

From the outset of the curriculum change, an iterative process of faculty development activities (e.g. working groups, workshops, medical education rounds and skill building sessions) was aimed at the faculty members in general and at teachers with specific roles, as described by Steinert et al. (2005, 2007). This allowed for input from the faculty and buy-in, as well as building faculty capacity for teaching and assessing professionalism. For example, a series of faculty development workshops that mirrored the students' work was provided to prepare and support the Physician Apprenticeship faculty preceptors (Steinert et al. 2010). For any interested faculty member, activities to increase knowledge, provide a common vocabulary and improve specific skills (e.g. role modeling, feedback) were provided. The concurrent student learning and faculty development programs are linked and have

Table 13.2 Faculty development for the competency of Professionalism, at the individual learner and teacher level[a]

Learner knowledge and skills	Learning strategies	Assessment strategies	Faculty knowledge, skills & attitudes needed	Faculty development activities & strategies
Core knowledge of professionalism	Lecture Small group discussion	Written exams	Professionalism principles; core knowledge, 'vocabulary'	Working groups & workshops on core knowledge Workshops on small group facilitation
Application in progressively realistic contexts	Case vignettes discussed in groups. Simulated patients	OSCE	Facilitation skills for small groups Simulation debriefing OSCE case development	Workshops on small group facilita- tion using vignettes Courses on debriefing Course on OSCE development
Development of professional behaviors and demonstration in practice	Experiential (work- based) learning Reflection Role models	Direct observation/ feedback Portfolios	Observation and feedback skills Facilitating reflection Role modeling	Feedback workshop Workshops on reflection, use of narrative Role modeling workshop

[a]This table shows the link between what the learners must learn, what the teachers must teach and assess, and how faculty development can foster this

included activities as outlined in Table 13.2. In this table the content for the student or resident can be learned and assessed using different strategies. The faculty must possess knowledge or skills to do this, and there are specific faculty development strategies and activities that can facilitate this.

13.5.3   Faculty Development at the Systems Level

Selected faculty members involved in leading curriculum change or evaluating its success also needed skills in these areas. As a result, a 4-day leadership development program was developed and activities to develop program evaluation and educational research skills were offered. Residency program directors participated in focused activities aimed at improving their skills in recognizing all fundamental competencies, designing relevant curricula, and implementing appropriate assessment methods. The faculty leaders were very supportive of both the curriculum change and the faculty development program. Table 13.3 depicts the link between the organization or system goals, the changes needed in faculty to achieve these goals, and the faculty development activities that facilitated this.

Table 13.3 Faculty development for the competency of professionalism, at the institution and systems level

Institutional goal	Faculty knowledge, skills & attitudes needed	Faculty development activities & strategies
Selection of professional traits in entering trainees using multiple mini-interviews (MMI)	MMI construction	MMI station development training
Ensuring faculty buy-in, motivation, consensus and knowledge	Ensuring faculty buy-in and motivation	'Think tanks' on teaching & assessing professionalism
	Ensuring consensus on content, teaching & assessment strategies; stimulating discussion about feasibility	Invitational workshops on teaching & on assessing professionalism
	Developing a group of skilled, knowledgeable faculty members	Faculty-wide workshops on teaching & on assessing professionalism
Provide skills to program directors	Knowledge about core competencies	Focused day-long workshops on teaching and assessing core competencies, curriculum development, developing and using new assessment tools
	Curriculum models	
	Assessment tools	
Evaluation of curriculum change & faculty development initiatives	Education research skills	Peer mentoring and capacity building sessions for education research and program evaluation methods
Developing leaders for change	Leadership skills, change management skills	Faculty leadership development program

13.5.4   Results of the Faculty Development Program

The evaluation of the various faculty development components showed that the faculty members were:

> … able to expand their teaching of professionalism, in part because they had become more knowledgeable about the cognitive base underlying professionalism, strategies for teaching this subject matter, and methods of evaluation. Secondly, the initiative allowed the medical school to agree on the cognitive base of professionalism, the attributes and characteristics of a professional, and the behaviors to be encouraged in students, residents and faculty (Steinert et al. 2005, p. 134).

It also led to the development of better methods of evaluating professional behavior. Finally, the initiative showed that faculty development can be a powerful tool in initiating and setting the direction for curriculum change. This initiative raised awareness, channeled the faculty's efforts and stimulated desire for curriculum change and reform. 'Many of the educational initiatives currently underway would probably not have occurred as rapidly, or in their current form, without both the stimulus and the direction of this program' (Steinert et al. 2005, pp. 134–135). The specific faculty development program for the Physician Apprenticeship preceptors:

... increased teachers' perceptions of connection (and reconnection) to teaching, medical education, core professional values, and colleagues. It also demonstrated the benefits of a longitudinal faculty development course, rooted in both situated and work-based learning, which mirrored the students' experiences and helped to promote a community of practice (Steinert et al. 2010, p. 1248).

13.6   Conclusion

In this chapter, we have highlighted the link between faculty development and curriculum change and used a case study to illustrate a number of 'best practices'. As we noted, there is a reciprocal relationship between curriculum change and faculty development. Faculty development can be used as a tool to engage the faculty in curriculum change and promote capacity building. Curriculum change can, and probably should, be a 'bottom-up' as well as a 'top-down' process. Some aspects of curriculum change might be viewed as more 'difficult' to implement (e.g. implementing teaching about health advocacy frequently provokes resistance to change). Engaging faculty members early in the change process is essential to promote buy-in; it can also assist in developing applicable tools for teaching and assessing learners and in educating faculty about their use. Faculty development is important for attitude change and consensus-building around change. Second, programs should address faculty needs; in a curriculum change, these needs may include education about unfamiliar content and curriculum models as well as about teaching and assessment methods. Third, skill building must go beyond teaching and assessment: leadership, change management and education scholarship must also be addressed. Support from leaders is important, but developing new leaders with the skills to lead change is equally so. Finally, faculty development in the context of curriculum change can have effects on the organization or system. The case study is an example of faculty development leading to change as well as supporting it. It illustrates what Steinert et al. (2007) noted; in the context of curriculum change or renewal, faculty development 'can help to build consensus, generate support and enthusiasm, and implement a change initiative; it can also help to change the culture within the institution by altering the formal, informal, and hidden curricula' (p. 1057). In fact, as Jolly has stated: 'Modifying a curriculum is likely to be difficult. Without faculty development, it may well be impossible' (p. 945).

13.7   Key Messages

- There is a reciprocal relationship between curriculum change and faculty development. Faculty development is a tool to both engage the faculty in curriculum change and to promote capacity building.
- Faculty members should be engaged early in the curriculum change process to promote buy-in, to develop tools for teaching and assessment of learners, and to educate faculty about their use.

- Faculty development programs should address content that may be unfamiliar to faculty members. It can also assist faculty understand and use new curriculum approaches.
- Skill building should also address leadership abilities, change management and education scholarship.
- Faculty development is important for attitude change and consensus-building around change.
- Faculty development in the context of curriculum change can have effects on the organization or system.

References

Boillat, M., Bethune, C., Ohle, E., Razack, S., & Steinert, Y. (2012). Twelve tips for using the Objective Structured Teaching Exercise for faculty development. *Medical Teacher, 34*(4), 269–273.

Carraccio, C., Wolfsthal, S. D., Englander, R., Ferentz, K., & Martin, C. (2002). Shifting paradigms: From Flexner to competencies. *Academic Medicine, 77*(5), 361–367.

Cruess, R. L., Cruess, S. R., Kearney, R., Snell, L., & Steinert, Y. (2009). *CanMEDS Train-the-Trainer (TTT) Program on Professionalism.* Ottawa, ON: The Royal College of Physicians and Surgeons of Canada.

Cruess, S. R., Cruess, R. L., & Steinert, Y. (2008). Role modeling: Making the most of a powerful teaching strategy. *BMJ, 336*(7646), 718–721.

Dath, D. & Iobst, W. (2010). The importance of faculty development in the transition to competency-based medical education. *Medical Teacher, 32*(8), 683–686.

Dannefer, E. F. & Henson, L. C. (2007). The portfolio approach to competency-based assessment at the Cleveland Clinic Lerner College of Medicine. *Academic Medicine, 82*(5), 493–502.

Farmer, E. A. (2004). Faculty development for problem-based learning. *European Journal of Dental Education, 8*(2), 59–66.

Frank, J. R. & Danoff, D. (2007). The CanMEDS initiative: Implementing an outcomes-based framework of physician competencies. *Medical Teacher, 29*(7), 642–647.

Frank, J. R., Mungroo, R., Ahmad, Y., Wang, M., De Rossi, S., & Horsley, T. (2010a). Toward a definition of competency-based education in medicine: A systematic review of published definitions. *Medical Teacher, 32*(8), 631–637.

Frank, J. R., Snell, L. S., Ten Cate, O., Holmboe, E. S., Carraccio, C., Swing, S. R., et al. (2010b). Competency-based medical education: Theory to practice. *Medical Teacher, 32*(8), 638–645.

Grand'Maison, P. & Des Marchais, J. E. (1991). Preparing faculty to teach in a problem-based learning curriculum: The Sherbrooke experience. *CMAJ, 144*(5), 557–562.

Harris, P., Snell, L., Talbot, M., & Harden, R. M. (2010). Competency-based medical education: Implications for undergraduate programs. *Medical Teacher, 32*(8), 646–650.

Holmboe, E. S., Sherbino, J., Long, D. M., Swing, S. R., & Frank, J. R. (2010). The role of assessment in competency-based medical education. *Medical Teacher, 32*(8), 676–682.

Holmboe, E. S. & Snell, L. (2011). Principles of competency-based education: Better preparation of learners for practice. In J. Sherbino & J. Frank (Eds.), *Educational design: A CanMEDS guide for the health professions,* (pp. 7–12). Ottawa, ON: The Royal College of Physicians and Surgeons of Canada.

Iobst, W. F., Sherbino, J., Ten Cate, O., Richardson, D. L., Dath, D., Swing, S. R., et al. (2010). Competency-based medical education in postgraduate medical education. *Medical Teacher, 32*(8), 651–656.

Jolly, B. C. (2002). Faculty development for curriculum implementation. In G. Norman, C. van der Vleuten, & D. Newble (Eds.), *International handbook of research in medical education,* (pp. 945–967). Dordrecht, NL: Kluwer Academic Publishers.

Kusurkar, R. A., Croiset, G., Mann, K. V., Custers, E., & Ten Cate, O. (2012). Have motivation theories guided the development and reform of medical education curricula? A review of the literature. *Academic Medicine, 87*(6), 735–743.

Laan, R. F. J. M., Leunissen, R. R. M., & van Herwaarden, C. L. A. (on behalf of the Project Group). (2010). The 2009 framework for undergraduate medical education in the Netherlands. *GMS Zeitschrift für Medizinische Ausbildung, 27*(2), Doc35. Available from: http://www.ncbi. nlm.nih.gov/pmc/articles/PMC3140367/

Lanphear, J. H. & Cardiff, R. D. (1987). Faculty development: An essential consideration in curriculum change. *Archives of Pathology & Laboratory Medicine, 111*(5), 487–491.

Licari, F. W. (2007). Faculty development to support curriculum change and ensure the future vitality of dental education. *Journal of Dental Education, 71*(12), 1509–1512.

Musick, D. W. (2006). A conceptual model for program evaluation in graduate medical education. *Academic Medicine, 81*(8), 759–765.

Nayer, M. (1995). Faculty development for problem-based learning programs. *Teaching & Learning in Medicine, 7*(3), 138–148.

Physicians for the Twenty First Century. (1984) *The GPEP report: Report of the Panel on the General Professional Education of the Physician and College Preparation for Medicine.* Washington, DC: Association of American Medical Colleges.

Scheele, F., Teunissen, P., Van Luijk, S., Heineman, E., Fluit, L., Mulder, H., et al. (2008). Introducing competency-based postgraduate medical education in the Netherlands. *Medical Teacher, 30*(3), 248–253.

Sherbino, J., Frank, J., Flynn, L., & Snell, L. (2011). 'Intrinsic Roles' rather than 'armour': Renaming the 'non-medical expert roles' of the CanMEDS framework to match their intent. *Advances in Health Sciences Education, 16*(5), 695–697.

Simpson, J. G., Furnace, J., Crosby, J., Cumming, A. D., Evans, P. A., Friedman Ben-David, M., et al. (2002). The Scottish doctor – Learning outcomes for the medical undergraduate in Scotland: A foundation for competent and reflective practitioners. *Medical Teacher, 24*(2), 136–143.

Snell, L. S. & Frank, J. R. (2010). Competencies, the tea bag model, and the end of time. *Medical Teacher, 32*(8), 629–630.

Snell, L.S., Mann, K., Bhanji, F., Dandavino, M., Frank, J. R., LeBlanc, C., et al. (2010). *Resident teaching STARs: Improving residents' skills as teachers. A CanMEDS scholar role Train-the-Trainer Program.* Ottawa, ON: The Royal College of Physicians and Surgeons of Canada.

Steinert, Y. (2011a). Commentary: Faculty development: The road less traveled. *Academic Medicine, 86*(4), 409–411.

Steinert, Y. (2011b). *Faculty development for postgraduate education: The road ahead.* The Future of Medical Education in Canada: Postgraduate Project. Retrieved July 10th, 2012, from http:// www.afmc.ca/pdf/fmec/21_Steinert_Faculty%20Development.pdf

Steinert, Y., Boudreau, J. D., Boillat, M., Slapcoff, B., Dawson, D., Briggs, A., et al. (2010). The Osler Fellowship: An apprenticeship for medical educators. *Academic Medicine, 85*(7), 1242–1249.

Steinert, Y., Cruess, R. L., Cruess, S. R., Boudreau, J. D., & Fuks, A. (2007). Faculty development as an instrument of change: A case study on teaching professionalism. *Academic Medicine, 82*(11), 1057–1064.

Steinert, Y., Cruess, S., Cruess, R., & Snell, L. (2005). Faculty development for teaching and evaluating professionalism: From programme design to curriculum change. *Medical Education, 39*(2), 127–136.

Swanwick, T. (2008). See one, do one, then what? Faculty development in postgraduate medical education. *Postgraduate Medical Journal, 84*(993), 339–343.

Swing, S. R. (2007). The ACGME outcome project: Retrospective and prospective. *Medical Teacher, 29*(7), 648–654.

Taber, S., Frank, J. R., Harris, K. A., Glasgow, N. J., Iobst, W., & Talbot, M. (2010). Identifying the policy implications of competency-based education. *Medical Teacher, 32*(8), 687–691.

Todhunter, S., Cruess, S. R., Cruess, R. L., Young, M., & Steinert, Y. (2011). Developing and piloting a form for student assessment of faculty professionalism. *Advances in Health Sciences Education, 16*(2), 223–238.

Verma, S., Broers, T., Paterson, M., Schroder, C., Medves, J. M., & Morrison, C. (2009). Core competencies: The next generation. Comparison of a common framework for multiple professions. *Journal of Allied Health, 38*(1), 47–53.

Verma, S., Paterson, M., & Medves, J. (2006). Core competencies for health care professionals: What medicine, nursing, occupational therapy and physiotherapy share. *Journal of Allied Health, 35*(2), 109–115.

Wadey, V. M., Dev, P., Buckley, R., Walker, D., & Hedden, D. (2009). Competencies for a Canadian orthopaedic surgery core curriculum. *Journal of Bone and Joint Surgery – British Volume, 91*(12), 1618–1622.

Zaidi, Z., Zaidi, S. M., Razzaq, Z., Luqman, M., & Moin, S. (2010). Training workshops in problem-based learning: Changing faculty attitudes and perceptions in a Pakistani medical college. *Education for Health, 23*(3), 440.

Chapter 14
Faculty Development for Interprofessional Education and Practice

Liz Anderson, Sarah Hean, Cath O'Halloran, Richard Pitt, and Marilyn Hammick

14.1 Introduction

> Interprofessional education occurs when students from two or more professions learn about, from and with each other to enable effective collaboration and improve health outcomes (WHO 2010, p. 7).

Interprofessional education (IPE) is a response to specific changes within health and social care delivery in the twenty first century, aimed at facilitating the delivery of integrated services and patient-focused care. IPE is shaped by a commitment to safe, patient-centered collaborative practice by national governments worldwide, including the United Kingdom (Department of Health 2000), Canada

L. Anderson, Ph.D. (✉)
Department of Medical and Social Care Education, University of Leicester, Leicester, UK
e-mail: esa1@le.ac.uk

S. Hean, Ph.D.
In-2-Theory: Interprofessional Theory and Scholarship Network, School of Health and Social Care, Bournemouth University, Bournemouth, Dorset, UK
e-mail: shean@bournemouth.ac.uk

C. O'Halloran, Ph.D., M.Sc.
Department of Health Sciences, School of Human and Health Sciences,
University of Huddersfield, Queensgate, Huddersfield, UK
e-mail: coh@hud.ac.uk

R. Pitt, M.Phil.
Interprofessional Learning, Law and Ethics Interest Group for Health and Social Care,
School of Nursing, Midwifery and Physiotherapy, Queens Medical Centre Campus,
University of Nottingham, Nottingham, UK
e-mail: richard.pitt@nottingham.ac.uk

M. Hammick, M.Sc., Ed.D.
The Best Evidence Medical Education Collaboration, Dundee, Scotland, UK
e-mail: mhammick@gmail.com

Y. Steinert (ed.), *Faculty Development in the Health Professions: A Focus on Research and Practice*, Innovation and Change in Professional Education 11, DOI 10.1007/978-94-007-7612-8_14, © Springer Science+Business Media Dordrecht 2014

(Health Canada 2001), Australia (Australian Council for Safety and Quality in Health Care 2005) and the United States of America (Cerra and Brandt 2011), and global workforce policy (WHO 2010).

In this chapter, we will look at how faculty development can prepare faculty to deliver a workable curriculum[1] for the local context and in the process advance faculty members' skills to teach, implement and offer IPE that assures student engagement. In addition, we explore how IPE has the potential to involve practitioners in deeper reflection and analysis of their collaborative working. This, in turn, enhances patient care. Our examples are mainly drawn from undergraduate curriculum development, but they apply equally to post-graduate, classroom and practice-based IPE. We acknowledge the challenges educators face in the development and delivery of effective IPE, outlining how these can be overcome. Using a theoretical curriculum model, we show how these challenges can be managed and how we can bring IPE practitioners together as a community of practice.

14.2 The Challenges of Developing and Delivering Interprofessional Education

We have identified five challenges associated with the development and delivery of an interprofessional curriculum. Our position is that faculty development is essential to address these challenges, establish interprofessional learning (IPL) throughout a professional curriculum and promote effective interprofessional practice (IPP).

Challenge 1: *Crossing professional boundaries*
Curriculum development and other educational activities within a single discipline are complex and nonlinear endeavors. This complexity can be articulated at a professional/school level through the use of Engeström's activity theory (2001), and diagrammatically as a triangle representing a single activity system (Fig. 14.1). The diagram summarizes the many factors within the profession/school that surround and mediate curriculum development. These phenomena include the tools that may mediate this activity (e.g. means of assessment), the rules or social norms that may govern how the profession and its training is managed, as well as the range of individuals (e.g. teachers, students, administrators) who may be involved and the manner in which different roles are allocated amongst them.

This complexity increases when faculty from different activity systems or disciplines collaborate to develop an interprofessional curriculum, as shown in Fig. 14.1. To work effectively together, faculty members must learn to understand each other's activity system and work together to create new shared understandings and ways of working. Without an understanding and empathy for the activity system of the other,

---

[1] We use curriculum to mean the content and processes of a learning opportunity; this might be a lengthy undergraduate programme or short continuing professional development workshop.

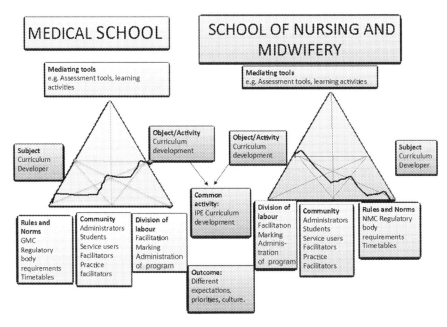

Fig. 14.1 Education as an activity system: Interprofessional integration. The diagram is adapted from Engeström (2001) and shows the activity systems of a nursing and medical school coming together to form an Interprofessional Education Curriculum. The *thick black line* across each activity system represents a contradiction within each system (the requirement by the regulator to deliver IPE) that is resolved if the two systems interact successfully. If unresolved, different cultures, priorities and expectations prevail

contradictions within their shared activity remain unidentified and unresolved. This allows the different expectations, priorities and cultures of each system to remain unexplored, and for poor intergroup attitudes and a lack of cooperation to grow (Hean et al. 2012a).

Challenge 2: *Integrating interprofessional education into each profession's existing curricula*
If the IPE curriculum remains separate to existing curricula it can become an add-on activity; subsequently, students can lose motivation and faculty members can prioritize other subjects. The challenge is the integration and alignment of the IPE curriculum so students and faculty members appreciate its fit with profession-specific curricula, its contribution to student learning, and its role as a valid part of the educational experience.

Challenge 3: *Paying attention to the theoretical rigor and the evidence base for IPE*
Interprofessional education has been accused of lacking sound theoretical underpinnings (Reeves and Hean 2013). The design and evaluation of IPE curricula are said to be superficial, descriptive and lacking in rigor. There has been limited understanding of the outcomes or processes at work within IPE (Hean et al. 2009). A growing

number of interprofessional educators, evaluators and practitioners now identify and apply theories from sociology, psychology and education in their work (Hean et al. 2012b). Striving to understand and apply theory needs encouragement, with faculty supported in work that pays attention (and gives time) to the development of theoretically sound and evidence-based IPE.

Challenge 4: *Managing the changeable and unpredictable nature of interprofessional education development and delivery*
Aligning uniprofessional and IPE elements of a curriculum needs a flexible and adaptable team, able to collaborate and continually learn about, from and with each other. Faculty members need to be comfortable with the concept of expansive learning and be able to cope with uncertainty and change (Engeström 2001).

Challenge 5: *Recognizing that interprofessional learning is complex and different*
IPE produces diverse learning groups. The students vary not only through their personal traits but through adherence to values which have shaped their career choice and become further molded as they take on a professional identity during training (Anderson et al. 2009). One role for faculty development includes critical reflective work to appreciate the unique properties of these mixed student groups and to equip educators with the skills to support students to learn about, from and with each other. Faculty development should aim to support everyone involved in the design and delivery of IPE curriculum as they re-analyze their personal teaching repertoires and become competent in managing interprofessional learning groups.

14.3 The Interprofessional Education Curriculum: Modeling Its Complexity

We have borrowed Coles and Grant's (1985) curriculum model to identify the IPE faculty constituency and unpack the development needs associated with the roles different faculty members have in establishing and assuring a credible IPE curriculum.

The curriculum model (Fig. 14.2) comprises three components – the curriculum-on-paper, the curriculum-in-action, and the curriculum experienced by the learners. There is always some incoherence between these components; not everything in the curriculum-on-paper will be translated into action by those responsible for curriculum delivery, and learners, with their unique knowledge and skills, will experience different versions of the curriculum. The model recognizes the dynamic nature of a curriculum and can usefully guide faculty development through attention to the need to maximize, as much as possible, component coherence. It is particularly useful in health professions learning, where courses include practice experiences, often including unplanned, opportunistic learning.

The IPE curriculum is not only influenced by the contributions and interplay of its three different components but additionally by the different professions working in IPE and the diversity of the IPL students. In the following sections, we discuss faculty

Fig. 14.2 Model of curriculum design (adapted from Coles and Grant 1985). Written for curriculum evaluation purposes, we have taken the original concepts from Coles and Grant's paper (1985) of the curriculum as three distinct overlapping circles; the curriculum-on-paper (A), the curriculum-in-action (B), and the curriculum experienced by the students (C). We have not addressed those parts of the circles which overlap

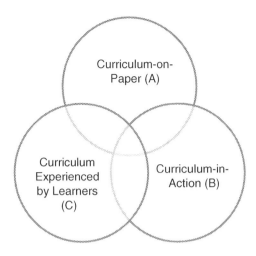

development initiatives for faculty members responsible for maximizing the coherence of the three components of the IPE curriculum and thus, for ensuring effective IPL.

14.4   The Interprofessional Faculty

Faculty development initiatives need to be available to all involved in the planning and delivery of the IPE curriculum, and the design of the initiatives needs to reflect the different roles for faculty members. This is a priority for those in roles that are essential to the success of an IPE curriculum which we will define and explore in detail: namely, the *IPE Champion*, the *IPE Professional Leads* and *IPE Facilitators*. Table 14.1, shows there are many other individuals involved in IPE curricula whose contribution to IPE will be enhanced by interprofessional faculty development.

The local *IPE Champion* can be defined as the leader and ambassador for both the strategic and operational aspects of the curriculum with management and research responsibilities (Barker et al. 2005; Oandasan and Reeves 2005). Their major task is to maintain strong partnerships across professions, organizations and institutions (Bjørke and Haavie 2006; Gilbert 2005). Mostly there is one *IPE Champion*, a sole voice who is responsible for the early vision for IPE and for initi-ating the local IPE curriculum. In addition, each profession may appoint an *IPE Professional Lead,* with in-depth understanding about their profession-specific cur-riculum, to work alongside the champion.

Those involved in the IPE curriculum-in-action are *IPE Facilitators*. The title reflects the mode of interprofessional learning where the educator assists the prog-ress of learning, paving the way for students to construct meaning through debate, discussion and shared reflection (Reeves et al. 2011). *IPE Facilitators* are usually university academics or practitioners who teach in practice (also known as precep-tors, mentors, clinical or practice teachers). They may also be patients/service users and students with a teaching role (McKeown et al. 2010; Selby et al. 2011).

Table 14.1 Faculty members involved in an interprofessional education curriculum

Curriculum areas	Faculty members involved
The curriculum-on-paper	External experts involved in curriculum approval (e.g. senior clinicians, managers or representatives from licensing bodies)
	Deans, Heads of School
	Faculty committee decision-making members
	IPE champion(s)
	IPE leads (profession-specific)
	Students involved in curriculum development
	Patient/service user reference groups
	Administrators
The curriculum-in-action	IPE champion(s)
	IPE leads
	Facilitators from academia and practice
	Administrators
The curriculum experienced by learners	External reference group (e.g. external examiners, external advisors to the research group)
	IPE lead researcher(s)
	Evaluators responsible for IPE quality control mechanisms
	Student feedback groups
	University assessment committee members
	Administrators

14.5   The Purpose of Interprofessional Faculty Development Initiatives

The purpose of interprofessional faculty development is to align more closely the different IPE curriculum components (e.g. written, in-action and experienced). Outcomes should assure a vibrant community of highly competent teachers who advance their practice and student learning through evidenced-based teaching. To reach such goals, faculty development must address the five challenges we outlined for developing an IPE curriculum. We continue by exploring the 'when', 'where', 'what' and 'how' of initiatives designed to achieve this.

14.5.1   Faculty Development and the Interprofessional Education Curriculum-on-Paper

Faculty development events that bring together members of different professions to work together on curriculum development provide opportunities to model interprofessional learning. They promote group work and the formation of a new community of practice. The function of team building cannot be understated (Steinert 2005). Initially we suggest organizing 'away days' or 'time-out' events for faculty members; the aim here is to encourage ownership of the curriculum-on-paper. The environment for these events needs to be versatile, enabling interactive debate and discussion towards consensus agreements. A series of events may be necessary to address some or all of the aims of this faculty development, as detailed below.

14.5.1.1   Gain an Understanding of the Education Context of the Other Professions Involved in Developing the IPE Curriculum (Challenge 1)

Early activities should include opportunities for interaction and sharing of professional programs and underpinning education values. This can be achieved through group work that enables participants to find out about each other, their courses, and their interest in IPE development. The end-point of these activities would be the sharing of course documentation, professional body standards, and other relevant materials, as a starting point for identifying the common ground for IPE development and preliminary agreement about the local IPE curriculum strategy.

14.5.1.2   Confirm Common Ground in Professional Curricula Where IPE Could Be Developed (Challenge 2)

Patient safety is an example of a topic that provides common ground for the design of IPE. The seminal document within the USA on patient safety, *To Err is Human* (Kohn et al. 2000), mirrored in the UK by the Department of Health's *An Organisation with a Memory* (Donaldson 2000), emphasizes the importance of patient-centered team-working in practice. The World Health Organization (WHO) has a comprehensive guide to including patient safety in health professions curricula with methods for teaching and assessing patient safety interprofessionally (WHO 2011).

14.5.1.3   Write Interprofessional Learning Outcomes (Challenges 2 and 3)

The goal here is for participants to experiment with writing interprofessional learning outcomes. This means translating the broader philosophical issues discussed in earlier sessions into learning outcomes that are coherent with the IPE curriculum rationale and resonate with curriculum documentation conventions in the academic institutions involved. Intended learning outcomes have been described and include: patient-centered team-working, the different roles and responsibilities of health and social care professionals, interprofessional communication, interprofessional reflection, patient safety and human behavior, and ethical aspects of shared practice (Thistlethwaite and Moran 2010).

14.5.1.4   Design Theoretically Sound and Evidence Informed Interprofessional Learning Activities (Challenge 3)

Faculty development should expose participants to the wide range of theories that have been applied in IPE and encourage them to use these to design effective IPL. We recommend that this event draws on the emerging research literature which can provide pre-reading material for the session. Syntheses of useful theories for IPE are available (Colyer et al. 2005; Hean et al. 2009, 2012b) to encourage debate that focuses on theories that reflect, explain or hypothesize the means to promote social learning (learning about, from and with each other) which is achieved in groups and mediated by social actors. These theoretical frameworks underpin the guidance to curriculum developers as shown in Table 14.2.

14.5.1.5   Select Appropriate Methods for Assessing IPL (Challenge 1, 3 and 4)

This involves sharing the assessment regimes for each profession and (finally) agreeing upon an interprofessional assessment strategy. The following are areas to consider:

- Decide if the assessment will measure learning in action (e.g. how students behave during interprofessional learning) or the attainment of learning outcomes (knowledge recall). There has been a recent growth in the use of competence frameworks to assess the knowledge, skills and attitudinal components of IPL (Reeves 2012; Wilhelmsson et al. 2012). Consider also capability frameworks (Gordon and Walsh 2005).
- An assessment strategy where interpretation offers some flexibility because it can be used for the IPE assessment while satisfying profession-specific requirements. For example, a case study report or essay following patient-centered, practice-based IPE could both fulfill the professional requirements and the agreed local IPE assessment strategy.
- A trajectory of assessments to show progression over time, for example, a Professional Portfolio. A progressive accumulation of learning can show student development along the continuum from novice to expert. Also, the use of a Professional Portfolio is now popular across the professions gaining increased importance in medicine (Buckley et al. 2009). As there is overlap between the aspects of learning for professionalism and interprofessionalism, a Professional Portfolio can combine both of these assessments (McNair 2005).
- The value of practical examinations to reveal student performance. Today, in health and social care, it is common to combine performance examinations with written examinations. Miller has drawn attention to the need to assess student knowledge ('*Knows*'), competence ('*Knows how*'), how this knowledge is applied ('*Shows how*'), and the more challenging aspect of what students do with this learning when in practice ('*Does*') (Miller 1990).

Table 14.2 Guidance for curriculum developers (Adapted from O'Halloran et al. 2006)

Questions to be asked of all IPL activities
Will the activity provide the students with a productive learning experience? Is it relevant and will it allow students to meet the learning outcomes?
Is it sufficiently challenging? (e.g. Is it based on realistic cases from practice; is it at the correct academic level?)
Is there adequate support in place? (e.g. Are appropriate learning or technical resources available; will access to a facilitator be needed?)
Will students have control over their own work? If the activity is overly prescribed, the group will have no freedom to decide how to tackle the task
Does it require students to formulate questions and seek the help of other group members?
Does the group have to produce something (e.g. a report, a presentation, public information)?
Does it only require students to act as representatives of their profession in a way that is appropriate to their stage in their program? (e.g. Final-year students can be expected to provide an informed professional perspective on a practice problem, but first-year students could be asked to research which professions would be involved.)
Will the activity generate genuine interdependence? Do the students have to depend on each other to complete the exercise successfully?
Does it allow division of work between members of the group? When the work is divided are there enough tasks and roles to ensure everyone has an essential contribution to make?
Will it allow group members to contribute unique skills that will enable the group to achieve goals that the individuals otherwise could not? These may be professional (e.g. negotiation skills, data analysis) or non-professional (e.g. artistic ability, IT skills)
Will it require students to share resources such as information, meanings, concepts and conclusions?
Does the assessment reinforce the inter-dependence? Are the students assessed as individuals or as a group? Is everyone in the group subject to the same assessment? Are the consequences of passing or failing the same for each profession in the group?
Will the activity foster differentiation and mutual inter-group differentiation? Will the activity allow students to explore the differences as well as the similarities in the professions they represent?
Will each profession be able to contribute something special to the exercise?
Will the contributions to be made by each profession encourage the students to acknowledge and value the strengths of other professions?
Will the activity allow equal contribution? Will the activity allow all members of the team to invest in the success of the project?
Will it allow the group to generate shared goals? The patient is the reason why health and social care professions work together and so activities based on practice scenarios, clinical cases, service improvement, patient safety or public health challenges are helpful
Will all members have equal status? Activities must not favor one professional group over another

It is wise to seek students' views on assessment and encourage their involvement in the assessment process, for example, on the use of peer assessment. Remember to also ask for patient/service user views on work-based assessments of interprofessional behaviors within practice settings (Frankel et al. 2007; Freeman and McKenzie 2002).

14.5.1.6 Ensure Curriculum Alignment and Integration Within Core Profession-Specific Curricula (Challenge 2, 3 and 4)

Finally, the group needs to agree how to align and integrate IPE throughout profession specific curricula (Biggs and Tang 2007; Stone 2010). This requires debate on whether IPE is to be placed within modules at set times, versus approaches where IPE is included as small group activities that can be easily run at different times. We suggest avoiding too much rigidity and focusing on a pathway of learning that starts with theory and knowledge and progresses to application for understanding in practice. Experiential learning to appreciate the complexity of effective team-based collaborative practice, based in practice, should be included as soon as students are familiar with learning alongside other student professions.

To achieve this understanding, faculty development activities should include mapping exercises to ensure that all faculty members can articulate how the IPE curriculum-on-paper has been (vertically and horizontally) aligned and integrated for coherence within the core profession-specific curriculum of participating professions. Engeström's activity theory is a useful way of looking at alignment and unpacking the interplay of systems, and can lead to a pictorial understanding of alignment (Engeström 2001). Figure 14.3 shows the result of a faculty development activity that looked at how IPL informs uniprofessional learning and vice-versa.

The IPE curriculum-on-paper may be subject to formal approval, and for faculty members involved in approval processes we suggest a seminar to assist their understanding of these challenges. Do try to include (or invite) a diverse audience including academics or senior clinicians involved in university course approval, professional and regulatory body representatives, and senior academics (e.g. Deans with resource allocation responsibility). More specifically, this type of seminar should aim to:

1. Explain the policy drivers for IPE relevant to the approving institution(s).
2. Discuss options for the alignment of learning intentions and how this might appear in course documentation.
3. Explain the importance of stakeholder involvement and what to look for in course documentation.
4. Discuss the importance of leadership and how to recognize whether this has been considered by those developing the curriculum.
5. Explain the resource implications of undertaking IPE and questions the panel should ask about funding, faculty capacity and capability.

14.5.2 Faculty Development and the Interprofessional Education Curriculum-in-Action

We move on to consider faculty development for translating aspirations into reality, to the 'IPE curriculum-in-action' overseen by the *IPE Champion* and the *IPE Leads*. The IPE curriculum-in-action is what faculty members involved in assigning resources and teaching IPE 'do' with the *IPE curriculum-on-paper*. This includes

Fig. 14.3 Alignment of the IPE curriculum within the core profession-specific curriculum. The *cylinder* represents the core profession-specific curriculum with interprofessional curriculum running through as a theme of learning, here with three distinct learning episodes. The *arrows* from the IPE events link to uniprofessional learning as students, helped by faculty members, integrate and align their learning within their professional training program

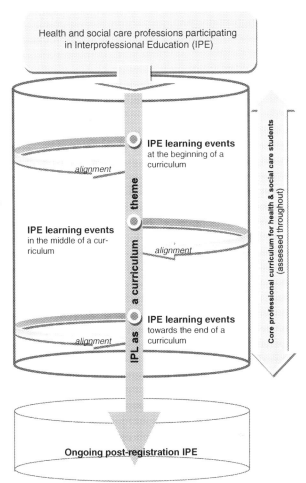

ensuring that sufficient time is available in the timetable, deciding whether student learning groups meet physically in classrooms or in practice, virtually or both, the size and professional mix of the learning groups, the number of appropriately trained facilitators needed, what learning tasks are developed, and the administration of the learning events. The translation of the curriculum aspirations heavily depends upon faculty support for the *IPE Champion*, *IPE Leads* and the *IPE Facilitators*.

14.5.2.1 Faculty Development to Lead and Teach on Interprofessional Education Events

The *IPE Champion* requires a unique skill set (Table 14.3) and we suggest that this person attends leadership and change management courses and is supported to work with national and international IPE organizations. (See Chap. 3 for more information

Table 14.3 Unpacking the skill set of the interprofessional education champion

Aptitudes that IPE champions should seek through faculty development
Core aptitudes
Credibility: From both the local and national IPE community which is underpinned by educational research and androgogy which aspires others to follow
Capability: To lead and initiate the necessary steps for faculty development and to work alongside relevant colleagues to steer the emerging joint vision
Authority: To use wisely within the IPE Community of Practice. This authority is not just that bestowed from Heads of Faculty for chairing meetings but earned through scholarship and professional behavior
Other aptitudes
Problem solver: Able to tackle the key obstacles in a collegial way which assures solutions
Communicator: To work closely with others using excellent communication strategies which aim to assure the delivery of the local IPE aspirations, while ensuring to listen to all viewpoints, to seek compromise. And to remain non-judgmental
Scholar: Through the application and alignment of theoretical thinking to curriculum design, development and research/evaluation
Political: To be aware of linked systems and issues which could undermine IPE and to assure solutions to sustain IPE when challenged. Seeks relevant external reference group support in these endeavors
Reflective: Able to see things from many viewpoints and especially using second order interprofessional reflection (Wackerhausen 2009)
Economical: Aware of financial pressures and resource issues seeking internal and external funding where necessary

about faculty development and leadership opportunities). This would include attending local and international conferences, for example, the conference series All Together Better Health (ATBH VI, on-going) and Collaboration Across Borders (CAB IV, on-going). Skill development can also be enhanced through mentoring opportunities from within the IPE national and international community of practice. With the support and benefits of their own professional development, the *IPE Champion* can subsequently lead the development of *IPE Professional Leads* and *IPE Facilitators*.

Developing skilled *IPE Facilitators* is an important faculty development role. IPE facilitation is a complex skill; it cannot be assumed that an experienced educator, from practice or academia, will seamlessly become a skilled *IPE Facilitator* (Anderson and Thorpe 2010; Anderson et al. 2011; Hammick 1998; Howkins and Bray 2008). Our experience is that IPE facilitators need preparation and development for their role. We offer a model to guide the faculty developer to achieve the combination of skills required (outlined in Fig. 14.4).

Educators usually develop an understanding of the interprofessional course content quickly. Skilled IPE facilitation means recognizing the primacy of learning rather than teaching *and* the ability to appreciate and reflect from multiple professional perspectives (Wackerhausen 2009). It also demands the desire to facilitate through understanding and managing the complexity of interprofessional group dynamics in a learning context. Faculty development should assist faculty members to achieve an in-depth understanding of these elements of mixed profession group teaching relevant to IPE. As previously acknowledged, interprofessional student

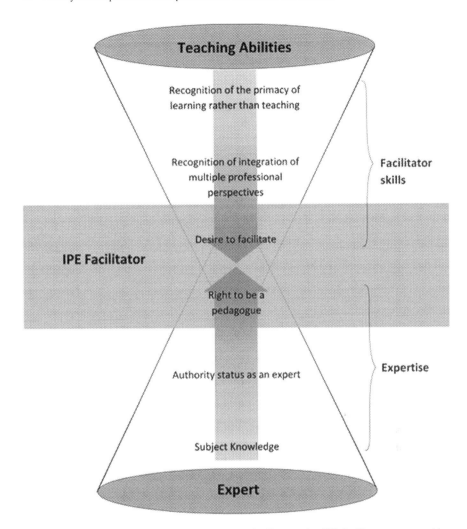

Fig. 14.4 Developing interprofessional education facilitators. An IPE facilitator must combine being an **Expert** (a full understanding of the aspects of teaching for learning to become a pedagogue) with competent **Teaching Abilities** (facilitation skills for managing small mixed-professional IPE students groups underpinned with interprofessional values) for the management of effective learning

groups are more diverse than many other learning groups, different not just by age, gender or academic profile, but in respect of their reasons for choosing their profession and over time through the process of taking on a professional identity (Anderson et al. 2009). It follows that there can be tensions that need to be managed as the different individuals come together to learn together, for example, when a student from one profession thinks the approach from another profession is wrong, or where a student feels the medical student is dominant, taking on the leadership role unnecessarily. *IPE Facilitators* can be helped in this regard through appreciation of the psychological and sociological principles of team working and learning, which we will explore further in Sect. 14.5.3.

IPE facilitation development may include regular in-house teaching events or certificated programs. Examples of successful local programs are available (Deutschlander and Suter 2011; Freeman et al. 2010; Freeth et al. 2005; Howkins and Bray 2008). Successful faculty development programs develop a range of teaching competencies and bring together mixed professional academic and practice faculty working in small groups to mirror the student IPE experience (Anderson et al. 2009). In this way, expert stances are shared between practice and academia, and facilitation skill sets are exchanged. See Table 14.4 for a possible framework for facilitator faculty development. This could be set up as a credited course or a series of certificated workshops. The framework offers an assessment process to assure competent *IPE Facilitators* who are confident to work in pairs, to team teach, and to support student interprofessional learning. *IPE Facilitators* who are skeptics should be offered opportunities to observe the teaching in action, working with positive role models as this can positively change attitudes to favor IPE (Anderson et al. 2011).

14.5.2.2 Developing a Community of Practice

Putting the curriculum into action demands more than IPE champions and skilled facilitators. It needs a community with a common interest in the development, delivery and evaluation of IPE. Through their practice as facilitators, curriculum developers, IPE champions or researchers, faculty members face complex challenges and often, great uncertainty. Forming a recognized Community of Practice (CoP) that adopts the principles presented by Wenger et al. (2002) is a valuable way for colleagues from different professions to learn to deliver collaboratively a successful IPE curriculum. Table 14.5 includes more details of how to do this.

A Community of Practice is particularly important in the delivery of practice-based IPE where it has been shown to enable professional exchanges and enhance service delivery (Lennox and Anderson 2012). Sustaining practice-based IPE is dependent upon strong networks (Armitage et al. 2009). Note also that the IPE CoP should, where possible, include patients/service users and students whose needs for support may be time consuming, demanding similar processes of befriending, and development as outlined above (Anderson and Ford 2012; Furness et al. 2012).

14.5.3 Faculty Development and the Experienced Interprofessional Curriculum

We mostly learn about the IPE curriculum experienced by learners or, put another way, the students' lived experience of IPE, through evaluations and/or research conducted for faculty committees. These data may identify issues where faculty

Table 14.4 A faculty development framework for preparing IPE facilitators[a]

Competencies for IPE facilitation (Freeth et al. 2005, p. 106)	Proposed faculty development activities	How to assess IPE facilitators' competence (Anderson et al. 2009)
A commitment to IPE and IPP	• *Knowledge exchange*: Ask the group to map the national and international IPE policy requirements (e.g. on patient safety) and link research evidence on poor team working and collaborative practice to outcomes • *Showcase* the literature on how team working enhances patient care	(a) **Informal feedback** The IPE Champion/IPE Lead asks questions and seeks clarification for understanding from attendees (b) **Formative** Faculty members are helped to practice and work through problems receiving feedback from both peers and the session leaders (c) **Summative** The attending faculty members seeking to become IPE Facilitators complete an IPE Teaching Portfolio, containing: (i) Theory applied to IPE events in which they participate (e.g. why this design?) (ii) Reflections on how the teaching event was facilitated (e.g. Could they have acted differently to support student learning, were there problems? What could have been done differently and why?) (iii) A reflection on observer feedback to include a personal critical analysis on their performance
Credibility in relation to the particular focus of the IPE to which the educator contributes	• Explore collaborative practice in modern health and social care • Ask faculty members to share their experience and expertise (e.g. within mental health, child and elderly care, acute adult hospital care, public health and other sectors) • Faculty members with expertise in research and education (non-clinical staff) can share their expert stances (e.g. application of theory to practice in education and health and social care delivery, educational research approaches suitable to evaluate IPE)	
Positive role modeling	• IPE Champion/IPE Leads who run the sessions should role model what is required. In this way, the leads should team-teach and come from different professional backgrounds • Place participants in small and interprofessional working groups. Discuss group tensions throughout	

(continued)

Table 14.4 (continued)

Competencies for IPE facilitation (Freeth et al. 2005. p. 106)	Proposed faculty development activities	How to assess IPE facilitators' competence (Anderson et al. 2009)
An in-depth understanding of interactive learning methods and confidence in application	• Relate adult learning theories to IPE • Ask groups to design IPE using interactive teaching methods • Explore psychological and sociological theories of power and difference (e.g. stereotypes)	
A knowledge of group dynamics	• Consider how to set ground rules at the start of IPL • Ask participants to practice managing poorly functioning groups by working through real examples from IPE events. Ensure facilitators understand how to remain non-judgmental and to motivate group work and encourage student group discussions	
Valuing diversity and unique contributions	• Share medical and social models of health • Share the value base of the professions	
Balancing the needs of individuals and groups	• Discuss patient/service user-centered care • Set up debates and discussions on corrupting factors in team working, leadership battles, etc • Explore Belbin's (1993) model of group roles	
Inner conviction and good humor in the face of difficulties	• De-brief on how those leading the session role model IPE facilitation. Share examples within the group • Explore the use of humor to dissipate group tension	

[a]The competencies for IPE facilitation are adopted from the literature as shown

Table 14.5 Developing an interprofessional community of practice (CoP)

Principles of designing a community of practice (from Wenger et al. 2002)	Strategies for application
Treat the development and delivery of an IPE committee as an evolutionary process	Allow facilitators, curriculum developers, IPE champions and researchers, practitioners from different professions, faculties and institutions to share their interests. The IPE agenda evolves from the CoP participants
Create an open dialogue between people inside and outside of the CoP	Enable a dialogue between the members of the CoP themselves and those outside (e.g. students, academics from other disciplines-education, psychology, and external reference groups such as: the UK Centre for Interprofessional Education (CAIPE); Canadian Interprofessional Health Collaborative (CIHC); Australasian Interprofessional Practice and Education Network (AIPPEN); American Interprofessional Health Collaborative (AIHC)
Invite different levels of participation	There are three levels of participation in a CoP. The core group forms the active membership and peripheral membership. The core group forms the strategic and operational committees, those engaged in IPE while the peripheral members may in the future take on this role if they are helped to perceive the benefits. Although active participation is encouraged, it should not be forced. Different faculty members may play different roles at different stages of development. Faculty members may begin as facilitators when they first enter the community but progress to greater involvement as curriculum designers and eventually IPE champions as their skills and confidence develop
Focus on value	Involvement in the CoP must have an active value for its members who can perceive benefits (Anderson et al. 2011)
Develop both public and private community spaces	A CoP is about building strong individual relationships between its members. Public spaces may include seminars, workshops, facebook pages, blogs and discussion forums open to all faculties to attend and discuss. Private spaces are more protected and include confidential spaces such as emails between selected individuals or special interest groups engaged in more discrete or focused activity
Combine familiarity and excitement	The CoP should mix a set of activities to generate comfort and familiarity, while novel activities such as away days need to be included to maintain vibrancy
Create a rhythm for the community	A regular pattern of activity should be established in the IPE CoP. This could include a schedule of working meetings, a seminar program to promote sharing of ideas, teleconferences focused on particular projects, with a central tenet that during these activities participants learn about, from and with each other

development has worked and also where it is failing to achieve its goals. This should lead to an assessment of what further faculty development is needed and/or may help identify small issues for immediate short-term attention.

Student assessment outcomes can similarly alert faculty to concerns that warrant a review of faculty development. The faculty development leadership team needs to ensure on-going faculty meetings to work through each issue. Involvement of a student consultative group and/or researcher(s) able to analyze and collate random samples of uniprofessional student focus group material will ensure clarity of the priority of student concerns. Faculty away days provide opportunities for *IPE Champion*(s)/*Leads* from participating professions to have protected time to re-explore and review the IPE strategy, leading to a redesigned curriculum-on-paper and in-action that takes account of student experiences of IPL.

We have already highlighted how learning within IPE sessions is different for every learner because of what each of them brings to the learning context. Our experience, supported by the literature (Anderson and Thorpe 2010; Carpenter and Hewstone 1996; Hean et al. 2006), is that there are some common issues within interprofessional learning groups. These include what students feel during the IPE experience, such as negative stereotyping, and may depend on how well students are prepared for the difference of IPL to uniprofessional learning and the perceived relevance of the session and how it relates to practice (Freeth et al. 2005). Table 14.6 offers some ideas for faculty development relating to these issues.

The underpinning differences between student groups can be easily understood by considering social capital theory described as 'an unceasing effort of sociability, a continuous series of exchanges in which recognition is endlessly affirmed and reaffirmed' (Bourdieu 1997, pp. 51–52). The learning, skills and trust of other professional groups created within this exchange is cumulative in nature, constituting social capital, and encourages the learner to reinvest and build future collaborations when joining interprofessional teams in practice. The advantage gained through this social network may be afforded to some but denied to others. Similarly, not all professionals come to the IPE learning group on a level playing field. Students may bring in social capital (and other forms of capital such as human capital) from their professional groups (or other networks) that afford them greater status, skills and/or experiences. This enables them to take advantage of the knowledge transfer that happens in the IPE group to a greater degree than other learners denied these networks.

Student engagement by faculty members should be encouraged with greater understanding of the local possibilities and constraints for IPE. Students can become peer-teachers and support the development of the IPE curriculum where a collegiate approach is taken.

14.6 Conclusion

There is growing evidence of the value of interprofessional faculty development (Simmons et al. 2011). Preparing tomorrow's workforce for interprofessional practice requires IPE to be carefully woven into health and social care professional education

Table 14.6 Listening to the students' experiences of interprofessional education: messages for faculty development

Issues which might hinder student learning	Proposed faculty development activities
Students arrive unprepared for the IPE activity	Design written materials (handbooks) and verbal materials (virtual or actual presentations) for preparing students for IPE. These could be shared within the IPE faculty community using blogs and wikis (e-technology). Design other educational tools (e.g. short films) to help orientate students see: http://youtu.be/Fh7tIr4Tl1o
	The TIGER Open educational resources have materials for re-purposing to help students to get the most out of group learning (TIGER 2012)
	Ensure student preparation for IPE is part of the IPE Facilitator training. Ensure IPE facilitators have the skills to engage all students at the beginning of any event using relevant ice breakers and developing ground rules
	The IPE Champion may need to convene a meeting with all IPE Leads to ensure the same approach is followed for student preparation by all schools
Students fail to learn because of the location and the environment	IPE Champion and IPE Leads will need to revisit the location and reflect on student insights. Change venues where they are not conducive for IPE
	Develop partnerships with students so that they better understand why certain environments are chosen for IPE and seek their help to get the environment right. This may mean students representatives at IPE faculty curriculum meetings
	Re-assess all materials that inform students about the 'place' for IPE and prepare design materials to help orientate students to the location
	Agree upon a neutral learning environment where an emphasis is placed on equality between participants
	IPE Champion and IPE Leads work to develop relevant clinical sites for IPE in practice
Students are overwhelmed by the status, power and territory of some or one of the participating student professions	Reflect on the content of IPE facilitation to ensure IPE Facilitators can recognize these issues and deal with them in a collegial way during the sessions. This may include engaging students in debate on power and territory in health and social care practice
	Run events with facilitators to enhance their understanding of these issues from a theoretical perspective using, for example, social capital theory (Bourdieu 1997)
Students fail to recognize the learning content as it does not apply to their future work (e.g. authenticity of the event)	The IPE Champion and Leads should review the curriculum map for each school(s) to ensure the content of IPE has relevance for all students participating in the IPE curriculum
	Liaise with clinical practitioners to ensure participating students are aware of how the IPE is appropriate for their learning requirements
	Run a student focus group to seek their views on orientation for, and engagement in, IPE

curricula. This, in turn, is dependent upon effective faculty development for all faculty members involved.

In this chapter, we have suggested how to best achieve faculty development across the diverse faculty groups involved in IPE, planning and delivery. Our aim has been to highlight effective ways to move the three IPE curriculum components, the curriculum-on-paper, the curriculum-in-action and the curriculum experienced by the learner, into closer harmony. A future challenge for faculty development is to ensure that faculty members are able to correctly direct the pace and direction of movement of each component. The question of what should move where will only be answered when all three are based on sound theory, shaped by evidence, and faculty members can apply this understanding to their teaching.

For long lasting acceptance of the curriculum-on-paper there is a need for opportunities for faculty from the different professions to learn to continue to work together. In this way, the separate professional education activity systems embed an IPE curriculum that is likely to endure. Sustainability is also enhanced through the development of a Community of Practice. Here, a learning environment built on strong interpersonal relationships between faculty, alongside students and patients/service users, supports its members through the complexities of IPE development, delivery and review.

The IPE curriculum needs to maintain credibility and nowhere is this more so than within practice. The current trend is to develop practice-based IPL that is focused on learning within already effective team-based care (e.g. rehabilitation, cancer care, mental health, further enriching faculty and benefitting patients) (Kinnair et al. 2012). This enables students to see interprofessional practice (IPP) at its best. Other clinical settings where teams are more fluid and practice is fraught with challenges are marginalized. They miss the potential to transform their practice and improve health and social care outcomes. These practice settings present new challenges for faculty members developing the interprofessional curriculum-on-paper and for faculty development initiatives aimed at supporting their work.

A successful curriculum-in-action requires the development of leaders and team members who understand how to best deliver the curriculum-on-paper. Here, faculty development aims to develop in faculty members the same interprofessional competencies set for students: team working skills, an understanding of other faculty roles and responsibilities, the ability to communicate across professional, faculty and institutional barriers, and dealing with uncertainty. These are always likely to feature in interprofessional faculty development initiatives, but in the future we will need facilitators who are in tune with twenty-first century learning. This means greater use of information technology and social media, and recognizing the role of individual learning. We will need facilitators who can empower and support students as they translate the curriculum-on-paper into their own curriculum-in-action, especially in practice settings. 'In situ' faculty development, as suggested by Silver and Leslie (2009), may well suit emergent IPE practitioners already used to interprofessional learning and keen to guide practice-based interprofessional learning in their work settings.

The curriculum experienced by learners offers important clues to tailoring faculty development following implementation of the planned IPE curriculum.

But, in writing this chapter, we have realized the lack of material from the learner experienced curriculum available to guide faculty development initiatives. In the future, we would hope for enhanced use of program evaluations and robust research to identify key mechanisms for bringing the experience of interprofessional learning closer to the curriculum-on-paper, and for ensuring that this is driven by student learning needs.

The curriculum model used in this chapter offers a theoretical basis for research into the mechanisms needed for effective and sustainable interprofessional faculty development. In turn, this will lead to an evidence base for faculty development for IPE and IPP. There is an on-going need to refresh interprofessional faculty development as emerging practitioners who have experienced IPL in pre-registration programs and continued professional development courses shape and naturally develop IPE opportunities within practice. We suggest that future faculty development needs to be continually shaped by the views of patients, service users and students, the fresh insights offered by developments in the theory of interprofessional learning and practice, and the growing evidence base of IPE and IPP.

14.7 Key Messages

- Faculty development for interprofessional education involves building strong partnerships with diverse stakeholders, including students, clinicians and colleagues from external organizations.
- Interprofessional faculty development aims to enable faculty members to understand the work and values of colleagues from other professions and institutions.
- As interprofessional education becomes a key part of professional curricula, faculty development has a role in helping faculty adapt and extend their teaching skills repertoire.
- Interprofessional faculty development is an opportunity for faculty to experience and understand the processes of interprofessional learning and practice.
- Well planned interprofessional faculty development has the potential to enrich and enhance all teaching, learning and research activities across university and related practice settings.

Acknowledgements The authors wish to thank Dr. Deborah Craddock (formerly of the University of Southampton) for her contribution to the early ideas of this chapter.

References

Anderson, E. S., Cox, D., & Thorpe, L. N. (2009). Preparation of educators involved in interprofessional education. *Journal of Interprofessional Care, 23*(1), 81–94.

Anderson, E. S. & Ford, J. (2012). *Enabling service users to lead interprofessional workshops to improve student listening skills.* Higher Education Mini Grant Project No: MP220. Newcastle

University, School of Medical Sciences Education Development. Available from: http://www.medev.ac.uk/funding/7/22/funded/

Anderson, E. S. & Thorpe, L. N. (2010). Interprofessional educator ambassadors: An empirical study of motivation and added value. *Medical Teacher, 32*(11), e492–e500.

Anderson, E. S., Thorpe, L. N., & Hammick, M. (2011). Interprofessional staff development: Changing attitudes and winning hearts and minds. *Journal of Interprofessional Care, 25*(1), 11–17.

Armitage, H., Pitt, R., & Jinks, A. (2009). Initial findings from the TUILIP (Trent Universities Interprofessional Learning in Practice) project. *Journal of Interprofessional Care, 23*(1), 101–103.

Australian Council for Safety and Quality in Health Care. (2005). *National patient safety education framework.* University of Sydney: The Centre for Innovation in Professional Health Education. Available from: http://www.safetyandquality.gov.au/wp-content/uploads/2012/01/framework0705.pdf

Barker, K. K., Bosco, C., & Oandasan, I. F. (2005). Factors in implementing interprofessional education and collaborative practice initiatives: Findings from key informant interviews. *Journal of Interprofessional Care, 19*(Suppl. 1), 166–176.

Belbin, R. M. (1993). *Team roles at work.* London, UK: Butterworth-Heinemann.

Biggs, J. & Tang, C. (2007). *Teaching for quality learning at university,* (3rd Ed.). Berkshire, UK: Open University Press.

Bjørke, G. & Haavie, N. E. (2006). Crossing boundaries: Implementing an interprofessional module into uniprofessional Bachelor programmes. *Journal of Interprofessional Care, 20*(6), 641–653.

Bourdieu, P. (1997). The forms of capital. In A. H. Halsey, H. Lauder, P. Brown, & A. Stuart Wells (Eds.), *Education: Culture, economy, and society,* (pp. 46–58). Oxford, UK: Oxford University Press.

Buckley, S., Coleman, J., Davison, I., Khan, K. S., Zamora, J., Malick, S., et al. (2009). The educational effects of portfolios on undergraduate student learning: A Best Evidence Medical Education (BEME) systematic review. BEME Guide No. 11. *Medical Teacher, 31*(4), 282–298.

Carpenter, J. & Hewstone, M. (1996). Shared learning for doctors and social workers: Evaluation of a programme. *British Journal of Social Work, 26*(2), 239–257.

Cerra, F. & Brandt, B. (2011). Renewed focus in the United States links interprofessional education with redesigning health care. *Journal of Interprofessional Care, 25*(6), 394–396.

Coles, C. R. & Grant, J. G. (1985). Curriculum evaluation in medical and health-care education. *Medical Education, 19*(5), 405–422.

Colyer, H., Helme, M., & Jones, I. (2005). *The theory-practice relationship in interprofessional education.* London, UK: Higher Education Academy Health Sciences and Practice.

Department of Health. (2000). *A health service of all the talents: Developing the NHS workforce.* London, UK: The Stationery Office. Available from: http://webarchive.nationalarchives.gov.uk/+/www.dh.gov.uk/en/Publicationsandstatistics/Publications/PublicationsPolicyAndGuidance/DH_4007967

Deutschlander, S. & Suter, E. (2011). *Interprofessional mentoring guide for supervisors, staff and students.* Alberta Health Services. Retrieved June 5th, 2012, from http://www.albertahealthservices.ca/careers/docs/WhereDoYouFit/wduf-stu-sp-ip-mentoring-guide.pdf

Donaldson, L. (2000). *An organisation with a memory.* London, UK: The Stationery Office. Retrieved May 30th, 2012, from http://webarchive.nationalarchives.gov.uk/20130107105354/http:/www.dh.gov.uk/prod_consum_dh/groups/dh_digitalassets/@dh/@en/documents/digitalasset/dh_4065086.pdf

Engeström, Y. (2001). Expansive learning at work: Toward an activity theoretical reconceptualization. *Journal of Education and Work, 14*(1), 133–156.

Frankel, A., Gardner, R., Maynard, L., & Kelly, A. (2007). Using the Communication And Teamwork Skills (CATS) assessment to measure health care team performance. *The Joint Commission Journal on Quality and Patient Safety, 33*(9), 549–558.

Freeman, M. & McKenzie, J. (2002). SPARK: A confidential web-based template for self and peer assessment of student teamwork: Benefits of evaluating across different subjects. *British Journal of Educational Technology, 33*(5), 551–569.

Freeman, S., Wright, A., & Lindqvist, S. (2010). Facilitator training for educators involved in interprofessional learning. *Journal of Interprofessional Care, 24*(4), 375–385.

Freeth, D., Hammick, M., Reeves, S., Koppel, I., & Barr, H. (2005). *Effective interprofessional education: Development, delivery and evaluation.* Oxford, UK: Blackwell.

Furness, P. J., Armitage H. R., & Pitt, R. (2012). Establishing and facilitating practice-based interprofessional learning: Experiences from the TUILIP project. *Nursing Reports, 2*(1), e5, 25–30.

Gilbert, J. (2005). Interprofessional learning and higher educational structural barriers. *Journal of Interprofessional Care, 19*(Suppl. 1), 87–106.

Gordon, F. & Walsh, C. (2005). A framework for interprofessional capability: Developing students of health and social care as collaborative workers. *Journal of Integrated Care, 13*(3), 26–33.

Hammick, M. (1998). Interprofessional education: Concept, theory and application. *Journal of Interprofessional Care, 12*(3), 323–332.

Health Canada. (2001). *Social accountability: A vision for Canadian medical schools.* Ottawa, ON: Health Canada. Available from: http://www.afmc.ca/pdf/pdf_sa_vision_canadian_medical_schools_en.pdf

Hean, S., Craddock, D., & Hammick, M. (2012a). Theoretical insights into interprofessional education: AMEE Guide No. 62, *Medical Teacher, 34*(2), e78–e101.

Hean, S., Craddock, D., & O'Halloran, C. (2009). Learning theories and interprofessional education: A user's guide. *Learning in Health and Social Care, 8*(4), 250–262.

Hean, S., Macleod-Clark, J., Adams, K., & Humphris, D. (2006). Will opposites attract? Similarities and differences in students' perceptions of the stereotype profiles of other health and social care professional groups. *Journal of Interprofessional Care, 20*(2), 162–181.

Hean, S., Staddon, S., Clapper, A., Fenge, L. A., Heaslip, V., & Jack, E. (2012b). *Interagency training to support the liaison and diversion agenda.* Poole, UK: Bournemouth University. Available from: http://www.caipe.org.uk/silo/files/interagency-report-december-2012.pdf

Howkins, E. & Bray, J. (2008). *Preparing for interprofessional teaching: Theory and practice.* Oxford, UK: Radcliffe Publishing.

Kinnair, D., Anderson E. S., & Thorpe, L. N. (2012). Development of interprofessional education in mental health practice: Adapting the Leicester model. *Journal of Interprofessional Care, 26*(3), 189–197.

Kohn, L. T., Corrigan, J. M., & Donaldson, M. S. (Eds.). (2000). *To err is human: Building a safer health system.* Washington, DC: Institute of Medicine National Academy Press.

Lennox, A. & Anderson, E. S. (2012). Delivering quality improvements in patient care: The application of the Leicester model of interprofessional education. *Quality in Primary Care, 20*(3), 219–226.

McKeown, M., Malihi-Shoja, L., & Downe, S. (2010). *Service user and carer involvement in education for health and social care: Promoting partnership for health.* Oxford, UK: Blackwell Publishing.

McNair, R. P. (2005). The case for educating health care students in professionalism as the core content of interprofessional education. *Medical Education, 39*(5), 456–464.

Miller, G. E. (1990). The assessment of clinical skills/competence/performance. *Academic Medicine, 65*(9 Suppl.), S63–S67.

Oandasan, I. & Reeves, S. (2005). Key elements of interprofessional education. Part 2: Factors, processes and outcomes. *Journal of Interprofessional Care, 19*(Suppl. 1), 39–48.

O'Halloran, C., Hean, S., Humphris, D., & Macleod-Clark, J. (2006). Developing common learning: The new generation project undergraduate curriculum model. *Journal of Interprofessional Care, 20*(1), 12–28.

Reeves, S. (2012). The rise and rise of interprofessional competence. *Journal of Interprofessional Care, 26*(4), 253–255.

Reeves, S., Goldman, J., Gilbert, J., Tepper, J., Silver, I., Suter, E., et al. (2011). A scoping review to improve conceptual clarity of interprofessional interventions. *Journal of Interprofessional Care, 25*(3), 167–174.

Reeves, S. & Hean, S. (2013). Why we need theory to help us better understand the nature of interprofessional education, practice and care. *Journal of Interprofessional Care, 27*(1), 1–3.

Selby, J. P., Fulford-Smith, L., King, A., Pitt, R., & Knox, R. (2011). Piloting the use of an interprofessional stroke care learning package created by and for students. *Journal of Interprofessional Care, 25*(4), 294–295.

Silver, I. L. & Leslie, K. (2009). Faculty development for continuing interprofessional education and collaborative practice. *Journal of Continuing Education in the Health Professions, 29*(3), 172–177.

Simmons, B., Oandasan, I., Soklaradis, S., Esdaile, M., Barker, K., Kwan, D., et al. (2011). Evaluating the effectiveness of an interprofessional education faculty development course: The transfer of interprofessional learning to the academic and clinical practice setting. *Journal of Interprofessional Care, 25*(2), 156–157.

Steinert, Y. (2005). Learning together to teach together: Interprofessional education and faculty development. *Journal of Interprofessional Care, 19*(Suppl. 1), 60–75.

Stone, J. (2010). Moving interprofessional learning forward through formal assessment. *Medical Education, 44*(4), 396–403.

TIGER. (2012). Transforming Interprofessional Groups through Educational Resources. Available from: http://tiger.library.dmu.ac.uk

Thistlethwaite, J. & Moran, M. (2010). Learning outcomes for Interprofessional Education (IPE): Literature review and synthesis. *Journal of Interprofessional Care, 24*(5), 503–513.

Wackerhausen, S. (2009). Collaboration, professional identity and reflection across boundaries. *Journal of Interprofessional Care, 23*(5), 455–473.

Wenger, E., McDermott, R., & Snyder, W. M. (2002). *Cultivating communities of practice*. Boston, MA: Harvard Business School Press.

Wilhelmsson, M., Pelling, S., Uhlin, L., Owe-Dahlgren, L., Faresjö, T., & Forslund, K. (2012). How to think about interprofessional competence: A metacognitive model. *Journal of Interprofessional Care, 26*(2), 85–91.

World Health Organization. (2010). *Framework for action on interprofessional education & collaborative practice*. Geneva, CH: WHO Press. Available from: http://whqlibdoc.who.int/hq/2010/WHO_HRH_HPN_10.3_eng.pdf

World Health Organization. (2011). *Patient safety curriculum guide multi-professional edition*. Geneva, CH: WHO Press. Retrieved May 30th, 2012, from http://www.who.int/patientsafety/education/curriculum/en/index.html

Chapter 15
International Faculty Development Partnerships

Stacey Friedman, Francois Cilliers, Ara Tekian, and John Norcini

15.1 Introduction

International faculty development partnerships are relationships that form for mutual benefit and seek to achieve shared, and sometimes complex, goals such as improved health care. They are motivated by a desire to achieve specific goals more effectively than any partner could independently (Kolars et al. 2012; Leffers and Mitchell 2011). They are also a response to the globalization of health professions education, research, and practice (Marchal and Kegels 2003). Globalization includes conceptualizing health professions education in global terms, with cross-border integration and exchange of ideas and resources (Hodges et al. 2009). International faculty development partnerships have variously been called collaborations, networks, coalitions, alliances, consortia, task forces, joint-working, and twinning (Dowling et al. 2004). The term partnership will be used for the purposes of this chapter.

S. Friedman, Ph.D. (✉)
Foundation for Advancement of International Medical
Education and Research (FAIMER), Philadelphia, PA, USA
e-mail: sfriedman@faimer.org

F. Cilliers, M.B., Ch.B., M.Phil., Ph.D.
Education Development Unit, Faculty of Health Sciences,
University of Cape Town, Cape Town, South Africa
e-mail: francois.cilliers@uct.ac.za

A. Tekian, Ph.D., MHPE
Department of Medical Education, College of Medicine,
University of Illinois at Chicago, Chicago, IL, USA
e-mail: tekian@uic.edu

J. Norcini, Ph.D.
Foundation for Advancement of International Medical
Education and Research (FAIMER), Philadelphia, PA, USA
e-mail: jnorcini@faimer.org

Y. Steinert (ed.), *Faculty Development in the Health Professions: A Focus on Research and Practice*, Innovation and Change in Professional Education 11, DOI 10.1007/978-94-007-7612-8_15, © Springer Science+Business Media Dordrecht 2014

For institutions that participate, partnerships may build global awareness of the institution, improve student recruitment and faculty retention, and provide a resource for students, faculty members, and alumni (Kanter 2010). Well-functioning partnerships allow faculty to be exposed to different methods of teaching and learning, expanded opportunities for research, and clinical contexts, materials, and methods that they may not encounter locally (McAuliffe and Cohen 2005). Moreover, they allow faculty to expand their networks of collaborators and the communities of scholarship in which they work. There are similar advantages for students in the schools that are involved in faculty development partnerships, realized either indirectly via faculty exposure or directly where student exchanges are part of the faculty development partnership, allowing students to experience different patient populations, develop cultural sensitivities, and learn about other healthcare systems.

International faculty development partnerships arise in response to a range of needs and opportunities, but they all seek to enhance the quality and relevance of education as a means of achieving their goals. One of the biggest needs some faculty development partnerships seek to contribute toward addressing is that of inadequate quality, quantity, and/or distribution of health care workers in both high and low income countries (Norcini and Banda 2011; WHO 2008). One dimension of this need is the production of enough health workers with basic and advanced qualifications that are relevant to the needs of the community (Scheffler et al. 2009). Another dimension is the ability to offer faculty members adequate and appropriate opportunities for professional growth in their own institutions and a satisfactory local environment in which to function (Marchal and Kegels 2003). Professional and personal factors that may influence faculty decisions to relocate to a different institution, country, or region include remuneration, access to equipment and advanced technology, career and training opportunities, skills development, professional network creation, opportunities for career advancement, work environment, opportunity for experience in a different environment, regional politics of health care, desire to improve medicine in region, social conditions, personal safety, degree of personal freedom, and family issues (Burch et al. 2011; Burdick et al. 2006).

As illustrated by the examples in this chapter, international faculty development partnerships differ (and evolve over time) in structures and purposes, and in the corresponding degree of organizational independence (Gajda 2004). Organizational independence can be conceptualized along a continuum from cooperation (where fully independent organizations share information) to coordination (where independent organizations align activities or co-sponsor events) to collaboration (where organizations give up some independence to achieve mutual goals).

Partnerships also vary in terms of partner resources and needs. The nature of partner contributions and benefits differ in part depending on partner resources and needs. For partnerships between relatively well-resourced and resource-limited institutions, the well-resourced may in part be motivated by altruism, as well as the potential for enhanced reputation, influence, and broadened perspectives and knowledge. The ideal partnership would be one in which there were equal, if distinct, benefits to each partner involved. Einterz et al. (2007) argue that equity, rather than equality, should be a characteristic of productive relationships, given that 'medical systems in the developed and developing world are inherently unequal' (Einterz et al. 2007, p. 813). Partnerships are supported by mutual contributions and benefits. This entails empowerment of all partners and a focus on fostering institutional strength.

In this chapter we will describe: (1) individual, institutional, system, societal, and relationship benefits of international faculty development partnerships; (2) ways in which international partnerships to date have been structured, of which we will provide examples; and (3) factors that support the quality and strength of partner relationships.

15.2 What Are the Benefits of International Faculty Development Partnerships?

There are inevitably multiple stakeholders in international faculty development partnerships, each operating within a different context and each with unique needs and strengths. Stakeholders include individuals, their institutions, and the societies and systems – including national healthcare and education systems – in which these institutions are situated (see Fig. 15.1). Organizations providing funding for partnership programs may also have an interest in partnership outcomes.

Each category of stakeholder (individuals, institutions, systems) derives different benefits from partnerships, as shown in Table 15.1. In addition, there are benefits distinctly related to the relationships between stakeholders. Achievement of any of the benefits will depend on well-functioning relationships, and so these are shown as central in Fig. 15.1. Faculty development evaluation has often focused

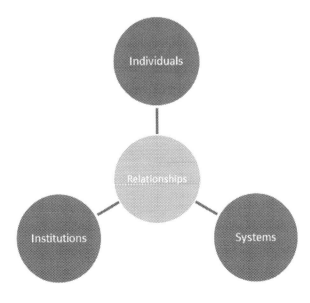

Fig. 15.1 Components of international faculty development partnerships

Table 15.1 Benefits of international faculty development partnerships

A. Individual benefits
New/expanded learning opportunities for faculty and students, resulting in knowledge/skill/ attitude/behavior changes
Broadened perspectives on health professions education (learning about healthcare and education practices and values in different countries and cultures)
Increased faculty preparedness for teaching, leadership, and other roles (broadly, or in educational areas)
B. Institutional benefits
Enhanced institutional reputation (by being seen as innovative, involved in global health)
Financial/resource benefits; strengthened institutional financial status; funding (resource sharing between partner institutions, resources from third parties external to partner institutions)
Development of sustainable capacity for ongoing faculty development
Education innovations or improvements
C. System and societal benefits
Strengthened education system (broadly, or in specific specialty areas)
Strengthened health care (broadly, or for specific health issues)
Enrichment of international practice of medicine and health professions education as well as health sciences and health professions education knowledge
Movement toward consideration of global standards/competencies as applicable
D. Relationship benefits
Development of, or improvements in, relationships between faculty members (through development of and participation in programs)
Development of an international community of health professions educators

on individual-level outcomes; however, there is increasing recognition of the need to examine 'relationship' aspects of faculty development (Asthana et al. 2002; El Ansari et al. 2001; Halliday et al. 2004; O'Sullivan and Irby 2011).

15.2.1 Individual Benefits

Potential benefits to those involved in any faculty development program will vary with the nature of the program being offered, and such benefits have been extensively treated in other chapters in this book. However, some benefits are particular to individual faculty members participating in an international program. Exposure to faculty and ideas from other countries, as well as to health care and culture in new contexts, can be motivating to faculty (Kanter 2010). Participation in partnerships can contribute to faculty and student growth by enhancing their knowledge about illness and wellness in different cultures and can thereby enrich their practice of both health professions education and health care (Brook et al. 2010; Kanter 2010). Benefits might also include enhanced work satisfaction accrued from participating in innovations in health professions education in low resource settings (Kolars et al. 2012). Greater professional recognition and advancement may also accrue to individuals for involvement in such partnerships (Tekian and Dwyer 1998).

15.2.2 Institutional Benefits

Most faculty development initiatives are intended to increase capacity and improve the quality of education at the participating institutions. These benefits should in turn extend to student learning and health care. Ideally, these benefits should be such that they are sustained beyond the duration of the faculty development partnership. The design of the initiative would be one crucial factor among several in determining whether any benefit accrues beyond participating individuals (Grossman and Salas 2011; Holton et al. 2003).

Involvement in partnerships can result in resource sharing or development by partners. These resources could be materials or access to facilities or exposure to a disease profile not common to one or the other institution. Involvement in partnerships can also generate access to funding that allows the development of capacity that would not otherwise be possible in resource-constrained environments (Kanter 2010; Kolars et al. 2012). Institutions involved may benefit from funding of external agencies (such as grant funding) that is channeled through their institutions. This funding may augment departmental and/or institutional resources by buying out faculty time for their involvement in the partnership.

When the faculty development partnership is between institutions from high and low income countries, the value proposition for partners from high income nations may be in part altruistic (Kolars et al. 2012). Helping to improve the quality of health professions education or health in resource constrained settings can enhance the reputation of institutions from high income countries (Kanter 2010).

Moreover, the reputation of all partners can be enhanced through collaboration and development of innovations (Kanter 2010). Involvement in international collaborations can gain credibility for partners with influential role players like legislators and national, regional, and international funding agencies (Conaboy et al. 2005; Tekian and Dwyer 1998). Over the longer term, benefits such as these could strengthen institutions by allowing them to attract better faculty and students (Kanter 2010).

15.2.3 System and Societal Benefits

The ultimate goal of many international faculty development partnerships is strengthening health care in their countries, typically by way of strengthening educational systems (Kanter 2010). The focus of international partnerships may be on a major illness, an area of specialty training, or more general areas of education. Faculty development that enhances education in partners' countries may contribute to the retention of health workers, especially where health care worker migration is an issue (Burch et al. 2011; Clinton et al. 2010). Stemming this migration, both between countries and from underserved (often rural) areas within countries, potentially reduces the costs of meeting the health needs of a nation (Kanter 2010).

Relatively small faculty development initiatives cannot hope to address major societal issues such as the small number of universities graduating health professionals and the small number of graduates they deliver. However, issues like faculty preparedness to teach, curriculum development skills, the ability to network with other health professions educators, and preparation to assume leadership and management roles in the health care system (Kolars et al. 2012) can be addressed by such initiatives.

Faculty development partners from high income countries may benefit to some degree by contributing to the realization of humanitarian goals like improving the quality of health professions education around the world (Guo et al. 2009), enhancing health in a district or nation where resources are limited, and helping solve pressing health problems by improving the quality and relevance of the education of health professionals (Kanter 2010; Kolars et al. 2012). Strengthening health care and enhancing health in lower income countries may have benefits that extend to all partners. For instance, this could contribute to decreasing the spread of illness from one country to another (Kanter 2010). As importantly, much can be learned from the solutions to challenges encountered in low resource environments. Finally, mutual engagement across cultural and resourcing divides can build knowledge about the practice of medicine and of health professions education that can enrich these practices internationally.

15.2.4 Relationship Benefits

It may sound obvious to say that partnerships are about relationships, but in fact there are distinct benefits related to a partnership comprised of well-functioning relationships. Partnerships can build teams and strengthen networks (Kolars et al. 2012). Lessons learned about facilitators and challenges of relationship sustainability and success can be applied to strengthen and expand international partnerships (Tekian and Dwyer 1998). Extended partnerships can contribute to the development and strengthening of international communities of health professions educators.

15.3 Examples of International Faculty Development Partnership Programs

Each international faculty development partnership has arisen from a unique set of perceived needs and available resources. This section will briefly describe some partnership programs. It is important to note that one partnership may yield multiple programs. Likewise, faculty development may be one component of an international collaboration (e.g. a collaboration to start a new medical school that includes faculty development as one component). Programs in this section have been selected on the basis that faculty development through sustained institutional partnerships is a substantive component of the overall program. Not included here are international and regional conferences, consortia, committees, and task forces such as those supported by the Association for Medical Education in Europe (AMEE), the World Health Organization (WHO), and the World Federation for Medical Education (WFME), all of which have broader health professions education oversight and improvement goals (e.g. Conaboy et al. 2005). Examples were also selected based on the availability of information about the program.

The following sections offer a few examples of varied partnership program structures that include coordinating organizations with multi-institution participation; health professions education degree- and diploma-conferring institutions; and two-institution partnerships. They are not intended as an exhaustive listing of partnerships. Each program's 'desired benefits' are those identified in the literature, and may not include all levels of benefits described in the previous section of this chapter.

15.3.1 Coordinating Organization with Multi-institution Participation

International partnership programs that involve a central coordinating organization with multi-institution participation are capable of global reach. The following two examples illustrate this geographic breadth.

One example of a program run by a coordinating organization is **The Harvard Macy Institute: Program for Educators in Health Professions** (http://www.harvardmacy.org; Armstrong et al. 2003; Armstrong and Barsion 2006; Armstrong 2007). Program faculty come from a range of institutions and countries. Some program alumni are involved as faculty. International participants are healthcare professionals with a role as educators. The program was established with a grant from the Josiah Macy Jr. Foundation, and additional funding comes from tuition fees paid by participants. Additional support comes from faculty and staff time from Harvard and other institutions.

The program consists of two residential sessions about 4 months apart. There are five curricular themes: learning and teaching, curriculum, evaluation, leadership, and information technology. Participants undertake an educational project (e.g. revision of curriculum or implementation of a faculty development program in the participant's home institution). The informal curriculum is noted to be as important as the formal curriculum (i.e. largely ad hoc interpersonal interactions between and among students and faculty are as important to the achievement of program goals as the formally stated and intended curriculum).

Desired benefits of the program include enhancing the professional development of health professionals as educators, supporting institutional changes via changes in participant teaching behaviors and professional activities, and developing communities of practice across disciplines and institutions. Evidence of goal achievement includes participants' (learners') report of:

- Increased awareness and use of a greater array of teaching methods; increased knowledge about and comfort with active learning.
- Increased enthusiasm for and commitment to medical education as a primary career direction and stronger identity and confidence as a medical educator.
- New understanding of, and appreciation for, ways in which medical education is implemented in institutions nationally and globally (i.e. broadened perspectives).
- Evidence of organizational change via participant behaviors (e.g. additional projects, joining educational committees, educational grant applications).
- Creation/expansion of a global network of resources and connections, including support from like-minded colleagues.

The **Foundation for Advancement of International Medical Education and Research (FAIMER): FAIMER Institute and FAIMER Regional Institutes** are also examples of programs with a coordinating organization (http://www.faimer. org; Burdick et al. 2006, 2007, 2010, 2011, 2012; Norcini et al. 2005). The FAIMER Institute program has on-site sessions based in the USA with international participants; FAIMER Regional Institutes have on-site sessions and participants based in their regions (including programs based in India, Brazil, China, and South Africa). The core program faculty and leadership include FAIMER personnel, alumni of the fellowships (including local alumni for the Regional Institutes), and other international faculty. Health professions educators apply in a competitive process to participate in the fellowship programs, with evidence of institutional support as part of the application process. FAIMER provides partial funding and in-kind support for the fellowships. Regional Institutes provide in-kind support. The Brazil program is largely funded by the Brazil Ministry of Health. Fellows and their institutions share costs of the program, with each program working on a slightly different cost sharing model. Fellows and alumni are occasionally funded to attend national and international health professions education conferences, based upon advancing collaborative projects.

The FAIMER programs are 2-year fellowships, with two residential sessions (at the start of each year) interspersed with an 11-month intersession of learning at a distance. An educational innovation project is central as an opportunity for hands-on application of fellowship learning and work towards institutional or regional change in health professions education. Community building occurs via extensive interaction during residential sessions, overlap of the on-site sessions of year 1 and 2 fellows, and continued engagement with program alumni.

Desired benefits of the programs include strengthening fellows' skills in health professions education methods, leadership, management, research, and scholarship. At the institutional level, there is the desire to improve health professions education in the fellows' home institutions and countries/regions, stimulate growth in the field of health professions education, and improve opportunities for professional advancement. The programs also aim to build a transnational community of practice by creating a critical mass of health professions educators and facilitating interaction, resource sharing, and collaboration. Evidence of goal achievement includes the following:

- Fellows have reported applying knowledge and skills gained from the fellowship experience in their home institutions, including achievement of a range of project outcomes.
- The majority of fellows have reported that their educational innovation projects have been incorporated into the curriculum or institutional policy, and/or replicated in their institution or another setting.
- Follow-up data indicate that fellowship program alumni have health professions education career paths, produce education scholarship, engage in collaborative projects, and serve as resource experts in health professions education.
- Fellows have reported a community of practice characterized by support, shared learning and problem solving, and a network of expanded breadth in terms of geographic diversity and expertise.

As the above examples illustrate, the coordinating organization model of international faculty development programs is distinguished by not only geographic breadth of reach but also a desire to build international communities of practice. This latter distinction also may involve on-going relationships with program graduates.

15.3.2 Health Professions Education Degree- and Diploma-Conferring Institutions

International partnerships for health professions education degree/diploma programs (Tekian and Harris 2012) vary in the roles of each partner institution (including degree conferral), and plans for long-term sustainability (e.g. joint degree program versus capacity building for program administered by one partner institution). Two examples are offered here in order to illustrate this variation.

The **Joint Master of Health Professions Education (JMHPE) Maastricht University – Suez Canal University** (http://www.maastrichtuniversity.nl/web/show/id=449891/langid=42; http://www.themedfomscu.org; Mohamed et al. 2012) involves core program faculty and leadership from both Maastricht and Suez Canal Universities. Global faculty are chosen from program graduates. Participants are graduates of any health professions education institution (e.g. medicine, nursing, dentistry, pharmacy, health sciences, physiotherapy, and speech therapy). Participants include presidents of universities, deans and vice deans of health professions education institutions and full professors.

The program is a 1 year (9 blocks) Master program, conducted entirely via distance learning. By the end of the program a master degree is jointly granted, and the certificate is co-signed by both Maastricht and Suez Canal Universities.

There is WHO sponsorship for the program. Most participants are either self-funded and pay the full tuition fees, or get partial fellowship funding from the WHO and pay part of the fee. A few participants get a full fellowship from the WHO that covers all program expenses including the full tuition fees and travel costs to attend their graduation. Some participants share costs of the program with their institutions. JMHPE Management provides limited full/partial funding for joining the program.

Desired benefits of the programs include equipping participants with the knowledge and skills required for a career in health professions education and research, and developing critical masses of graduates who can actively participate in the enhancement of medical education in their home institutions. Evidence of goal achievement includes the following:

- Program graduates and participants (learners) report that the program supports increased knowledge of health professions education as well as enhanced capacity building and career development at the national, regional, and international levels.
- The Medical Education Department of Suez Canal University was awarded a Leadership and Management Award in 2010 by Management Sciences for Health, an international non-profit organization working with individuals, communities and institutions in developing nations to build stronger health systems, improve health services, and respond to priority health problems.

Another example of a degree- or diploma-conferring partnership is the **University of Illinois at Chicago (UIC) and KLE University in Belgaum, India – Diploma and Masters in Health Professions Education (MScHPE) program** (http://www.kleuniversity.edu.in/udeph/index.html; A. Tekian, personal communication, August 22, 2012). The core teaching faculty for this program come from UIC and are full-time professors. There are other local faculty as well who were trained at UIC. All the participants come from India. Priority is given to KLE University faculty members; however, a few health professionals from neighboring provinces are accepted as well. All participants are health professionals, with the majority from medicine, dentistry, and nursing.

This is a 2-year program, with mandatory week-long courses offered at regular intervals. All course material is developed at UIC taking into consideration the Indian context of education and culture. Completion of the program requires a capstone. The primary advisor is from UIC and the thesis committee consists of three faculty members. All capstone projects are presented at an Annual Conference in health professions education held in Belgaum. Diplomas and degrees are offered by KLE University.

The program is funded by KLE University and is housed at the University Department of Education for Health Professionals (UDEHP). UDEHP provides in-kind support for the daily operation of the program, including coordination of communication, educational resources such as handouts, and the physical facility. KLE University provides lodging accommodations located on campus for all international teaching faculty. Tuition fees are subsidized and participants are supported by their institutions, or pay themselves.

Desired benefits of the program include acquisition and improvement in knowledge and proficiency in essential skills in medical education, including teaching and learning, curriculum development, scholarship, and leadership. It is also hoped that program participants will act as change agents and resources within their colleges and departments, promote collaboration institution wide, and help to create an educational climate within the institution that fosters excellence in education and scholarship. On a systems level, it is hoped that the program will strengthen the educational system nation-wide by fostering dissemination of educational innovations within the country's higher education system, within institutions associated with the Ministries of Health and Education, and through professional societies. The program also aims to support relationships among participants in order to create a community of practice among health professionals who exchange ideas and share resources; to create working relationships and collaborations among institutions to share data and conduct inter-institutional scholarship; and to prepare and submit multi-institutional grant proposals to fund research. Evidence of goal achievement includes the following:

- Participants of the program have been involved in introducing education changes at their institutions (primarily KLE) and have published and presented education scholarship. For example, the concept of competency-based curriculum has been introduced for the first time in the College of Dentistry.
- Faculty development activities in medical education are organized and conducted by the participants of the program. UDEHP and a few participants of the program organized the first medical education conference in Belgaum in 2012.
- A select number of participants have been asked to serve as educational consultants to committees that guide national policies.
- Networking among the participants has initiated multi-institutional projects attracting research funding.

The examples above illustrate different models for partnership capacity building – i.e. creation of a joint degree program (Suez-Maastricht) versus enhancing capacity of one partner institution to independently offer degree/diploma conferral (KLE-UIC). There are also differences in whether the degree/diploma program is focused on faculty from one of the partner institutions (e.g. KLE University) or whether it is geared to more broad dissemination (e.g. Suez–Maastricht, which also uses distance learning to broaden its reach).

15.3.3   Two-Institution Partnerships

There are several documented examples of partnerships between two institutions in different countries. These programs vary in their structures and goals, including faculty development as part of a larger initiative such as development of a new residency program (e.g. Alem et al. 2010), bilateral exchange of faculty and students (e.g. Wong and Agisheva 2004, 2007), and long-term institutional partnerships (twinning, e.g. Lacey-Haun and Whitehead 2009; Tache et al. 2008). The following offers some examples, not an exhaustive survey, of programs based on the Indiana-Moi twinning partnership. This partnership includes multiple components, and has evolved and grown over the course of about 20 years.

The **Indiana University – Moi University (IU-Moi) Partnership** (Einterz et al. 2007) involves collaboration between virtually all disciplines at both schools and relationships at both individual and department levels.

Desired benefits of the partnership include achieving mutual, equitable benefits for both partner institutions and their individual participants; developing leaders in healthcare for the United States and Kenya; and fostering the values of the medical profession and promoting health through collaboration and education.

One program based on the Indiana-Moi partnership is the Academic Research Ethics Partnership (AREP). AREP has developed two Master's degree programs, one at Indiana University-Purdue University Indianapolis (IUPUI) and one at Moi University. These programs have common components, joint advisory committees, and a practicum experience partly taken at the counterpart university. Each AREP partner convenes an annual Teaching Skills in International Research Ethics (TaSkR) workshop to provide training to approximately 50 faculty and students each year. AREP is funded by a $940,000 4-year grant from the Fogarty International Center at the National Institutes of Health.

A second program based on the Indiana-Moi partnership is the Academic Model for the Prevention and Treatment of HIV/AIDS (AMPATH). AMPATH partners include Moi University, Moi Teaching and Referral Hospital, and a consortium of North American academic health centers led by Indiana University, working in partnership with the Government of Kenya. AMPATH has established a comprehensive HIV-care system that serves over 40,000 patients and their communities. AMPATH has been supported by grants from multiple sources, including the United States Agency for International Development, President's Emergency Plan for HIV/AIDS Relief, U.S. Centers for Disease Control and Prevention, Maternal to Child Transmission Plus Initiative, Gates Foundation, and other private philanthropy.

Evidence of goal achievement includes establishment of initiatives such as AREP and AMPATH, and the achievements of these programs including the opportunities and services offered to faculty, students, and patients.

Partnerships such as the above example are distinguished by having multiple components (e.g. student and faculty exchanges, faculty development, joint programs), evolution over time in response to partner needs (e.g. focusing on HIV pandemic) and collaboration with additional partners (medical institutions and hospitals, government institutions, communities, funders) to achieve specific goals.

15.4 Descriptors of International Faculty Development Partnerships

The previous examples illustrate some of the variations in international faculty development partnerships. The descriptors in Table 15.2 attempt to more systematically illustrate potential variations in partnership programs. Generally there is a collaborative relationship (i.e. partners giving up some independence) between two or more institutions at the core of program delivery. However, there are often other cooperative and coordinating relationships – either with additional institutions or between the partner institutions but for other purposes. For example, the Foundation for Advancement of International Medical Education and Research (FAIMER)

Table 15.2 Descriptors of international faculty development programs

Descriptor	Explanation
Degree of organizational independence	While partnerships generally involve collaboration (where organizations give up some independence to achieve mutual goals), they may also involve cooperation (where fully independent organizations share information) and coordination (where independent organizations align activities or co-sponsor events)
Partners and their roles	Backgrounds and selection of faculty development program faculty and participants (e.g. geographic representation, participation of program alumni as faculty for the program, program faculty, and participants internal/external to partner institutions)
Desired benefits/goals	Purpose, change or goal that program seeks to achieve (see Table 15.1)
Programs and processes	Timing of program (longitudinal ongoing, at regular intervals, at varying intervals depending on need). This refers to the timing of faculty development programs; partnerships would by definition be long-term
	Credentialing (source of any degree/diploma conferral – e.g. 'home' institution confers degree with technical/resource support from external institution; degree conferred by external institution)
	Process and content (e.g. curricular themes; education methods)
Resourcing	Funding and other resources from external third party, one/some/all partners, program participants

programs involve collaboration with the institutions hosting and providing in-kind resources for regional faculty development programs as well as cooperative relationships with the institutions from which participants come. The Indiana-Moi partnership has also led to the development of a consortium of North American academic health centers led by Indiana University, working in partnership with the Government of Kenya.

Thus, partnerships can be conceptualized as a set of relationships that evolve over time in structure, purpose, and degree of independence in order to meet changing needs and respond to emerging opportunities.

15.5 Factors That Facilitate Successful Partnerships

While there is a need for more research on success factors for international faculty development partnerships (El Ansari et al. 2001; Glendinning 2002; Halliday et al. 2004; O'Sullivan and Irby 2011), existing literature on successful partnerships, including international collaborations in medical education, point to relevant factors for international faculty development partnerships (Kolars et al. 2012; Tekian and Dwyer 1998).

'Success' is defined by both the process and outcomes of the partnership. Indicators of process success include high engagement and commitment of the partners, agreement about the purpose and need for the partnership, high levels of trust and respect, supportive surrounding environments (financial climate, institutional and

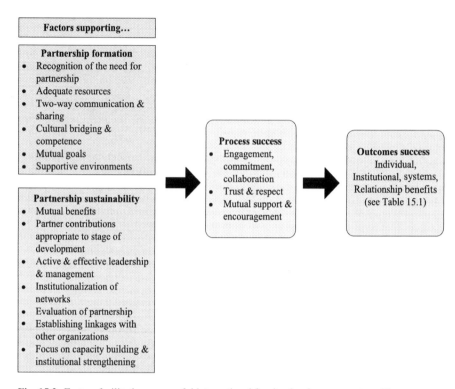

Fig. 15.2 Factors facilitating successful international faculty development partnerships

legal structures, broader inter-organizational relationship), adequate monitoring and evaluation of the partnership, and active and effective leadership and management (Dowling et al. 2004).

Process success can further be divided into success with partnership formation and success with sustaining partnerships over time (Leffers and Mitchell 2011). Outcome success indicators relate to achievement of the individual, institutional, system, and relationship benefits described earlier in this chapter. These may include positive changes in the partner institutions (e.g. quality of teaching) as well as the community being served (e.g. competence of graduates, health of community). Outcome success is dependent upon process success in forming and sustaining the partnership.

Figure 15.2 represents our synthesis and adaptation of ideas from the multiple sources cited in this chapter regarding definitions and facilitators of partnership success.

15.5.1 Partnership Formation

Three key elements in the establishment of partnerships are the respective partners; certain human, financial, and material resources; and a process of engagement (Leffers and Mitchell 2011). Recognition and acceptance of the need for partnership, frequent and two-way communication, mutual goal setting, adequate resources (including not only tangible assets but also time, expertise, trust, and understanding of each other), knowledge and information sharing, and cultural competence are cited as factors supporting the establishment of partnership relationships (Asthana et al. 2002; Gajda 2004; Kolars et al. 2012; Leffers and Mitchell 2011; Tekian and Dwyer 1998).

Incorporating these factors into a partnership requires mindful planning. For example, there is a need to recognize and minimize organizational barriers that may impede sharing information between institutions (e.g. policies restricting information sharing). Mutual goal setting is important to ensure that all partners benefit; it also helps to avoid the potential fostering of dependency of one partner on the other (Kolars et al. 2012).

Cultural competence includes being open to and valuing differences, with cultural differences arising also from differences in organizational cultures (Asthana et al. 2002). Addressing language differences may be part of this (Wong and Agisheva 2007), along with cultural awareness, knowledge, and skills (Tekian and Dwyer 1998; Campinha-Bacote 2002). The bridging of cultures also extends to educational cultures (Wong and Agisheva 2007). Faculty in one setting may not be accustomed to being subjected to teaching strategies in the course of faculty development activities that are commonplace in another setting.

In a comparison of international partnerships to establish Masters programs in Health Professions Education (MHPE) in China and Egypt, Tekian and Dwyer (1998) highlight the importance of effective communication and the challenges of language differences. This includes potential difficulty with faculty members communicating with each other and with students (in the absence of translators), and limited use of literature in languages where faculty and students have limited fluency. Cultural awareness, understanding of accepted values, political climate, and the socioeconomic status of the country are important when developing international faculty development partnerships. Thus, partners need to work toward understanding each other's contexts, needs, resources, and priorities, and using this awareness as a basis for developing the partnership agenda.

Strategies to achieve cultural competence may include seeking culturally-friendly teaching and assessment tools, resisting stereo-types, discussing features of culture with others, reviewing the literature on identity, and participating in professional development that addresses cultural competence (Willis 1999). Careful preparation, including molding and tailoring a program to local needs and adapting and supplementing the content with examples and case studies appropriate to local environments, is also imperative to success (Tekian and Dwyer 1998).

Cultural perspectives, personal attributes, personal expectations, and knowledge of the partner country all play a role in the development of the partner relationship. Careful selection of faculty who are willing to teach in a different culture improves the productivity and contribution of the faculty. Additionally, sufficient time should be devoted for preparing faculty interested in undertaking international assignments in order to minimize cultural misunderstandings and increase tolerance to seeing the world through multiple lenses (Tekian and Dwyer 1998).

Citing various papers, Leffers and Mitchell (2011, p. 99) highlight the role of various attributes for effective partnerships, including the following: 'agreement to partner; collegial relationships that include reciprocity, communication, mutual support, mutual trust, respect, equality and conflict management; interdependency that involves sharing, cooperation, and synergy between professionals; frequent feedback; and power and leadership that is consensual and egalitarian'.

Effective communication, shared decision making, and negotiation are important skills for effective collaboration (Kolars et al. 2012; Leffers and Mitchell 2011; Tekian and Dwyer 1998). This is aided by face-to-face meetings between collaborators (Kolars et al. 2012). Establishing mutually-agreed goals is part of the on-going process of exchange. Implicit in this process is the development of a shared set of values.

Setting a clear agenda for both what constitute appropriate goals and how those goals will be measured may help ensure an effective partnership. One way of achieving this is devising and undertaking a needs assessment process together (Guo et al. 2009). One collective of partnerships between North America and sub-Saharan African institutions devised ten learning questions to inform their discussions and a framework of desired evidence at the outset (Kolars et al. 2012). Taking this a step further, robust approaches need to be developed to assess potential benefits and risks so that parties engaging in a collaboration are both informed about and optimally able to address relevant issues (Kanter 2010).

15.5.2 Partnership Sustainability

As discussed in the beginning of this chapter, partnership structures and goals may evolve over time. Mutual support and encouragement are important at all stages of partnerships. Partners contributing energy at different stages of the process can be important for sustainability, as are mutual benefits. Altruism alone is not a sufficient condition for maintaining a partnership (Einterz et al. 2007).

Active and effective leadership and management and shared project ownership have been noted to support sustainability of partnerships (Asthana et al. 2002; Leffers and Mitchell 2011). For relationships to be sustainable, there is a need to transcend dependence on specific individuals (since the specific individuals involved are likely to change over time). Institutionalizing networks so that relationships and values are part of the structure and process of how the partnership operates may support this (Asthana et al. 2002). Evaluation of partnerships may also provide information and accountability that is useful for improving and sustaining the partnership (Asthana et al. 2002).

Establishing linkages with other organizations engaged in related work may strengthen the success and sustainability of partnerships (Asthana et al. 2002). Large collaborations may be effectively established by first establishing relationships at personal, departmental, and institutional levels, before involving universities, government ministries, and central governments (Einterz et al. 2007).

Attention to sustainability is in itself of great importance so that partners focus on institutional strengthening rather than transitory relationships and benefits (Kolars et al. 2012). This sort of capacity building may entail attention to champions, leadership, expertise structures, policies, procedures, and resources (Leffers and

Mitchell 2011). Depending on the ultimate partnership goals, success over time may involve transfer of program ownership from joint to one partner, once sufficient capacity exists. There has also been a call for government and philanthropic funders to direct support to the establishment of long-term institutional partnerships so as to increase the likelihood of impact on building developing countries' health systems (Einterz et al. 2007).

15.6 Conclusion

International faculty development partnerships are often comprised of a set of relationships that evolve over time in structure, purpose, and degree of independence in order to meet changing needs and respond to emerging opportunities. The potential benefits of these partnerships, and means to achieve benefits, are varied. General factors that support successful partnership formation include frequent two-way communication, mutual goal setting, setting a clear agenda, adequate resources, and cultural competence. Partnership sustainability is supported by realization of mutual benefits, effective leadership and management, shared project ownership, establishment of linkages with other organizations, and institutional strengthening and capacity building.

15.7 Key Messages

- Building relationships is crucial for productive, sustained international faculty development partnerships.
- Well-functioning partnerships allow faculty exposure to methods, materials, opportunities, contexts, and contacts/networks that they may not encounter locally.
- Cultural bridging, effective and frequent communication, and mutual goal setting are important to partnership success.
- Success in partnerships is defined by both process and outcomes success, and rests on attention to and planning for not only partnership formation but also sustainability.
- International faculty development partnerships vary in their structures and purposes, with both potentially evolving over time in response to partner needs and goals.

References

Alem, A., Pain, C., Araya, M., & Hodges, B. D. (2010). Co-creating a psychiatric resident program with Ethiopians, for Ethiopians, in Ethiopia: The Toronto Addis Ababa Psychiatry Project (TAAPP). *Academic Psychiatry, 34*(6), 424–432.

Armstrong, E. G. (2007). An outcomes approach to evaluate professional development programmes for medical educators. *Annals of the Academy of Medicine, Singapore, 36*(8), 619–621.

Armstrong, E. G. & Barsion, S. J. (2006). Using an outcomes-logic-model approach to evaluate a faculty development program for medical educators. *Academic Medicine, 81*(5), 483–488.

Armstrong, E. G., Doyle, J., & Bennett, N. L. (2003). Transformative professional development of physicians as educators: Assessment of a model. *Academic Medicine, 78*(7), 702–708.

Asthana, S., Richardson, S., & Halliday, J. (2002). Partnership working in public policy provision: A framework for evaluation. *Social Policy & Administration, 36*(7), 780–795.

Brook, S., Robertson, D., Makuwaza, T., & Hodges, B. D. (2010). Canadian residents teaching and learning psychiatry in Ethiopia: A grounded theory analysis focusing on their experiences. *Academic Psychiatry, 34*(6), 433–437.

Burch, V. C., McKinley, D., van Wyk, J., Kiguli-Walube, S., Cameron, D., Cilliers, F. J., et al. (2011). Career intentions of medical students trained in six sub-Saharan African countries. *Education for Health, 24*(3), Art. 614.

Burdick, W. P., Amaral, E., Campos, H., & Norcini, J. (2011). A model for linkage between health professions education and health: FAIMER international faculty development initiatives. *Medical Teacher, 33*(8), 632–637.

Burdick, W. P., Diserens, D., Friedman, S. R., Morahan, P. S., Kalishman, S., Eklund, M. A., et al. (2010). Measuring the effects of an international health professions faculty development fellowship: The FAIMER Institute. *Medical Teacher, 32*(5), 414–421.

Burdick, W. P., Friedman, S. R., & Diserens, D. (2012). Faculty development projects for international health professions educators: Vehicles for institutional change? *Medical Teacher, 34*(1), 38–44.

Burdick, W. P., Morahan, P. S., & Norcini, J. J. (2006). Slowing the brain drain: FAIMER education programs. *Medical Teacher, 28*(7), 631–634.

Burdick, W. P., Morahan, P. S., & Norcini, J. J. (2007). Capacity building in medical education and health outcomes in developing countries: The missing link. *Education for Health, 20*(3), 65.

Campinha-Bacote, J. (2002). The process of cultural competence in the delivery of healthcare services: A model of care. *Journal of Transcultural Nursing, 13*(3), 181–184.

Clinton, Y., Anderson, F. W., & Kwawukume, E. Y. (2010). Factors related to retention of postgraduate trainees in obstetrics-gynecology at the Korle-Bu Teaching Hospital in Ghana. *Academic Medicine, 85*(10), 1564–1570.

Conaboy, K. A., Nugmanova, Z., Yeguebaeva, S., Jaeger, F., & Daugherty, R. M. (2005). Central Asian republics: A case study for medical education reform. *Journal of Continuing Education in the Health Professions, 25*(1), 52–64.

Dowling, B., Powell, M., & Glendinning, C. (2004). Conceptualising successful partnerships. *Health and Social Care in the Community, 12*(4), 309–317.

Einterz, R. M., Kimaiyo, S., Mengech, H. N. K., Khwa-Otsyula, B. O., Esamai, F., Quigley, F., et al. (2007). Responding to the HIV pandemic: The power of an academic medical partnership. *Academic Medicine, 82*(8), 812–818.

El Ansari, W., Phillips, C. J., & Hammick, M. (2001). Collaboration and partnerships: Developing the evidence base. *Health & Social Care in the Community, 9*(4), 215–227.

Gajda, R. (2004). Utilizing collaboration theory to evaluate strategic alliances. *American Journal of Evaluation, 25*(1), 65–77.

Glendinning, C. (2002). Partnerships between health and social services: Developing a framework for evaluation. *Policy & Politics, 30*(1), 115–127.

Grossman, R. & Salas, E. (2011). The transfer of training: What really matters. *International Journal of Training and Development, 15*(2), 103–120.

Guo, Y., Sippola, E., Feng, X., Dong, Z., Wang, D., Moyer, C. A., et al. (2009). International medical school faculty development: The results of a needs assessment survey among medical educators in China. *Advances in Health Sciences Education, 14*(1), 91–102.

Halliday, J., Asthana, S. N. M., & Richardson, S. (2004). Evaluating partnership: The role of formal assessment tools. *Evaluation, 10*(3), 285–303.

Hodges, B. D., Maniate, J. M., Martimianakis, M. A., Alsuwaidan, M., & Segouin, C. (2009). Cracks and crevices: Globalization discourse and medical education. *Medical Teacher, 31*(10), 910–917.

Holton, E. F., Chen, H-C., & Naquin, S. S. (2003). An examination of learning transfer system characteristics across organizational settings. *Human Resource Development Quarterly, 14*(4), 459–482.

Kanter, S. L. (2010). International collaborations between medical schools: What are the benefits and risks? *Academic Medicine, 85*(10), 1547–1548.

Kolars, J. C., Cahill, K., Donkor, P., Kaaya, E., Lawson, A., Serwadda, D., et al. (2012). Perspective: Partnering for medical education in Sub-Saharan Africa: Seeking the evidence for effective collaborations. *Academic Medicine, 87*(2), 216–220.

Lacey-Haun, L. C. & Whitehead, T. D. (2009). Leading change through an international faculty development programme. *Journal of Nursing Management, 17*(8), 917–930.

Leffers, J. & Mitchell, E. (2011). Conceptual model for partnership and sustainability in global health. *Public Health Nursing, 28*(1), 91–102.

Marchal, B. & Kegels, G. (2003). Health workforce imbalances in times of globalization: Brain drain or professional mobility? *The International Journal of Health Planning and Management, 18*(Suppl 1), S89–S101.

McAuliffe, M. S. & Cohen, M. Z. (2005). International nursing research and educational exchanges: A review of the literature. *Nursing Outlook, 53*(1), 21–25.

Mohamed, A. A., Yousef, W. T., Hamam, A. M., & Khamis, N. N. (2012). *Evaluation of the Joint Master of Health Professions Education: A distance learning program – between Suez Canal University, Egypt, and Maastricht University, The Netherlands.* Unpublished manuscript, Suez Canal University.

Norcini, J. J. & Banda, S. S. (2011). Increasing the quality and capacity of education: The challenge for the 21st century. *Medical Education, 45*(1), 81–86.

Norcini, J. J., Burdick, W. P., & Morahan, P. (2005). The FAIMER Institute: Creating international networks of medical educators. *Medical Teacher, 27*(3), 214–218.

O'Sullivan, P. S. & Irby, D. M. (2011). Reframing research on faculty development. *Academic Medicine, 86*(4), 421–428.

Scheffler, R. M., Mahoney, C. B., Fulton, B. D., Dal Poz, M. R., & Preker, A. S. (2009). Estimates of health care professional shortages in Sub-Saharan Africa by 2015. *Health Affairs, 28*(5), w849–w862.

Tache, S., Kaaya, E., Omer, S., Mkony, C. A., Lyamuya, E., Pallangyo, K., et al. (2008). University partnership to address the shortage of healthcare professionals in Africa. *Global Public Health, 3*(2), 137–148.

Tekian, A. & Dwyer, M. (1998). Lessons for the future: Comparison and contrasts of the Master of Health Professions Education programs offered in China and Egypt. *Teaching and Learning in Medicine, 10*(3), 190–195.

Tekian, A. & Harris, I. (2012). Preparing health professions education leaders worldwide: A description of masters-level programs. *Medical Teacher, 34*(1), 52–58.

Willis, W. O. (1999). Culturally competent nursing care during the perinatal period. *The Journal of Perinatal & Neonatal Nursing, 13*(3), 45–59.

Wong, J. G. & Agisheva, K. (2004). Cross-cultural faculty development: Initial report of an American/Russian experience. *Teaching and Learning in Medicine, 16*(4), 376–380.

Wong, J. G. & Agisheva, K. (2007). Developing teaching skills for medical educators in Russia: A cross-cultural faculty development project. *Medical Education, 41*(3), 318–324.

World Health Organization, Global Health Workforce Alliance: Taskforce on Scaling up Education and Training (2008). *Scaling up, saving lives.* Available from: http://www.who.int/workforcealliance/documents/Global_Health%20FINAL%20REPORT.pdf

Chapter 16
Starting a Faculty Development Program

Ivan Silver

16.1 Introduction

Faculty development programs in medical and other health professions schools, specialty societies, and colleges have grown steadily over the past 20 years (Al-Wardy 2008; McLeod and Steinert 2010). This surge in growth has been precipitated by the acknowledgement that support for faculty in their roles as teachers, educators, researchers and administrators is essential for a vibrant academic community and culture (Steinert et al. 2006).

For the purposes of this chapter, faculty development is defined as:

> The broad range of activities that institutions use to renew or assist faculty members in their multiple roles. Faculty development activities include programs to enhance teaching and education, research and scholarly activity, academic leadership and management, and faculty affairs, including faculty recruitment, advancement, retention, and vitality. The intent of these activities is to assist faculty members in their roles as teachers, educators, leaders, administrators and researchers (1st International Conference on Faculty Development in the Health Professions 2011).

Faculty development programs have also grown in complexity in response to recent trends and changes in health professions education. Some of these key trends include the professionalism of health professions education, competency-based education, technology-enhanced learning, social accountability, increasingly sophisticated and standardized selection of students and assessment processes, work-based learning, academic leadership development, interprofessional education, the use of simulation, patient safety and quality improvement, transitions curricula, and continuing

I. Silver, MD, M.Ed., FRCP(C) (✉)
Department of Psychiatry, Centre for Addiction and Mental Health,
Faculty of Medicine, University of Toronto, Toronto, ON, Canada
e-mail: ivan.silver@camh.ca

Y. Steinert (ed.), *Faculty Development in the Health Professions: A Focus on Research and Practice*, Innovation and Change in Professional Education 11, DOI 10.1007/978-94-007-7612-8_16, © Springer Science+Business Media Dordrecht 2014

personal and professional development for certification purposes (Association of Faculties of Medicine of Canada 2010, 2012; General Medical Council 2009; Medical Deans Australia and New Zealand 2009; Patricio and Harden 2010). These trends are also shaping the form in which faculty development is being offered.

Starting a faculty development program can be challenging for health professions educators and administrators. The purpose of this chapter is to outline an approach for starting a faculty development program—whether it is initiating a single hospital department-based program addressing a focused faculty development issue, building a program in a hospital, specialty society or college, or starting a program that is faculty-wide, national or international. Guided by change theory and other theoretical approaches and related models and guidelines that can inform faculty development, we will describe the developmental steps required (Steinert et al. 2005; Steinert and Mann 2006; Wilkerson 1984).

16.2   Initial Steps in Designing a Faculty Development Program

16.2.1   Accept the Challenge

Being asked or taking the initiative to start a faculty development program in an organization is the very first step. The leader needs to be convinced that there is a strong institutional willingness and support to engage in these activities, that there are colleagues who will work with the leader, and that the program will have some resources attached to it. When organizations don't fully understand what might be needed for a faculty development program to succeed, the proposed leader of the program needs to take the time to meet with those she/he reports to, in order to secure the necessary resources. It is very possible to start a program successfully with modest resources, combined with strong institutional willingness for its success. For example, one of the most compelling ways to begin a program is to simply gather interested faculty and staff together to talk about teaching, career development or leadership (D'Eon et al. 2000). While this isn't a common institutional practice, don't be surprised to hear participants say, 'I don't understand why we haven't done this before. When are we meeting again?'

16.2.2   Understand the Institutional and Organizational Culture

Understanding the institutional and organizational culture allows the faculty development program to be responsive to the organization's needs. This subject is crucial, since successful faculty development programs are situated contextually within organizations. See Chap. 6 for a further discussion of this topic.

Ideally, the faculty development leader is integrated into the organization's education leadership. In a small program, where the leader of faculty development may be the only faculty developer, this can take the form of representation on the faculty or society education or academic planning committee. In a larger faculty development program, this can take the form of mutual committee membership (i.e. representation of faculty developers on key curriculum committees and representation of university or society leadership on faculty development planning committees). Integrating the leaders of faculty development into the key decision-making bodies of an organization ensures alignment of the needs of the organization with program planning.

Curricular reform is an ideal time to situate or initiate a new faculty development program because there are more opportunities for new relationships, exchanges and collaborations to develop; funding for resources is also more often available (Rubeck and Witzke 1998). Health professions education is increasingly interprofessional, and this is reflected in several new faculty development programs (Brashers et al. 2012; Moaveni et al. 2008; Silver and Leslie 2009; Steinert 2005). Faculty development leaders need to address whether a program is oriented to single disciplines, interprofessional audiences or combinations of the two. Having permanent representatives from various health professions on faculty development planning committees can help faculty developers and educators anticipate and integrate new and cutting edge curricular innovations into the faculty development curricula and promote interprofessional education.

16.2.3 Develop a Change Strategy

Whether faculty developers or educational leaders are considering initiating a single faculty development program within a department or a system-wide program at a medical school, speciality society or college, it is easy to be intimidated by the challenge. Where do we start? Whom do we involve? How do we get our colleagues to be so excited about the change that they line up to help us succeed? Change strategies originating out of the leadership and change management literature can be very helpful. John Kotter (1996) describes a cogent eight-step process that can be directly applied to the context of a faculty development program. More specifically, Kotter emphasizes issues like creating a sense of urgency at a program's initiation, forming a powerful coalition of partners and collaborators, creating a vision for change that is well communicated, removing institutional obstacles, creating early wins for the program, consolidating gains and producing more change, and anchoring the change in institutional culture. Because this model can help to propel the initiation of a faculty development program, the reader is directed to Kotter and other change strategists for more information (Rogers 2003; Morrison 1998).

16.2.4 Form a Planning Committee

Gathering a group of like-minded individuals around the planning committee table is essential, whether the program is small or large. For smaller programs and initiatives, having members of the target audience and key stakeholders around the table is essential. For a larger program or centre, it is helpful to consider including representatives of the key curricular committees, leaders and change agents within the organization, as well as teachers, researchers and administrators who are opinion leaders. This committee can evolve into an ongoing management committee for the program as it develops and grows.

Faculty development programs at large medical schools might want to consider forming an additional governance committee made up of representatives of higher leadership within the organization, or if there are partner organizations involved, representatives from the various organizations. Examples of higher leadership include deans, vice-deans and associate deans, hospital chiefs (in education and faculty affairs), and department heads at medical schools. In specialty societies, they would include members of the organization's executive team, their lay advisory group, and key academic opinion leaders within the society. Medical schools and specialty societies should consider the inclusion of policy representatives from provincial or state associations to ensure alignment with human resource needs in the state or province. The purpose of a governance committee is to ensure alignment with the strategic plans of the host organization(s) and to ensure continuous infrastructure and funding support going forward.

Larger schools or programs may consider hiring an external change management consultant to assist with the planning and change process, since a consultant can be especially impartial during interviews and focus groups with stakeholders and participants, and can provide seasoned facilitation of the start-up process.

16.2.5 Conduct an Environmental Scan of Existing Programs

A literature search to find programs and education contexts similar to what we intend to build can be very helpful. Reviewing best practices in faculty development, such as systematic reviews and outcome studies, can establish which best practices should be incorporated into the program (Steinert et al. 2006). Website reviews are also helpful as many schools, specialty societies, and colleges highlight their faculty development programs online. Educators and administrators may make direct contact with other organizations to clarify details of their programs. This contact with the broader faculty development community can be a valuable part of relationship building.

16.2.6 Design and Execute a Needs Assessment

A needs assessment can establish the directions a program can take and elaborate the specific context and potential influence of the institution's stakeholders and potential participants. Case, Buhl and Lindquist (in Lindquist 1979) suggest some questions that institutions can utilize for a needs assessment:

- Will the institution's authorities champion a faculty development program?
- Who could influence the level of acceptance of the program?
- What resources related to faculty development are currently available?
- What has taken place already in faculty development in the institution? How was it received?
- Are the institution's goals and strategies known? Acted upon? Shared by all participants?
- What norms exist that might influence faculty participation?

Looking at subjective individual needs will help define the goals, identify the content and preferred learning methods, assure relevance, assess interest, and identify preferred timetables of activities. Common methods of conducting this assessment include surveys and individual interviews or focus groups with key informants, frontline teachers, researchers, administrators, students and patients (Blouin and Van Melle 2006). Objective data can be derived from student ratings of their teachers and supervisors, observing teaching in action, an accreditation report, or the faculty development literature. Needs assessment data may reveal unexpected observations that can help shape a program; for example, junior faculty will not perceive learning needs for academic development that more seasoned faculty may, and vice versa. Needs assessment data can also help translate goals into objectives for the program (Steinert et al. 2006).

16.2.7 Establish the Mission, Vision and Values of the Program

Establishing the mission, vision and values statements will bring the education community together for a common task. It is not unusual for these statements to take several months to write; it is a function of the process that advisory and organizing committees take to focus the program and establish the partnerships and culture that will characterize it. From personal experience, establishing the values statements can be the most meaningful of all the tasks undertaken by those establishing a new program in faculty development.

A **vision** statement describes what the program aspires to, what it wants to be, and its intended scope of influence:

> *Foundation for Advancement of International Medical Education and Research (FAIMER) Faculty Development Program:* To create and enhance educational resources for those

who teach physicians committed to improving and maintaining the health of the communities they serve (Foundation for Advancement of International Medical Education and Research 2012).

A **mission** statement states the purpose of the program and what it will do in the field, for example:

McGill University, Department of Family Medicine Faculty Development Office: The division of Faculty Development is committed to helping Family Medicine faculty, both in the University and in the community, improve their comfort and competence in the following areas: Teaching and learning, understanding research and stimulating interest, and research methods training (McGill University Department of Family Medicine 2011).
   Harvard University, Office of Faculty Development at Boston Children's Hospital (BCH): To facilitate the career advancement and satisfaction of Harvard Medical School (HMS) faculty at Boston Children's Hospital, fostering careers of all junior faculty, and increasing leadership opportunities for women and minorities (Boston Children's Hospital 2013).

Although it is rare for faculty development programs to have a specific values statement (i.e. we could not find another example of a specific values statement online, outside of our university), writing them can set the tone for a program at its inception. Bringing together the relevant stakeholders to do this can be an invigorating and inspiring experience. A **values** statement captures the culture the organization aspires to, for example:

University of Toronto, Centre for Faculty Development at St. Michael's Hospital: As leaders who are committed to excellence and the well-being of faculty, students and their patients, we embrace the following core values (Centre for Faculty Development n.d.):

- Learner centeredness.
- Inter-professional collaboration.
- Critical inquiry and scholarship.
- Innovation and creativity.
- Accessibility.
- Social accountability.

16.2.8 Describe the Purpose, Goals and Objectives of the Program

The purpose, goals and objectives should reflect institutional, departmental and individual issues. They are often derived from the results of a needs assessment (Wilkerson 1984). Crafting these statements carefully will be time well spent because they will influence the target audiences, the choice of program, the content and the formats of the faculty development program (Steinert and Mann 2006).

16.2.9 Create a Short List of Strategic Deliverables

Using the results of the needs assessment and the deliberations of the planning committee, two to three key strategic initiatives should be identified for delivery in the first year. More deliverables can be articulated and scheduled over a 3-year period, depending on the size of the program and available resources. When working groups are used, it is best to vet these initiatives first with the stakeholders who were previously consulted during the needs assessment. This will help ensure alignment of these initiatives with the vested interests and priorities of education leaders, curriculum committees and host institutions.

Clearly outlining each initiative's goals, objectives and implementation plan will make it clear to the institution's leaders where the faculty development program is going. In larger programs, working groups can be formed from interested stakeholders to flesh out the details of the program content, to identify how the program will be delivered and evaluated, and to determine the resources that might be needed over the 3-year period. The planning process is in itself a form of faculty development, as it helps to socialize a larger group of teachers, educators and researchers into a learning community. It also provides the leads of the working groups with leadership opportunities.

16.3 Establishing the Faculty Development Curriculum, Design and Method of Delivery

Having established the strategic needs of the organization or program, begin to develop faculty development curricula and identify how they will be designed and delivered. Nearly all programs worldwide have a strong focus on improving teaching effectiveness (Steinert 2000; Steinert and Mann 2006). A faculty development curriculum is often directed by the curriculum renewal process and by evolving trends in health professions education. Leadership and management programs are increasingly popular, especially with medical education associations, international foundations and medical schools (Gruppen et al. 2003; Lieff 2010; Swanwick and McKimm 2010). Organizational development is an equally important issue because it plays a critical part in creating an institutional culture that supports teaching excellence, education scholarship, innovation and leadership (Steinert and Mann 2006).

Changes in organizational systems are often necessary to provide these supports. For example, unless a medical school has aligned its policies on promotion to support promotion on the basis of teaching and education scholarship, faculty development programs will have difficulty recruiting participants, because the new skill sets learned by faculty members may not be rewarded. Career development, including orientation programs for junior faculty, specialized programs for mid-career and late career faculty, and programs with a special focus such as women and minority faculty, is seen as an essential component of support programs (Rust et al. 2006; Spickard et al. 2002).

Program developers need to choose the appropriate education formats to deliver faculty development curricula. Steinert (2010) has provided an excellent framework to guide the choice of these activities, ranging from formal to informal, and from individual to group. This framework includes workshops and seminars, mentoring, fellowships, longitudinal programs, online learning, peer coaching, peer and student feedback, work-based learning and communities of practice. Each of these formats has a rich literature that supports its efficacy (Fidler et al. 2007; Gruppen et al. 2006; Hatem et al. 2009; Lieff 2009; Pattison et al. 2012; Pololi et al. 2002; Steinert and McLeod 2006; Takagishi and Dabrow 2011; Thorndyke et al. 2008). Other formats could also be considered (depending on access to resources), including the use of co-teaching, simulation, and theatre techniques (Krautscheid et al. 2008; Kumagai et al. 2007; Orlander et al. 2000).

To get started, it may be more feasible to start small with a menu of activities that includes both formal and informal activities, such as workshops, rounds, seminars, co-teaching, mentoring, using peer and student feedback, and individual and group methods of work-based learning. Later, creating online learning, simulation, fellowships, longitudinal programs, and communities of practice can be added. Kotter's (1996) suggestion, of going for 'early wins', is relevant and practical in this context. Choosing an activity or a series of activities that will please or meet an urgent faculty development need in the organization can kick-start a program and create a 'buzz' about it. This could take the form of monthly grand rounds in education, a new academic leadership program for a speciality society or a journal club on supervision for postgraduate teachers.

16.3.1   Consider Theoretical Approaches and Related Models, Principles and Guidelines That Inform Faculty Development

No single comprehensive education theory explains how faculty develop academic skills, but several theories, guidelines, models and principles can help inform the planning of a faculty development program (Steinert 2011). The following is a summary of key approaches and their implications for initiating a new program.

16.3.1.1   Andragogy

Malcolm Knowles (1984) introduced the term 'andragogy' to describe key principles on how adults learn. These learner-centered principles have strongly influenced health professions education for almost three decades and provide a solid foundation for initiating a faculty development program:

- Setting a cooperative learning climate where learners feel safe.
- Creating mechanisms for mutual planning of curricula (by teachers and students).
- Arranging for a diagnosis of learner needs and interests.
- Enabling the formulation of learning objectives based on the diagnosed needs and interests.
- Designing sequential activities for achieving objectives.
- Executing the design by selecting methods, materials and resources.
- Evaluating the quality of the learning experience by having learners critically reflect on their learning.

16.3.1.2 Self-Directed Learning

Self-directed learning is a method of organizing teaching and learning so that learners are empowered to accept personal responsibility for their learning. Learners are provided a menu of learning formats to choose from and are encouraged to be autonomous. This approach to learning helps guide faculty development program leaders to structure learning in a manner that gives much of the responsibility to faculty learners. For example, to encourage faculty to be self-directed in their learning, it is suggested that learners have opportunities to critically appraise new information, to ask questions, to identify their own learning gaps by comparing these to education best-practice benchmarks, and to critically reflect on how and what they have learned (Lunyk-Child et al. 2001; Mamary and Charles 2003; Silén and Uhlin 2008). There are elaborate collaborative faculty development programs designed with this self-directed learning in mind (Sanders et al. 1997). Please see Chap. 11 on online faculty development for more examples.

16.3.1.3 Self-Efficacy

Self-efficacy theory was articulated by Albert Bandura (1986). His work in this area focused on how an individual's self-assessment of their ability is central to how they behave. It is very specific to a domain or specific tasks. Self-efficacy is the individual's perception of their ability to execute a certain task (or tasks) that predicts the level of the goals, the effort and the persistence they will demonstrate. Essentially, perceived success can raise our self-efficacy, while failures (especially if they are early in the learning process) can lower self-efficacy. Bandura wrote that these self-judgments are based on a combination of factors (in decreasing order of influence): the person's experience with the task; observational learning; verbal persuasion; and the individuals' physiological state. Self-efficacy is not a fixed perception; it can be changed through education and learning experiences. For example, when thinking about observational learning, this theory predicts that if we set up our faculty development programs so faculty members can be observed being successful with unfamiliar tasks, other faculty are more likely to feel that they can perform the tasks well too. Giving faculty members an opportunity to practice new skills, receive feedback and achieve some success can also be a powerful way in which to build a sense of self-efficacy.

16.3.1.4 Expectancy-Value Theory

Related to self-efficacy theory is a framework called expectancy-value theory (Fishbein and Ajzen 1975). According to this theory, a learner's motivation is determined by how much they value a goal and whether they expect to succeed with a task or activity. Heckhausen (1991) defined several types of expectancies that learners can have, including the subjective probability of obtaining a particular outcome with an activity, and the subjective probability of an outcome being associated with a specific consequence. These dynamics can often be at play in faculty development. For example, if clinical teachers anticipate that faculty development will enhance their professional development, and if they believe that these activities are relevant to them, they may be more likely to attend workshops and seminars on teaching improvement. In addition, the value they place on self-improvement and in their teaching activities may be self-motivating (Steinert 2010).

This theory has great potential to help faculty developers understand what motivates faculty to attend sessions. Educators need to understand why well-rated teachers or excellent administrators habitually attend faculty development work-shops, while faculty who might really need the faculty development do not attend. Seasoned faculty developers have also observed that it is sometimes difficult for faculty to move out of the safety of their own department, unit or area of speciality to attend workshops with faculty members from different specialities or health professions. These faculty members may not place much intrinsic value on interpro-fessional learning, or expect that it will not go well. However, it has been observed that expectancies and values can change after a single, well-taught interdisciplinary workshop (Pandachuck et al. 2004).

16.3.1.5   Constructivist Theory

Within a constructivist framework, learning involves the active construction of learning and mental processes (Fosnot 1996). Several theories of learning are constructivist. Within a faculty development context, this theory would predict that it is important to understand faculty's preconceptions and to build knowledge based on what has been learned already. It is also important to understand that individual faculty members will have different experiences, knowledge and values, and as a result, they may construct their understanding of their teaching, research and leadership behaviors in different ways. Faculty developers need to understand the specific contexts in which faculty members teach, conduct their research, and work in their organizations in order to construct learning sessions that are optimally relevant and useful.

Teachers and administrators will also change their behavior based on the learning that occurs in their teaching and organization's environments. Teaching more effectively results from gaining practical knowledge and skills from the teaching experience itself (i.e. constructing meaning and building on prior knowledge). Reconstructing actual teaching or administrative experiences during faculty development sessions, or reviewing videotapes of previous teaching sessions, are applications of construc-tivist theory in practice (Skeff et al. 1986).

16.3.1.6   Social-Cultural Theories

Social learning theories focus on how learning occurs with, and from, others and from the environment. These theories generally have two perspectives: the first deals with the learning that happens within an individual; the second focuses on the learning that happens through interactions with other individuals. Social-cultural theories belong to the second perspective.

Within the social-cultural learning framework, learning is thought of as socialization into a new knowledge community (Wilkerson and Irby 1998). In a faculty development context, knowledge is socially constructed through interaction with a peer group of faculty. Learning occurs through contact with faculty members who are role model teachers and educators, and via arranged peer-coaching learning opportunities. Learners are immersed in a community where teaching and learning is explored, beliefs are discussed, and roles are identified. This is one of the most important and effective methodologies in faculty development (Steinert et al. 2006). Two learning constructs are derived from social-cultural theory: communities of practice and situated learning (Lave and Wenger 1991).

D'Eon has described teaching as a social practice that is purposive, rational and situated within a community (D'Eon et al. 2000). Communities of practice have been defined as a 'persistent, sustained, social network of individuals who share and develop an overlapping knowledge base, set of beliefs, values, history and experiences focused on a common practice and/or mutual enterprise' (Barab et al. 2002, p. 7). Faculty developers have an important role in socializing faculty and staff into communities of practice based on their mutual interests. Moreover, these communities of practice can provide an important foundation for influencing the greater community of teachers, administrators or researchers in an organization (Vescio et al. 2008).

Situated learning is based on the notion that learning is situated in authentic contexts (Miller et al. 2010). When learning normally occurs, it is embedded within activities, context and culture. This theory highlights the fact that knowledge needs to be presented in authentic contexts—settings and situations where this knowledge would be applied. In a faculty development context, case-based learning, role-playing and the use of simulation are teaching modalities that support this theory.

16.3.1.7 Reflective Practice

Donald Schön (1987) argued that formal learning theories were not adequate to explain the everyday messy problems of practice. He labeled professionals' automatic ways of responding to clinical situations in areas of superior competence as 'zones of mastery' or 'knowing in action'. When a clinician experiences a surprise situation in their practice, they 'reflect[s]-in-action' while the patient might still be in their office. The clinician would problem solve within the situation and make the best-educated formulation of the problem and come to a decision. Schön (1987) perceived this situation as an experiment based on the clinician's best hypothesis. Later in the day, the clinician might 'reflect-on-action' about what had happened. As a result, the clinician might consult other colleagues, a text, or the Internet to further understand the 'surprising' situation. Moreover, as a result of the 'reflection-on-action,' the clinician would learn something new, and this would become a new part of their zone of mastery.

Applied to a faculty development context, this model for learning would predict that the encouragement of mindfulness toward metacognitions, connected to teaching surprises and challenges, would be a helpful way to access narratives for sharing between teachers. In a teaching context, faculty developers could reconstruct these situations with other faculty members through role-playing and by assisting faculty to move along the continuum from reflection-in-action, to experimentation, to reflection-on-action.

16.3.2 Develop an Evaluation Plan to Measure Program Impact and Outcomes

Establishing an evaluation strategy at the outset is important to build an accountability framework for the program. This will be viewed favorably by the funders of the program and will provide opportunities for education scholarship and research.

There have been a number of evaluation models used in faculty development, including simple methods such as post-activity self-report evaluations, student evaluations of teachers, retrospective pre/post assessments, perceived competence in teaching methods, and commitment to change strategies (Bandiera et al. 2005; Boerboom et al. 2009; McLeod et al. 2008; Myhre and Lockyer 2010; Pandachuck et al. 2004). Something as simple as a well-designed participant satisfaction rating scale continues to remain an important component of faculty development evaluation; if programs are well-rated, participants will tell their colleagues about it. These instruments also provide valuable feedback to program planners regarding the teaching and learning strategies and the relevance of the program (Steinert and Mann 2006).

More comprehensive and systems-based evaluation strategies have been applied to faculty development programs including an outcomes logic model, the Kirkpatrick framework, objective structured teaching evaluations (OSTEs), faculty achievement tracking tools, curriculum vitae analyses, and qualitative evaluation methods (Armstrong and Barsion 2006; Knight et al. 2007; Morzinski and Schubot 2000; Pettus et al. 2009; Wamsley et al. 2005). Evaluating the impact of faculty development is important on many levels: accountability to the funders, growing the program, and marketing the program to potential participants. Whether or not a program becomes a permanent feature at a school or institution ultimately depends on its demonstrated value and a positive answer to the question "Does it work?"

16.3.3 Establish a Program of Scholarship in Faculty Development

Even as a program is just getting established, it is prudent to be thinking of the program's potential for scholarship and research. Starting a program is a unique opportunity to create a scholarly community in faculty development and to charge those involved with academic goals and aspirations. Good principles to guide the process include focusing scholarship on the programs that will be delivered, engaging education researchers early in the program planning stage, and focusing scholarship in areas that are aligned with education goals and objectives of the funding organization. (See Chaps. 17 and 18 for a further discussion of this topic.)

16.3.4 Develop a Plan for Sustainability

Thinking of how to sustain a program is an important consideration at the inception of a faculty development program. One consideration is to look at advocacy for policy changes within a university or at a government level that will help sustain the program. For example, at a university, developing promotion policies that are aligned with leadership or scholarship training programs in education are important. Education scholarship including excellence in teaching will need to be included as key criteria for promotion if faculty development programs are focused on developing teachers, scholars and leaders. Developing policies that mandate faculty development for all faculty members as part of their performance review can help sustain a program. At a government level, advocating for funding for the support of academic leadership development and health professions education grants to support innovation in faculty development are important interventions.

Even at the start-up of a program, it is important to begin to consider the identification of future leaders in faculty development and how to enable their personal growth and development as the program grows. When resources are available, hiring an associate director for the program early on can quickly broaden the scope of the program and address the importance of succession planning.

16.3.5 Secure Infrastructure Funding and Staffing

Faculty development program planners need to take into consideration the budget available to produce a program of activities. At a medical school level, the school may fund these programs as part of its core budget, although this may vary considerably between schools. Starting a program may well begin with very modest financial support. Hospital or university department-specific programs and specialty societies or colleges may also allocate funds for faculty development. Many medical schools expect a faculty development office or centre to be partially self-sufficient financially. Program leaders need to assess the culture of their organization to understand the faculty's tolerance for paying for faculty development. It is not uncommon for departments or hospitals to financially sponsor faculty members who are participating in longitudinal programs such as fellowships and Teaching/ Education Scholars Programs.

Education leadership programs developed by colleges or large medical associations are often financed on a cost-recovery basis. For larger programs, it is advisable to establish a formal business plan that can project the growing needs of the program forward for several years. This process can formalize the necessary accountability that organizations will expect when funding a new faculty development program.

There are few guidelines available to recommend the necessary start-up staff needed to run these programs. At one academic teaching hospital, the initial infrastructure of the office for faculty development includes one full-time equivalent (FTE) director and a 1.0 FTE administrative assistant serving approximately 900 faculty (Emans et al. 2008). A Master Teacher Program in a large medical school's department of medicine has a 0.6 FTE director and a 0.2 FTE administrative assistant serving 1,160 faculty members (D. Panisko, personal communication, August 2012). When resources are scarce, it is also possible to do faculty development on a 'shoestring' budget (Palloff and Pratt 2011). For example, students or residents who are technologically savvy may be highly motivated to assist faculty with this aspect of their professional development. Education specialists from the Education or Informatics Faculties may be very interested in collaborating with the Faculty of Health Sciences by providing single faculty development sessions at minimal cost. Encouraging experienced teachers, administrators and researchers to assist novice faculty either formally or informally can be organized with minimal administrative assistance.

16.3.6 Market the Program

Marketing and branding a faculty development program can be very useful in the start-up phase. Creating a faculty development website is an essential marketing tool. It can advertise the program calendar, highlight the staff and faculty who administer and teach the program, and provide additional education resources. Creating a unique logo for the program can be an effective community-building exercise. The use of social media—from blogs to wikis to tweets—has become a new means by which faculty development programs can communicate, collaborate and teach.

16.4 Conclusion

Starting a faculty development program can be an exciting, even exhilarating, time in a health professional's career. It's a time of relationship- and network-building, risk-taking, experimentation and creativity. Once started, there are many issues and challenges that faculty development leaders will face, including engaging staff and administrators in faculty development, addressing the fact that leading a faculty development program often needs to be balanced with clinical work, fitting students and trainees in with the productivity demands of service, balancing formal vs. informal learning opportunities, resolving ongoing funding challenges, and of course, ensuring the sustainability of the program.

Having an organized approach based on theoretical assumptions, trends in health professions education, principles, goals and objectives, and a change and design strategy, will help overcome the many challenges that are part of the journey of getting a program off the ground. This chapter has outlined a number of layered approaches that educators, administrators and faculty developers can use to frame a plan of action. Starting a faculty development program provides a unique opportunity to influence the next generation of health professions teachers, administrators and researchers. Starting and leading a program can be one of the most gratifying academic activities in a career. We invite future faculty developers to take up the challenge today, to continue to build capacity in the field and to join our growing international community.

> Start by doing what's necessary; then do what's possible; and suddenly you are doing the impossible.
>
> —*Saint Francis of Assisi*

16.5 Key Messages

- Consider implementing a comprehensive faculty development program that will serve the multiple needs of teachers, educators, researchers and administrators.
- Theoretical approaches, and related models, principles and guidelines can inform the strategies used to plan, develop, implement and evaluate a faculty development program.
- Align the faculty development program with the strategic goals, objectives and culture of the institution that the program is serving.
- Create vision, mission and values statements for the program.
- If participating in the program creates a sense of community, enables faculty members to be promoted, is accessible and enjoyable, the program will be successful.

Acknowledgments I would like to thank Ms. Jacquelyn Waller-Vintar and Ms. Stevie Howell for their excellent editorial assistance.

References

1st International Conference on Faculty Development in the Health Professions. (2011). *Faculty development definition*. Retrieved November 27th, 2012, from http://www.facultydevelopment2011.com

Al-Wardy, N. M. (2008). Medical education units: History, functions, and organisation. *Sultan Qaboos University Medical Journal, 8*(2), 149–156.

Armstrong, E. G. & Barsion, S. J. (2006). Using an outcomes-logic-model approach to evaluate a faculty development program for medical educators. *Academic Medicine, 81*(5), 483–488.

Association of Faculties of Medicine of Canada. (2010). *The future of medical education in Canada (FMEC): A collective vision for MD education.* Retrieved November 26th, 2012, from http://www.afmc.ca/fmec/pdf/collective_vision.pdf

Association of Faculties of Medicine of Canada. (2012). *The future of medical education in Canada, postgraduate project: A collective vision for postgraduate medical education in Canada.* Retrieved November 26th, 2012, from http://www.afmc.ca/future-of-medical-education-in-canada/postgraduate-project/pdf/FMEC_PG_Final-Report_EN.pdf

Bandiera, G., Lee, S., & Tiberius, R. (2005). Creating effective learning in today's emergency departments: How accomplished teachers get it done. *Annals of Emergency Medicine, 45*(3), 253–261.

Bandura, A. (1986). *Social foundations of thought and action: A social cognitive theory.* Englewood Cliffs, NJ: Prentice-Hall.

Barab, S. A., Barnett, M., & Squire, K. (2002). Developing an empirical account of a community of practice: Characterizing the essential tensions. *The Journal of the Learning Sciences, 11*(4), 489–542.

Blouin, D. & Van Melle, E. (2006). *Faculty development needs of Ontario rural physician preceptors.* Retrieved December 27th, 2012, from http://healthsci.queensu.ca/assets/fd/rrpnareport.pdf

Boerboom, T. B., Dolmans, D. H., Muijtjens, A. M., Jaarsma, A. D., Van Beukelen, P., & Scherpbier, A. J. (2009). Does a faculty development programme improve teachers' perceived competence in different teacher roles? *Medical Teacher, 31*(11), 1030–1031.

Boston Children's Hospital. (2013). *Office of faculty development: Mission statement.* Retrieved January 3rd, 2013, from http://www.childrenshospital.org/clinician-resources/office-of-faculty-development

Brashers, V., Peterson, C., Tullmann, D., & Schmitt, M. (2012). The University of Virginia interprofessional education initiative: An approach to integrating competencies into medical and nursing education. *Journal of Interprofessional Care, 26*(1), 73–75.

Centre for Faculty Development, University of Toronto at St. Michael's Hospital. (n.d.). *About us: Vision, mission, and values.* Retrieved January 3rd, 2013, from http://www.cfd.med.utoronto.ca/aboutus/mission.html

D'Eon, M., Overgaard, V., & Harding, S. R. (2000). Teaching as a social practice: Implications for faculty development. *Advances in Health Sciences Education, 5*(2), 151–162.

Emans, S. J., Goldberg, C. T., Milstein, M. E., & Dobriner, J. (2008). Creating a faculty development office in an academic pediatric hospital: Challenges and successes. *Pediatrics, 121*(2), 390–401.

Fidler, D. C., Khakoo, R., & Miller, L. A. (2007). Teaching scholars programs: Faculty development for educators in the health professions. *Academic Psychiatry, 31*(6), 472–478.

Fishbein, M. & Ajzen, I. (1975). *Belief, attitude, intention, and behavior: An introduction to theory and research.* Reading, MA: Addison-Wesley.

Fosnot, C. T. (1996). *Constructivism: Theory, perspectives and practice.* New York, NY: Teachers College Press.

Foundation for Advancement of International Medical Education and Research. (2012). *Strategic plan.* Retrieved January 3rd, 2013, from http://www.faimer.org/about-strategic-plan.html

General Medical Council. (2009). *Tomorrow's doctors: Outcomes and standards for undergraduate medical education.* Retrieved November 25th, 2012, from http://www.gmc-uk.org/static/documents/content/GMC_TD_09__1.11.11.pdf

Gruppen, L. D., Frohna, A. Z., Anderson, R. M., & Lowe, K. D. (2003). Faculty development for educational leadership and scholarship. *Academic Medicine, 78*(2), 137–141.

Gruppen, L. D., Simpson, D., Searle, N. S., Robins, L., Irby, D. M., & Mullan, P. B. (2006). Educational fellowship programs: Common themes and overarching issues. *Academic Medicine, 81*(11), 990–994.

Hatem, C. J., Lown, B. A., & Newman, L. R. (2009). Strategies for creating a faculty fellowship in medical education: Report of a 10-year experience. *Academic Medicine, 84*(8), 1098–1103.

Heckhausen, H. (1991). *Motivation and action*. Berlin, DE: Springer-Verlag.

Knight, A. M., Carrese, J. A., & Wright, S. M. (2007). Qualitative assessment of the long-term impact of a faculty development programme in teaching skills. *Medical Education, 41*(6), 592–600.

Knowles, M. S. (1984). *Andragogy in action: Applying modern principles of adult learning*. San Francisco, CA: Jossey-Bass.

Kotter, J. P. (1996). *Leading change*. Boston, MA: Harvard Business School Press.

Krautscheid, L., Kaakinen, J., & Warner, J. R. (2008). Clinical faculty development: Using simulation to demonstrate and practice clinical teaching. *Journal of Nursing Education, 47*(9), 431–434.

Kumagai, A. K., White, C. B., Ross, P. T., Purkiss, J. A., O'Neal, C. M., & Steiger, J. A. (2007). Use of interactive theater for faculty development in multicultural medical education. *Medical Teacher, 29*(4), 335–340.

Lave, J. & Wenger, E. (1991). *Situated learning: Legitimate peripheral participation*. New York, NY: Cambridge University Press.

Lieff, S. J. (2009). Evolving curriculum design: A novel framework for continuous, timely, and relevant curriculum adaptation in faculty development. *Academic Medicine, 84*(1), 127–134.

Lieff, S. J. (2010). Faculty development: Yesterday, today and tomorrow: Guide supplement 33.2 - Viewpoint. *Medical Teacher, 32*(5), 429–431.

Lindquist, J. (1979). *Designing teaching improvement programs*. The Council for the Advancement of Small Colleges.

Lunyk-Child, O. I., Crooks, D., Ellis, P. J., Ofosu, C., O'Mara, L., & Rideout, E. (2001). Self-directed learning: Faculty and student perceptions. *Journal of Nursing Education, 40*(3), 116–123.

Mamary, E. & Charles, P. (2003). Promoting self-directed learning for continuing medical education. *Medical Education, 25*(2), 188–190.

McGill University Department of Family Medicine. (2011). *Faculty development: Mission statement*. Retrieved January 3rd, 2013, from http://www.mcgill.ca/familymed/education/facdev

McLeod, P. J., Brawer, J., Steinert, Y., Chalk, C., & McLeod, A. (2008). A pilot study designed to acquaint medical educators with basic pedagogic principles. *Medical Teacher, 30*(1), 92–93.

McLeod, P. J. & Steinert, Y. (2010). The evolution of faculty development in Canada since the 1980s: Coming of age or time for a change? *Medical Teacher, 32*(1), e31–e35.

Medical Deans Australia and New Zealand. (2009). Retrieved November 26th, 2012, from http://www.medicaldeans.org.au/

Miller, B. M., Moore, D. E. Jr., Stead, W. W., & Balser, J. R. (2010). Beyond Flexner: A new model for continuous learning in the health professions. *Academic Medicine, 85*(2), 266–272.

Moaveni, A., Nasmith, L., & Oandasan, I. (2008). Building best practice in faculty development for interprofessional collaboration in primary care. *Journal of Interprofessional Care, 22*(1 Suppl), 80–82.

Morrison, K. (1998). *Management theories for educational change*. London, UK: Sage Publications.

Morzinski, J. A. & Schubot, D. B. (2000). Evaluating faculty development outcomes by using curriculum vitae analysis. *Family Medicine, 32*(3), 185–189.

Myhre, D. L. & Lockyer, J. M. (2010). Using a commitment-to-change strategy to assess faculty development. *Medical Education, 44*(5), 516–517.

Orlander, J. D., Gupta, M., Fincke, B. G., Manning, M. E., & Hershman, W. (2000). Co-teaching: A faculty development strategy. *Medical Education, 34*(4), 257–265.

Palloff, R. & Pratt, K. (2011). *Excellent faculty development on a shoestring*. Jossey-Bass Online Teaching and Learning: Online Community. Retrieved December 27th, 2012, from http://www.onlineteachingandlearning.com/faculty-development-shoestring

Pandachuck, K., Harley, D., & Cook, D. (2004). Effectiveness of a brief workshop designed to improve teaching performance at the University of Alberta. *Academic Medicine, 79*(8), 798–804.

Patricio, M. & Harden, R. M. (2010). The Bologna Process - A global vision for the future of medical education. *Medical Teacher, 32*(4), 305–315.

Pattison, A. T., Sherwood, M., Lumsden, C. J., Gale, A., & Markides, M. (2012). Foundation observation of teaching project – A developmental model of peer observation of teaching. *Medical Teacher, 34*(2), e136–e142.

Pettus, S., Reifschneider, E., & Burruss, N. (2009). Faculty achievement tracking tool. *Journal of Nursing Education, 48*(3), 161–164.

Pololi, L. H., Knight, S. M., Dennis, K., & Frankel, R. M. (2002). Helping medical school faculty realize their dreams: An innovative, collaborative mentoring program. *Academic Medicine, 77*(5), 377–384.

Rogers, E. M. (2003). *Diffusion of innovations* (5th Ed.). New York, NY: Simon & Schuster Inc.

Rubeck, R. F. & Witzke, D. B. (1998). Faculty development: A field of dreams. *Academic Medicine, 73*(9 Suppl), S32–S37.

Rust, G., Taylor, V., Herbert-Carter, J., Smith, Q. T., Earles, K., & Kondwani, K. (2006). The Morehouse Faculty Development Program: Evolving methods and 10-year outcomes. *Family Medicine, 38*(1), 43–49.

Sanders, K., Carlson-Dakes, C., Dettinger, K., Hajnal, C., Laedtke, M., & Squire, L. (1997). A new starting point for faculty development in higher education: Creating a collaborative learning environment. *To Improve the Academy, 16*, 117–150. Paper 386. Retrieved November 27th, 2012, from http://digitalcommons.unl.edu/podimproveacad/386

Schön, D. A. (1987). *Educating the reflective practitioner: Toward a new design for teaching and learning in the professions.* San Francisco, CA: Jossey-Bass.

Silén, C. & Uhlin, L. (2008). Self-directed learning – A learning issue for students and faculty! *Teaching in Higher Education, 13*(4), 461–475.

Silver, I. L. & Leslie, K. (2009). Faculty development for continuing interprofessional education and collaborative practice. *Journal of Continuing Education in the Health Professions, 29*(3), 172–177.

Skeff, K. M., Stratos, G. A., Campbell, M., Cooke, M., & Jones, H. W., III. (1986). Evaluation of the seminar method to improve clinical teaching. *Journal of General Internal Medicine, 1*(5), 315–322.

Spickard, A. Jr., Gabbe, S. G., & Christensen, J. F. (2002). Mid-career burnout in generalist and specialist physicians. *JAMA, 288*(12), 1447–1450.

Steinert, Y. (2000). Faculty development in the new millennium: Key challenges and future directions. *Medical Teacher, 22*(1), 44–50.

Steinert, Y. (2005). Learning together to teach together: Interprofessional education and faculty development. *Journal of Interprofessional Care, 19*(Suppl. 1), 60–75.

Steinert, Y. (2010). Faculty development: From workshops to communities of practice. *Medical Teacher, 32*(5), 425–428.

Steinert, Y. (2011). Commentary: Faculty development: The road less traveled. *Academic Medicine, 86*(4), 409–411.

Steinert, Y., Cruess, S., Cruess, R., & Snell, L. (2005). Faculty development for teaching and evaluating professionalism: From programme design to curriculum change. *Medical Education, 39*(2), 127–136.

Steinert, Y. & Mann, K. (2006). Faculty development: Principles and practices. *Journal of Veterinary Medical Education, 33*(3), 317–324.

Steinert, Y., Mann, K., Centeno, A., Dolmans, D., Spencer, J., Gelula, M., et al. (2006). A systematic review of faculty development initiatives designed to improve teaching effectiveness in medical education: BEME Guide No. 8. *Medical Teacher, 28*(6), 497–526.

Steinert, Y. & McLeod, P. J. (2006). From novice to informed educator: The Teaching Scholars Program for Educators in the Health Sciences. *Academic Medicine, 81*(11), 969–974.

Swanwick, T. & McKimm, J. (2010). Educational leadership. In T. Swanwick (Ed.), *Understanding medical education: Evidence, theory and practice*, (pp. 419–438). Oxford, UK: Wiley-Blackwell.

Takagishi, J. & Dabrow, S. (2011). Mentorship programs for faculty development in academic general pediatric divisions. *International Journal of Pediatrics, 2011*, Art. 538616.

Thorndyke, L. E., Gusic, M. E., & Milner, R. J. (2008). Functional mentoring: A practical approach with multilevel outcomes. *Journal of Continuing Education in the Health Professions, 28*(3), 157–164.

Vescio, V., Ross, D., & Adams A. (2008). A review of research on the impact of professional learning communities on teaching practice and student learning. *Teaching and Teacher Education, 24*(1), 80–91.

Wamsley, M. A., Julian, K. A., Vener, M. H., & Morrison, E. H. (2005). Using an objective structured teaching evaluation for faculty development. *Medical Education, 39*(11), 1160–1161.

Wilkerson, L. (1984). Starting a faculty development program: Strategies and approaches. *To Improve the Academy, 3*, 27–48. Paper 72. Retrieved November 27th, 2012, from http://digitalcommons.unl.edu/podimproveacad/72/

Wilkerson, L. & Irby, D. M. (1998). Strategies for improving teaching practices: A comprehensive approach to faculty development. *Academic Medicine, 73*(4), 387–396.

Part V
Research and Scholarship in Faculty Development

Chapter 17
Faculty Development Research: The 'State of the Art' and Future Trends

John Spencer

17.1 Introduction

We all know that faculty development works. Of course it does. It stands to reason that teachers will teach more effectively, researchers will research more productively, and leaders will lead more effectively if they are presented with models of good practice and provided with opportunities for action and reflection, together with guidance and feedback. Why else would we put all that effort into the faculty development enterprise if we didn't think it was effective? Evaluations, on the whole, confirm our presuppositions, justify our efforts and use of resources, and further encourage us. The gains go beyond an individual's personal and professional development, with potential benefits for colleagues and organizations. The received wisdom, to quote two major authors in the field, is quite simply that 'faculty development targeted to the several roles of faculty members is the key to academic vitality' (Wilkerson and Irby 1998, p. 394).

That wisdom is now enshrined in both educational policy and practice. For example, in the United Kingdom, recent recommendations on undergraduate medical education from the profession's governing body, the General Medical Council, state that 'everyone involved in educating medical students will be appropriately selected, trained, supported and appraised' (GMC 2009a, p. 69). Moreover, medical schools' compliance with this will be monitored. This reflects the requirement that all doctors who are involved in teaching must 'develop the skills and practices of a competent teacher' as part of their personal and professional development (GMC 2009b, p. 14). In North America, medical school faculty are required by the Liaison Committee on Medical Education (2012) to be able to teach effectively, and the recently revised Maintenance of Certification Program in Canada recognizes faculty

J. Spencer, FRCGP (✉)
Primary Care and Clinical Education, School of Medical Sciences Education Development,
Faculty of Medical Sciences, Newcastle University, Newcastle upon Tyne, UK
e-mail: john.spencer@ncl.ac.uk

Y. Steinert (ed.), *Faculty Development in the Health Professions: A Focus on Research and Practice*, Innovation and Change in Professional Education 11, DOI 10.1007/978-94-007-7612-8_17, © Springer Science+Business Media Dordrecht 2014

development as an important element in maintaining professional standards (Royal College of Physicians and Surgeons of Canada 2011, p. 7). The wisdom is clearly ever-present.

Yet, although we have a sense of *what* works, in spite of a considerable literature describing and evaluating faculty development, both in health professions education and in the broader field of higher education, we have relatively little understanding about how, why and in what circumstances. This chapter will firstly review what we know about what works in faculty development, with reference to recently published systematic reviews. It will then discuss aspects of the 'state of the art' of research and scholarship in the field, highlighting some important challenges facing scholars. These include the similarities and differences between evaluation and research, evaluation of complex interventions, and the utility of particular outcome measures, notably Kirkpatrick's framework and self-report, placed in the broader context of concerns about the quality of medical education research. The chapter will conclude with some recommendations about future research in faculty development.

17.2   What Do We Know About What Works in Faculty Development?

In this section the findings of four systematic reviews will be discussed, focusing both on the impact and outcomes of faculty development, and on what methods are effective.

17.2.1   What Are the Impacts and Outcomes of Faculty Development?

The most recent systematic review of the faculty development literature in medical education was published in 2012 and looked at the development of leadership skills (Steinert et al. 2012). The review focused on 'the effects of faculty development interventions designed to improve leadership abilities on the knowledge, attitudes and skills of faculty members in medicine, and the institutions in which they work' (p. 485). The reviewers addressed three distinct categories of intervention: those with their main focus on leadership; those including leadership as a component of a more comprehensive development program; and those including leadership within a program focusing on academic career development. All study designs reporting findings beyond participant satisfaction were included.

A modified version of Kirkpatrick's framework (Table 17.1) was used to evaluate the impact of studies (the utility of Kirkpatrick's framework will be discussed in Sect. 17.4), as well as global judgments about strength of findings and the quality of

Table 17.1 Kirkpatrick's modified evaluation framework

Level 1	Reaction	Participants' views about the learning experience, its organization, presentation, content, methods, and quality of instruction
Level 2a	Learning – change in attitudes	Changes in attitudes or perceptions among participant groups towards teaching and learning
Level 2b	Learning – modification of knowledge or skills	Knowledge; acquisition of concepts, procedures and principles
		Skills: acquisition of thinking/problem-solving, psychomotor and social skills
Level 3	Behavior – change in behavior	Evidence of transfer of learning to the workplace or willingness of learners to apply new knowledge and skills
Level 4a	Results – change in the system or organizational practice	Wider changes in the organization, attributable to the intervention
Level 4b	Results – change among participants' learners or colleagues	Improvement in learners' perceptions, approaches to study, or performance as a direct result of the faculty development intervention

After Steinert et al. (2006)

the research. Findings were grouped by type of intervention (e.g. workshop, longitudinal fellowship).

Forty eight papers described 41 studies of 35 specific interventions. Most targeted clinical faculty and used a range of formats including workshops, short courses and fellowships. The findings can be considered under three headings: impact of interventions, key features of (apparently) successful programs, and the quality of the research methods used.

In terms of outcomes and impact, the reviewers identified the following:

- High levels of participant satisfaction (Level 1 – see Table 17.1) – both in terms of practical relevance and usefulness, and for both personal and professional development.
- Changes in attitudes towards leadership as well as the organization (Level 2a) – such as increased awareness of institutional goals or of participants' own strengths and weaknesses, intentions to change, and increased confidence in undertaking leadership roles.
- Gains in knowledge and skills (Level 2b) – such as knowledge about leadership concepts and understanding change management principles.
- Changes in behavior, both self-reported and observed (Levels 3a and 3b respectively) – including application of new knowledge, change in leadership styles, adoption of new roles and responsibilities, and creation of new collaborations.
- Changes in the organization (Level 4a) – although these aspects were not often investigated, reported changes included implementation of specific innovations, increased emphasis on scholarship, development of new programs, and establishment of new networks.

The review built on earlier work focused on interventions intended to improve teaching effectiveness (Steinert et al. 2006). Fifty three papers were critiqued and, as with the leadership review, a wide variety of interventions described. A range of changes were reported in attitudes (in this case towards both teaching and towards faculty development), acquisition of new knowledge and skills (for example, knowledge about educational theory, or developing specific teaching 'micro-skills' such as questioning skills), changes in behavior (reported both by participants and their learners), and changes in organizational practice and student learning, although these were rarely reported.

These two reviews showed remarkably similar findings in terms of both the variety of interventions used, and their impacts. There were concerns, however, about many aspects of research quality and thus the strength of the findings and what conclusions could confidently be drawn from them. These issues will be discussed in detail in Sect. 17.3 and recommendations will be made at the end of the chapter. Nonetheless, it is apparent that faculty development *does* 'work' and at many levels, although these reviews could only speculate as to how and why.

Stes et al. (2010) in the Netherlands undertook a systematic review of the broader higher education literature (i.e. not confined to medical education), focusing on what the authors termed 'instructional development', defined as 'any initiative specifically planned to enhance course design so that student learning is supported' (Stes et al. 2010, p. 25). They critiqued five previous reviews, covering literature from the mid-1960s, including Steinert et al. (2006), noting the consistency of observations about the variable quality of research and the often inconclusive results. They set out to address several unanswered questions, including whether interventions extending over time were more effective than 'one-time' events, and whether course-like instructional development had better outcomes than alternatives such as peer teaching and action research projects. Like Steinert et al. (2006, 2012), they used a modified version of Kirkpatrick's framework, excluding papers that solely used participant satisfaction as an outcome. However, rather than analyze by format of intervention, in addition to clustering studies by level of outcome, they analyzed according to research design (quantitative, qualitative or mixed approaches). Thirty-six papers were reviewed, the majority of which assessed impact on participants. Changes were noted at several levels: participants' attitudes (e.g. towards teaching, increased confidence), conceptions of teaching (e.g. about student-centered approaches), knowledge (e.g. about the role of technology in the classroom), skills (e.g. use of that technology) and behavior (e.g. adopting more student-centered, and/or use of innovative approaches). Few studies explored impacts on *learners*, but relevant outcomes included positive changes in study approaches (notably, increased collaboration) and specific learning outcomes. Finally, although less often measured, some changes at the institutional level were noted, including increased networking, spin-off activities and dissemination of ideas. There was also a suggestion that interventions extending over time were associated with more positive outcomes than one-off events, as were alternative or hybrid formats (e.g. peer coaching, or formal course plus coaching and project work, respectively) compared to more traditional approaches such as workshops.

At the time of writing, the most recently published systematic appraisal of the faculty development literature, from Australia, is what the authors termed a *conceptual* review (Amundsen and Wilson 2012). They wondered whether previous reviewers had been asking the right questions in addressing issues of cause and effect (i.e. 'What works?'). Driven by the questions 'How are educational development practices designed?' and 'What is the thinking underpinning such design?' the authors developed a framework based on the core characteristics of the initiatives. These included the stated intentions or goals, the processes and activities used to attain the goals, and the evidence collected to demonstrate attainment. Their framework comprised six categories of practice, and papers were analyzed according to their main focus.

The six categories (or 'conceptual clusters') were:

- Skills focus – acquisition or enhancement of observable teaching skills and techniques, the aim being to support change in specific behaviors.
- Method focus – mastery of a particular teaching method e.g. problem-based learning, both to use the method and to understand underlying concepts.
- Institutional focus – coordinated institutional plans to support teaching improvement and/or successful diffusion of ideas.
- Reflection focus – changes in individual teachers' conceptions of teaching and learning through support for individual reflection.
- Disciplinary focus – developing pedagogical knowledge based on the assumption that teaching varies between disciplines because the knowledge base is different.
- Action research focus – individuals or groups of faculty pursuing topics of interest to them.

The authors argued that the merit of this approach was that it focused on understanding the 'process' as opposed to analyzing results against pre-defined outcomes, as with previous reviews. In addition, they reflected on the assumptions that faculty developers make about the orientations of programs at three levels: institutional, intellectual and contextual. Institutional orientation refers to whether programs are 'centralized' (i.e. led by faculty developers based in an institution delivering workshops and other programs to participants who usually leave their own workplace to attend), 'decentralized' (i.e. based in the workplace with faculty developers taking on a more facilitative role), or a combination. Intellectual positioning refers to the intended learning, for example whether it is focused on specific content or on processes such as reflection that facilitate continuing professional development. Finally, contextual orientation refers to whether activities are focused on improving individuals' teaching practice, or whether they are intended to engage faculty in 'teaching enhancement as a socially situated practice' (Amundsen and Wilson 2012, p. 109). The authors discuss how informal learning experiences may have a more profound influence than organized and didactic interventions, and, related to this, contend that so-called 'event-based' initiatives need to complement *not* displace situated social learning.

Table 17.2 Key features of effective faculty development interventions

Key features
Well designed, needs-based interventions
Use of a range of instructional methods within a program – e.g. small group discussions, simulation, role play, interactive exercises
Experiential learning and reflective practice – e.g. being able to apply new learning in practice, and having opportunities to reflect on personal goals and learning
Provision of feedback – e.g. feedback about teaching skills
Project work – both individual and group projects
Fostering effective peer relationships – including collegial support and development of communities of practice
Mentorship – including innovative approaches such as peer-mentoring and co-mentoring
Interventions that extend over time – e.g. fellowships
Institutional support – identified as critical to success of many programs, including funding, protecting participants' time and involving senior faculty

After Amundsen and Wilson (2012), Steinert et al. (2006, 2012), and Stes et al. (2010)

This review is perhaps of more interest to scholars and researchers than faculty developers per se in offering a different way of conceptualizing and categorizing initiatives. In particular, echoing Steinert et al. (2006), the authors noted how rarely the context in which faculty members teach and educational development takes place is acknowledged by researchers. In their words, 'At this point in time we know more about how to design educational initiatives to improve individual teaching practice but less about how this learning is actualized and embedded in the academic workplace' (Amundsen and Wilson 2012, p. 111).

In summary, the four reviews (three of them systematic, one a conceptual review, and two discipline-specific) broadly agree about the impacts of faculty development in respect to changes in participants' attitudes, knowledge, skills and behavior, developments at the institutional level, and impact on student learning. The fact that similar conclusions were drawn despite the different ways authors organized and analyzed the data (i.e. by format, outcome, study design and/or type of practice) strengthens the veracity of the findings. In addition, similar concerns were voiced in all reviews about the variable quality of the research, and recommendations were made about further research, both of which will be discussed later in the chapter.

17.2.2   What Works in Faculty Development?

All the reviews highlighted key features of effective faculty development interventions that appeared to contribute to positive outcomes. These were remarkably consistent across the reviews and are summarized in Table 17.2.

Many of these features concur with the literature on continuing education, specifically that effective interventions ideally should involve needs assessments, use interactive techniques with opportunities to put new learning into practice, incorporate appropriately sequenced and multi-faceted activities, and facilitate reflection (Mazmanian and Davis 2002). When studies were grounded in a theoretical framework (approximately 50 % of papers), it was most often in relation to a small number of theories that have currency in health professions education, including adult learning, socio-cultural theories and experiential learning.

17.3 What Do We Know About the Quality of the Research into Faculty Development?

This section addresses the quality of research highlighted in the four reviews discussed above. Appraisal of methodological quality and rigor of the studies in all reviews showed consistent findings.

In the leadership review (Steinert et al. 2012) the majority of studies were quantitative, all of which had a quasi-experimental design. There were also five qualitative studies and 12 using a mixed-methods approach. Global judgments of the quality of research and strength of findings were made using a Likert scale of 1–5; for *study quality*, 1 = low, 5 = high; for *strength of findings*, anchor statements were also provided, with 1 = 'No clear conclusions can be drawn. Not significant' through to 5 = 'Results are unequivocal'. Mean quality ratings for the three categories of study were around 2.8 (range 1–5) and strength of findings around 3.0 (range 1–4).

A number of methodological issues were highlighted. Most studies were descriptive and involved single groups (i.e. there were no comparison groups, rendering generalization difficult). A wide range of data collection methods and instruments were used. However, these were often 'home grown', developed specifically for the study, and validation procedures and/or their psychometric properties were rarely described. The majority of studies used only post-intervention measures, as opposed to using a pre-test/post-test approach, relied on participants' self-report (the limitations of which will be discussed below), and data were often captured some considerable time after the intervention. In terms of research methods, rigorous qualitative approaches were infrequently used. Finally, although most articles defined specific objectives and adequately cited relevant literature, fewer were grounded in a theoretical or conceptual framework.

In the earlier BEME review of teaching effectiveness (Steinert et al. 2006), study designs were similarly predominately quasi-experimental (47/53) with just 6 randomized controlled trials. The mean global rating for quality of studies was 3.14 (range 1–5), and for strength of findings, the mean rating was around 3.0 (range 1–4). Stes et al.'s findings (2010) resonated with those of previous reviewers, in particular the fact that the majority of studies were based on self-report and used data collection instruments that were mainly self-constructed, with psychometric data infrequently provided. Further, few studies were comparative, and descriptions of the interventions were usually poor.

In summary, all four reviews identified broadly similar problems in terms of issues such as study design, methods, data instruments and outcome measures. Recommendations were made about how to improve the quality of research and these will be synthesized and summarized at the end of the chapter.

17.4 The Broader Context of Medical Education Research

The observations about the quality of the faculty development literature reflect similar concerns in relation to medical education research in general. For example, Todres et al. (2007) reviewed 387 papers published during 2004 and 2005 in two leading general medical journals (*BMJ & The Lancet*) and two major medical education journals (*Medical Education & Medical Teacher*). They felt that most of the studies lacked rigor, the majority being cross-sectional surveys; less than 10 % were longitudinal or before-and-after studies. Ten were randomized controlled trials (RCTs), although most of them would have failed to meet accepted criteria for publication of trials in the clinical arena (e.g. lack of a clear hypothesis; absence of a power calculation). Their review undoubtedly made a helpful contribution to the debate, but was criticized because of the seemingly positivist stance the authors adopted in their critique of methodologies and reflections on the nature of 'rigor' and evidence (Dornan et al. 2008; Rapid Responses, BMJ 2007).

Approaching the problem from another angle, Albert et al. (2007) interviewed 23 'influential figures' from the medical education research community, exploring three themes: strengths and weaknesses of current research; the role of research in medical education; and the usefulness of theory in knowledge development. The majority of respondents felt the overall quality of research remained poor, despite some progress. Several reasons were identified. Studies were often repetitions of other work because researchers appeared to have limited knowledge of the literature in the field, and were thus unable to fully contextualize their study. There was limited use of theory, with analysis often restricted to a descriptive level, hampering the creation of an integrated body of new knowledge. Related to this, some respondents also expressed concern that research was often subordinated to the demands of administrators and educators, which in their opinion limited development of works of a theoretical nature; as one interviewee put it '…if there is no theory permitting understanding of fundamental processes, how is it possible to predict and control for the effectiveness of interventions?' (Albert et al. 2007, p. 109). Research was often opportunistic, reactive to curricular demands and carried out on a small scale, and, in the words of one respondent, failed to address 'the truly big questions.' Several influencing factors were identified, including: the contention that clinical educators (which, for the purposes of this chapter, one could arguably read 'faculty developers') have a predominantly pragmatic orientation towards and a limited interest in the theoretical dimensions of research – 'what they want are results'; and the dominance of the 'biomedical' model, which influences the research process at every level from availability of funding to publication policy. In an accompanying editorial, Norman, argued that theory was often used to *justify* an approach, rather than as a source of testable hypotheses, with the result that 'theories remain inert and contribute nothing to growth of knowledge'. He also emphasized the crucial role that expert peer review has to play in the quality assurance of published research. In his words 'I believe that the expert, thoughtful, reviewer, who is prepared to put the time into a serious review, is a tremendous force for change, almost like having a free mentor on demand' (Norman 2007, p. 4).

Cook et al. (2007) undertook a systematic review of experimental studies published during 2003 and 2004 in four leading medical education journals (*Academic Medicine, Advances in Health Sciences Education, Medical Education and Teaching and Learning in Medicine*) and two US generalist journals (*Journal of General Internal Medicine* and *American Journal of Surgery*). The quality of reporting of the majority of the 105 studies reviewed was poor. Important elements were often missing including: a critical literature review (i.e. one that identified the research gap and how the study would contribute new knowledge); a conceptual framework (the absence of which, they argued, potentially limits selection of variables, meaningful interpretation of results, and either refinement of existing theories or development of new ones); an explicit statement about study design; description of a comparison or control group; and information about ethical approval.

Although they did not specifically evaluate study quality, they speculated that poor quality reporting 'may reflect sub-optimal research designs and methods, and a lack of attention to human subject rights' (Cook et al. 2007, p. 743). Like Norman (2007), they suggested that peer review and editorial policy 'have the best chances of improving reporting quality' (Cook et al. 2007, p. 738).

17.4.1   Problems of Experimental Research in Medical Education

Cook and Beckman followed up their earlier review with a paper in which they further discussed some of the problems of experimental research in medical education (Cook and Beckman 2010). These included:

- Limitations of randomization – arguing that randomization is not a panacea since it controls for only a subset of variables.
- Pre-tests weakening study design – challenging received wisdom that 'pre-test/post-test' is the gold standard; indeed they call it 'a myth', but listed the circumstances in which pre-tests *should* be used, for example when the pre-test is part of the intervention, or when sample size is small.
- Limitations of 'no intervention' or placebo-controlled studies – such so-called 'justification studies', focused on what works, do not always advance our understanding, in comparison to 'clarification studies' which ask 'how and why does this work?' (Cook et al. 2008; Cook 2012).

- Multi-factorial interventions are 'hopelessly confounded' and may have limited potential application in new settings – see Sect. 17.5.2 on complex interventions.
- Interventions themselves are often not well described, a deficiency noted by all previous reviewers.

Some of these issues will be revisited in Sect. 17.6.

17.5 What Challenges Might Researchers in Faculty Development Face?

This section discusses some of the potential challenges faced by researchers and scholars in faculty development. These particular areas have been chosen since, in the author's experience, as a researcher and former editor, they commonly challenge researchers, whether from a philosophical or practical perspective. The challenges are: recognizing the differences and similarities between evaluation and research; evaluating complex interventions; and problems with measuring outcomes. For further discussion about the limitations of positivism in researching faculty development, along with a description of alternative research paradigms and several novel research methods, see Chap. 18 by O'Sullivan and Irby.

17.5.1 Evaluation or Research?

This section will firstly define evaluation and consider its purposes; similarities and differences between evaluation and research will then be discussed; finally, key features of effective evaluation will be highlighted.

17.5.1.1 What Is Evaluation?

Evaluation, defined as 'the systematic acquisition and assessment of information to provide useful feedback about some object' (Trochim 2006, p. 1), plays a central role in education. The majority of faculty developers would consider it inconceivable to run a program without some sort of evaluation, indeed they are usually required to evaluate as part of quality improvement. Although the generic goal of evaluation is to provide 'useful feedback', it can operate at many levels (e.g. the institution, the program, the faculty developers or the participants). Moreover, its purposes fall into three general categories: for accountability; to generate new insights and understanding; and to support and guide development (Goldie 2006). It can be formative or summative. The former, also known as 'process evaluation', asks the question 'how are we doing?', and may be an on-going enterprise; whereas the latter, also known as 'outcomes' or 'impact' evaluation, asks 'how did we do?' and is usually undertaken at the end. In terms of focus, evaluation may be targeted at one or more levels, including policy, institution, curriculum, teaching, learning or assessment. Potential stakeholders might thus include policymakers, regulators, funders, curriculum designers, managers, teachers and learners (and in health care settings, patients), and evaluators may therefore need to tackle difficult and conflicting issues. To quote one author, evaluation 'may encompass competing criteria and purposes, and is situated in potentially sensitive political and ethical contexts' (Silver 2004, p. 2). Careful consideration of purpose, focus, level and stakeholders' needs will determine the questions to be asked and thus the data to be collected and methods used. For example a formative evaluation focused on learner experience might seek feedback about aspects of the course from both learners and teachers (i.e. in the context of this chapter, faculty developers) using survey methods or interviews and focus groups, whereas a summative evaluation at institutional level might wish to look at aspects of curriculum governance through documentary analysis.

17.5.1.2 What Are the Similarities and Differences Between Evaluation and Research?

The question often arises as to the difference(s) between evaluation and research. This is of more than passing interest, since data collected for evaluation purposes are often used as the basis of a study that may eventually be submitted for publication, with the aim of adding to the knowledge base. The main difference between the two, arguably, lies in their respective aims. On the whole, research aims to generate new knowledge and understanding, or to develop theory, usually for consumption by the academic community, whereas, as highlighted above, evaluation aims to provide 'useful feedback' to inform and/or influence decision-making within the community of practice. A moment's reflection will reveal that there is considerable overlap between the two processes.

The issue is continuously debated within the academic community, and although no firm conclusions seem likely to be reached, it is reminiscent of discussions about the difference(s) between research and clinical audit when the latter was first introduced into medical practice in the late 1980s/early 1990s. A useful, albeit simplistic perspective that helped clarify thinking was that research asked the question 'what is the right thing to do?', whereas audit – evaluation? – asks either 'are we doing the right thing?' or 'are we doing the thing right?' In this respect, evaluation, like audit, is parochial, pragmatic, often political and sometimes just a bit 'messy'. Evaluation by its very nature involves making value-laden decisions about all stages of the process from what questions are asked of whom, to how results are framed and disseminated. The important thing is that these values are acknowledged and articulated.

17.5.1.3 What Is Good Practice in Evaluation?

Unfortunately, evaluation is often included as an afterthought, and may not be afforded the depth of attention and methodological rigor it demands. As a consequence, effort and resources may be wasted, inaccurate or irrelevant conclusions drawn, and inappropriate decisions made. Guidelines for good practice in evaluation have been produced by a number of organizations including the American Evaluation Association (AEA) and the UK Evaluation Society (UKES). The AEA guidance is underpinned by the philosophy that, despite a diversity of approaches '….the common ground is that evaluators aspire to construct and provide the best possible information that might bear on the value of whatever is being evaluated' (American Evaluation Association 2004, p. 1), and is structured around five key principles. These are systematic inquiry, competence, integrity, respect for people and responsibility. Difficulties of producing generic guidelines are acknowledged: '….it is impossible to write guiding principles that neatly fit every context in which evaluators work, and some evaluators will work in contexts in which following a guideline cannot be done for good reason' (American Evaluation Association 2004, p. 1). The UK Evaluation Society approached the issue from a different perspective in attempting to capture 'a diverse set of principles for action' for different stakeholders. So for example, the guidelines propose that evaluators need to be explicit about the purpose, methods, intended outputs and outcomes, and to be realistic about what is feasible. Participants must have the process fully explained and be assured that outputs such as reports will be made available to them. Commissioners of evaluation should provide access to documentation and data, and establish clear principles for reporting and disseminating results. Finally, those undertaking self-evaluation must ensure the process is built into the structure and function of the institution, and that all involved are engaged from the start. At the heart of the guidelines is a philosophy of transparency about the expectations and requirements of all stakeholders, *whoever* they are (UKES 2013).

Guidance about evaluation, specifically in the medical education literature, has also been published. In a comprehensive review, Goldie (2006) outlined key issues in relation to the role of the evaluator, ethics of evaluation, choosing the 'right' questions, design and range of approaches, analysis and interpretation of findings, dissemination of results, and influencing decision-making. Cook (2010) offered 12 pragmatic tips to guide evaluation, arguing that the two most important questions to ask were 'Whose opinion matters?' and 'What would be really meaningful to them?' Other important issues include focusing on desired outcomes before selecting instruments, considering the validity or trustworthiness of the data, and pilot testing the evaluation process (Cook 2010).

Notwithstanding differences in aims and purposes, all are agreed that to be of any value, evaluation must follow broadly similar precepts to research. It must be as rigorous as possible, ask relevant questions using appropriate methods, adhere to ethical principles, and report and disseminate the findings honestly. As with research, there is no single 'correct' approach, only more (or less) appropriate ones.

17.5.2   Complex or Simple Intervention?

Related to the positivist paradigm that underpins much of the faculty development research to date is the notion of a linear causal chain, whereby one event, the intervention, leads to a specific outcome, with the educational event conceptualized as a 'simple' intervention, rather like treatment of a specific disorder with a drug. Experimental approaches, such as the randomized controlled trial, which aim to control for all variables, are the methods of choice in assessing such simple interventions.

Yet even an apparently simple one-off workshop – the mainstay of faculty development programs – may be surprisingly complex. Take for example a hypothetical 3 h training session for OSCE examiners in a regional medical school. Instructional design combines a training model (describe, demonstrate, put in context, deliberate practice with feedback, assessment) and an adult learning approach. There is pre-session reading and the workshop itself comprises didactic input from the facilitator, video demonstration, role play and group discussion, with access to supplementary on-line resources for further study. Four facilitators of varying experience deliver the session in ten teaching centers around the region to clinical faculty, themselves with a range of experience and from different specialties; the session is held at different times during the working day or evening depending on site. Medical students are recruited for role play when they are available. It can be seen that this intervention is *far* from simple, with many potential variables and confounders, some that could be predicted and *possibly* controlled for, others which are likely unknown or unpredictable. To ascribe cause and effect in terms of a simple outcome such as self-reported confidence in examining in an OSCE could be seen as overly simplistic. Further, although this may tell us something about *what* worked it would not necessarily be able to answer questions such as why it worked or not, and in what circumstances. Clearly alternative approaches to researching complex interventions such as this scenario need to be considered.

17.5.2.1   What Distinguishes a Complex Intervention from a Simple One?

Several features of a complex intervention have been defined:

- It is usually based on several hypotheses or working theories, some more well defined and/or evidence-based than others.
- It will usually involve a wide range of participants (e.g. faculty developers, administrators, course participants, learners).
- It may be a 'long journey' from design of the intervention to delivery, with success dependent upon integrity of a cumulative chain of events.
- The chain is usually non-linear, with multiple pathways and feedback loops.
- Complex interventions are embedded in multiple social systems.

In the words of Pawson et al. 'complex service interventions, therefore, can be conceptualised as dynamic complex systems thrust amidst complex systems, relentlessly subject to negotiation, resistance, adaptation, leak and borrow, bloom and fade....' (Pawson et al. 2005, S1:23). Acknowledging this, it can be seen that if we wished to research the effectiveness of the hypothetical training session described above, several approaches may be required to capture its complexities. As argued, simply assessing pre-determined outcomes will not allow us to ask questions such as 'Why did the intervention work here and not there?' and 'What is it about it that works for whom in what circumstances?' In this respect, Cook (2012) suggested three main reasons why researchers in medical education continue to address such basic 'what works?'-type questions (usually using single-group pre-test/post-test studies): because they *can;* because they seem important questions to ask; and because they see others doing it in the literature. In fact, an intervention, especially if it is new and innovative, will almost certainly work, at least for a time. McCoubrie (2007) has argued that innovations in education tend to be effective because of a number of factors. Firstly, there is the so-called 'Pygmalion effect', whereby people do better simply because they're expected to; secondly, we encounter the 'Hawthorne effect', whereby the act of observation (by the researcher) alters the behavior of those being observed; and lastly, there is the 'halo effect', whereby performance is different (though not necessarily always improved) simply because of the novelty of the situation. In addition, innovations are often well funded and are championed by an enthusiast and generally do well – until funding dries up or enthusiasm wanes (McCoubrie 2007). Thus, an evaluation of an innovative or novel intervention using participant satisfaction alone, whilst likely to show favorable results, will not address questions such as *why* the innovation was successful.

17.5.2.2   Good Practice in Studying Complex Interventions

The science of researching and evaluating complex interventions has evolved over the past decade. For example, the UK Medical Research Council published guidelines in 2000, which were updated in 2008 (Craig et al. 2008).

Key issues highlighted include:

- The importance of having a sound theoretical understanding of how the intervention might cause change.
- Recognizing that an intervention's apparent lack of effect may reflect implementation problems rather than lack of effectiveness per se, begging the need for a thorough process evaluation.
- Allowing for adaptation to local settings may be more appropriate than strict adherence to a standardized protocol.
- The need to carefully consider the trade-off between the importance of the intervention and constraints on what evidence can be gathered about it.
- The importance of combining evidence from a number of sources.

The essence of the guidance is summed up thus: 'Best practice is to develop interventions systematically, using the best available evidence and appropriate theory, then to test them using a carefully phased approach starting with pilot studies targeted at each of the key uncertainties in the design, and moving onto an exploratory and then a definitive evaluation.' (Craig et al. 2008, p. 8).

17.5.2.3   A Novel Approach to Evaluating Complex Interventions

Several novel approaches to evaluating complex interventions have been developed, an example being 'realist evaluation'. Its basic tenet is that, rather than seeing causality as 'X follows Y', and recognizing that underlying mechanisms may be hidden, it takes a so-called 'generative' view, i.e. to infer a causal relationship between two events, X and Y, one needs to understand not only the outcome, but also the mechanism(s), the context and the relationships between them. The underlying question changes from 'What works?' to 'What is it about this intervention that works for whom, and in what circumstances?' Realist evaluation emphasizes *interpretation* rather than measurement or prediction and thus has an explanatory as opposed to a judgmental purpose (Pawson and Tilley 1997; Pawson et al. 2005). The kind of question a realist evaluation would address includes 'What is it about the intervention, or component of the intervention, that leads to a particular outcome in a particular context?' and this would usually be approached using qualitative or mixed methods.

There is often no sharp distinction between simple and complex interventions. Indeed, it has been argued that complexity and simplicity sometimes reside more in the eye of the beholder than in reality. Further, many interventions may be equally open to simple *or* complex analysis, and Petticrew (2011) argued that complexity may be simplified for the purpose of assessing specific simple outcomes when it is helpful to see and analyze them as such; the important issue is the nature of the research question (Petticrew 2011).

17.5.3   Measuring Outcomes

Notwithstanding the importance of exploring process and context as discussed above, there is still a need to assess the impact of interventions. This involves assessing outcomes, whether intended and pre-defined, or unintended and 'discovered' outcomes. This section will discuss two important methodological issues in evaluating impact, namely Kirkpatrick's framework and the use of self-report measures.

17.5.3.1   Kirkpatrick's Framework

Kirkpatrick's framework (Table 17.1) has been widely used to evaluate both educational interventions and as a framework for systematic reviews. It was originally developed for use in the manufacturing industry, the intended aim being to provide managers with easily identifiable and easy-to-measure outcomes, metrics to which a market value could be ascribed. Interestingly, it was not Kirkpatrick's intention that it should be treated as a hierarchy, although that is how the framework is usually used, with participant reaction ascribed the 'lowest' level, and impact on learners (or, in healthcare, patients) the highest. Yardley and Dornan, building on previous authors' work, provide a detailed critique of Kirkpatrick in the context of medical education (Yardley and Dornan 2012). Key criticisms include the fact that the framework, or at least the way it tends to be used, assumes causal links (i.e. that attainment of a lower level is a pre-requisite for a higher one). Secondly, the different levels relate to different stakeholders (such as faculty developers, their learners and the organization). Furthermore, evaluating against *anticipated* outcomes may blind researchers to other (unintended or unexpected) outcomes, addressing the question 'was outcome X achieved?' rather than 'what were the outcomes of this intervention?' (A clinical analogy would be carrying out a drug trial looking only at expected outcomes and not at side-effects.) Finally, it was apparently never fully validated since it rapidly found widespread use (Yardley and Dornan 2012). However, it does serve a useful purpose in terms of categorizing the range of possible outcomes and as such it is likely that Kirkpatrick's framework, or variations thereof, will continue to be used in research and evaluation. Users need to recognize the practical and conceptual limitations, which if nothing else serves to remind us that effective evaluation needs to be multi-dimensional.

17.5.3.2   A Theoretical Model of Learning Outcomes

Kraiger et al. (1993) developed a theoretically-based model of learning outcomes, drawing on research and theory from a range of disciplines, including cognitive, social and educational psychology, and human factors. In effect they elaborated Kirkpatrick's Level 2, classifying outcomes under three headings: 'cognitive' (sub-classified hierarchically as verbal or declarative knowledge, organization of knowledge, and cognitive strategies such as meta-cognition); 'skills-based' (acknowledging the nature of skills development from initial acquisition, through 'compilation' to automaticity); and 'affective' outcomes (including attitudinal and motivational outcomes). They identified the learning constructs underpinning these outcome categories, highlighted relevant foci of measurement, and suggested potential evaluation methods. For example, measurements of verbal knowledge would focus on amount or accuracy of knowledge using tests of recall or recognition. On the other hand, skills-based outcomes would usually require observational measures, and affective outcomes some kind of self-report. The importance of ensuring measurement instruments are 'fit for purpose' in terms of characteristics such as validity and reliability cannot be over-emphasized (Cook 2010), although a degree of compromise may be necessary for pragmatic reasons.

17.5.3.3 The Limitations of Self-Report

Self-report is a mainstay of research and evaluation whether it is in health, education or social policy, and the faculty development literature is no exception. The majority of studies in the systematic reviews described earlier used self-report; indeed, this was often the *only* method used, for example asking participants whether they found a course useful, or about changes in attitudes, gains in knowledge and skills, or modification of behavior. Ultimately there is no other way to find out what people think or feel than to ask them. It is important, however, to recognize the limitations of self-report. A large body of research, much of it from cognitive psychology, has shown that self-report i.e. accessing information from so-called autobiographical (as opposed to semantic) memory, is notoriously flawed (Tourangeau 2000). Apart from error inherent in any measurement, major potential biases include social desirability of responding in a particular way and the pressures to mis-report, for example to preserve self-image. More fundamentally, however, every stage of the memory-making process, from encoding, through retrieval, to recall and what has been called 'reconstruction' (i.e. filling in the gaps), is prone to bias and error. This is so much the case that one author was moved to write 'What we retrieve from memory often consists of our current beliefs about an incident, beliefs that reflect what we actually experienced (and remember), what we did not experience but infer, and what we learned later on' (Tourangeau 2000). In particular, people often have problems with recalling dates, sequences, and frequencies (with a tendency to remember events as happening more frequently than they did). A further confounding variable comes to bear when people are asked to appraise their own performance. It is well recognized that people do not (and possibly cannot) self-assess with any degree of accuracy (Eva and Regehr 2005). Taken together, these issues beg the need for caution when interpreting data obtained from self-report and where possible to triangulate by using more objective methods.

17.6 Recommendations for Future Research and Evaluation in Faculty Development

The following list of issues for consideration has been distilled from the literature reviewed in this chapter and is divided into two areas, the research process and the content or focus of research. General recommendations for improving quality were remarkably consistent across the four reviews and include greater collaboration between educators and researchers and across disciplines, in particular with scholars based in the social sciences and humanities, better research training, and more rigorous peer review.

17.6.1   The Research Process

Key practical messages from the literature about the *process* (i.e. how we undertake research and evaluation) include the following:

- Ensure research is informed as much as possible by theory and evidence; this will make the research more robust (and thus more useful), and strengthen links between theory and practice.
- Focus on evaluating process and context as much as outcomes and impact; this will help illuminate the complexity that characterizes all but the most basic intervention.
- Undertake 'clarification' studies, as opposed to descriptive or 'justification' studies because addressing questions such as 'why does X work in this situation and not in that?' is likely to generate more useful answers than simply asking 'does X work?'
- Consider using qualitative or mixed methods approaches whilst ensuring there is congruence between study design, research questions, data collection methods and analysis.
- Recognize the limitations of the single group pre-test/post-test design, and consider using retrospective pre-post approaches (Skeff et al. 1992).
- Consider comparative studies, recognizing the need for larger samples, but noting that valid inferences can be drawn from well-designed *non*-randomized studies, striving to ensure that the most appropriate method is used to answer the questions posed.
- Where possible, use validated outcome measures, including newer methods of behavioral or performance-based assessment; if using a 'home-grown' instrument, make sure it is piloted and assess and endeavor to report its validity and reliability, as well as its strengths and limitations.
- Describe both the intervention and the context in more detail; this will help colleagues make sense of the findings and also enable further research.
- Explore the core characteristics of the initiative (e.g. its theoretical foundation, goals and content) as well as the educational features (such as duration and format).
- Consider collaborating with colleagues in other disciplines.

17.6.2   Content or Focus of the Research

Potential areas for further research in faculty development emerging from the reviews include:

- The consequences and impacts of interventions over longer time periods. Intuitively one would expect long-term interventions to have better and more sustained outcomes, but the evidence-base for this is currently slim.
- The social determinants of participation, such as the role of motivation and the factors influencing it, to inform development of appropriate interventions.
- Which combination of blended learning is effective and for what reasons? Use of blended learning approaches (i.e. combinations of face-to-face and on-line learning) is increasing; thus, it is important to understand what works for whom and in what situations.
- Inter-professional education at basic/pre-registration level is increasingly the norm. Given that faculty are diverse and often drawn from a range of professional backgrounds, it would be useful to know whether and how inter-professional faculty development 'works'.
- The relationship between organizational culture and faculty development, including impacts at the institutional level.
- Development and sustainability of communities of practice and their role in promoting professional development.
- The impact of different interventions, of varied duration or format.

17.7   Conclusion

This chapter has described and discussed the findings of recent reviews of research into faculty development. Key features of effective interventions and strengths and weaknesses of the research were highlighted, and a number of important issues related to improving the quality of research were discussed. In their 2006 review, Steinert et al. (2006) predicted there would be an increase in the number of well-designed studies looking at objectively measured behavioral and systems-level outcomes in the early twenty-first century. Encouragingly, there is some evidence that this is the case. At the time of writing, a further systematic review is in process looking at the literature on faculty development for teaching effectiveness published since 2002. Preliminary analysis of around 130 papers has revealed more rigorous study designs, a diversity of methods, and use of more robust outcome measures. Despite concerns about quality, it would appear that the 'state of the art' is (to mix metaphors) 'alive and well.'

17.8 Key Messages

- Systematic reviews have demonstrated the effectiveness of faculty development interventions in terms of participant satisfaction, changes in attitudes, knowledge, skills and behavior, developments at the institutional level, and impact on student learning.
- Key features of effective faculty development include needs assessments, interactive techniques and collaborative approaches, opportunities for practice with feedback, appropriately sequenced and multi-faceted activities, reflective practice, and long-term interventions.
- Whereas research and evaluation differ in focus, aims and purpose, both approaches must be rigorous and systematic, ask relevant questions using appropriate methods, adhere to ethical principles, and report and disseminate findings honestly.
- Most faculty development initiatives are 'complex interventions' and novel approaches to their evaluation, such as 'realist evaluation', should be considered.
- Although Kirkpatrick's framework is useful in evaluating outcomes, its limitations should be recognized; similarly, the limitations of self-report measures should be acknowledged.
- With both research and evaluation, there is no single 'correct' approach, only more (or less) appropriate ones.

References

Amundsen, C. & Wilson, M. (2012). Are we asking the right questions? A conceptual review of the educational development literature in higher education. *Review of Educational Research, 82*(1), 90–126.

Albert, M., Hodges, B., & Regehr, G. (2007). Research in medical education: Balancing service and science. *Advances in Health Sciences Education, 12*(1), 103–115.

American Evaluation Association. (2004). Guiding principles for evaluators. Retrieved August, 2012, from http://www.eval.org/p/cm/ld/fid=51

Cook, D. A. (2010). Twelve tips for evaluating educational programs. *Medical Teacher, 32*(4), 296–301.

Cook, D. A. (2012). If you teach them, they will learn: Why medical education needs comparative effectiveness research. *Advances in Health Sciences Education, 17*(3), 305–310.

Cook, D. A. & Beckman, T. J. (2010). Reflections on experimental research in medical education. *Advances in Health Sciences Education, 15*(3), 455–464.

Cook, D. A., Beckman, T. J., & Bordage, G. (2007). Quality of reporting of experimental studies in medical education: A systematic review. *Medical Education, 41*(8), 737–745.

Cook, D. A., Bordage, G., & Schmidt, H. G. (2008). Description, justification and clarification: A framework for classifying the purposes of research in medical education. *Medical Education 42*(2), 128–133.

Craig, P., Dieppe, P., Macintyre, S., Michie, S., Nazareth, I., & Petticrew, M. (2008). Developing and evaluating complex interventions: The new Medical Research Council guidance. *BMJ, 337*(a1655), 979–983.

Dornan, T., Peile, E., & Spencer, J. (2008). On 'evidence'. *Medical Education, 42*(3), 232–234.

Eva, K. W. & Regehr, G. (2005). Self-assessment in the health professions: A reformulation and research agenda. *Academic Medicine, 80*(10 Suppl.), S46–S54.

General Medical Council. (2009a). *Tomorrow's Doctors: Outcomes and standards for undergraduate medical education.* Available from: http://www.gmc-uk.org/education/undergraduate/tomorrows_doctors.asp

General Medical Council. (2009b). *Good Medical Practice.* London, UK: GMC. Retrieved August, 2012, from http://www.gmc-uk.org/

Goldie, J. (2006). AMEE Education Guide No. 29: Evaluating educational programmes. *Medical Teacher, 28*(3), 210–224.

Kraiger, K., Ford, J. K., & Salas, E. (1993). Application of cognitive, skill-based and affective theories of learning outcomes to new methods of training evaluation. *Journal of Applied Psychology, 78*(2), 311–328.

Liaison Committee on Medical Education. (2012). *Functions and structure of a medical school: Standards for accreditation of medical education programs leading to the M.D. degree.* Available from: https://www.lcme.org/publications/functions2012may.pdf

Mazmanian, P. E. & Davis, D. A. (2002). Continuing medical education and the physician as a learner: Guide to the evidence. *JAMA, 288*(9), 1057–1060.

McCoubrie, P. (2007). Innovation in medical education: More than meets the eye. *The Clinical Teacher, 4*(1), 51–54.

Norman, G. (2007). Editorial - How bad is medical education research anyway? *Advances in Health Sciences Education, 12*(1), 1–5.

Pawson, R., Greenhalgh, T., Harvey, G., & Walshe, K. (2005). Realist review: A new method of systematic review designed for complex policy interventions. *Journal of Health Services Research & Policy, 10*(Suppl. 1), S1:21–S1:34.

Pawson, R. & Tilley, N. (1997). *Realistic evaluation.* London, UK: Sage.

Petticrew, M. (2011). When are complex interventions 'complex'? When are simple interventions 'simple'? *European Journal of Public Health, 21*(4), 397–398.

Rapid Responses, BMJ. (2007). Rapid responses to: Medical education research remains the poor relation, *BMJ, 335*(7615), 333–335. Available from: http://www.bmj.com/content/335/7615/333?tab=responses

Royal College of Physicians and Surgeons of Canada. (2011). *A continuing commitment to lifelong learning: A concise guide to Maintenance of Certification.* Retrieved August, 2012, from http://www.royalcollege.ca/portal/page/portal/rc/common/documents/moc_program/moc_short_guide_e.pdf

Silver, H. (2004). *Evaluation research in education.* Retrieved August, 2012, from http://www.edu.plymouth.ac.uk/resined/evaluation/index.htm

Skeff, K. M., Stratos, G. A., & Bergen, M. R. (1992). Evaluation of a medical faculty development program: A comparison of traditional pre/post and retrospective pre/post self-assessment ratings. *Evaluation and the Health Professions, 15*(3), 350–366.

Steinert, Y., Mann, K., Centeno, A., Dolmans, D., Spencer, J., Gelula, M., et al. (2006). A systematic review of faculty development initiatives designed to improve teaching effectiveness in medical education: BEME Guide No. 8. *Medical Teacher, 28*(6), 497–526.

Steinert, Y., Naismith, L., & Mann, K. (2012). Faculty development initiatives designed to promote leadership in medical education. A BEME systematic review: BEME Guide No. 19. *Medical Teacher, 34*(6), 483–503.

Stes, A., Min-Leliveld, M., Gijbels, D., & van Petegem, P. (2010). The impact of instructional development in higher education: The state-of-the-art of the research. *Educational Research Review, 5*(1), 25–49.

Todres, M., Stephenson, A., & Jones, R. (2007). Medical education research remains the poor relation. *BMJ, 335*(7615), 333–335.

Tourangeau, R. (2000). Remembering what happened: Memory errors and survey reports. In A. A. Stone, J. S. Turkkan, C. A. Bachrach, J. B. Jobe, H. S. Kurtzman, & V. S. Cain (Eds.),

The science of self-report: Implications for research and practice. Mahwah, NJ: Taylor & Francis (e-book).

Trochim, W. (2006). *Research methods knowledge base: Introduction to evaluation.* Cornell Office for Research on Evaluation: Web Center for Social Research Methods. Retrieved August, 2012, from http://www.socialresearchmethods.net/kb/intreval.php

UK Evaluation Society. (2013). *Guidelines for good practice in evaluation.* London, UK: UK Evaluation Society. Retrieved August 2012 from https://www.evaluation.org.uk/assets/UKES%20Guidelines%20for%20Good%20Practice%20January%202013.pdf

Wilkerson, L. & Irby, D. M. (1998). Strategies for improving teaching practices: A comprehensive approach to faculty development. *Academic Medicine, 73*(4), 387–396.

Yardley, S. & Dornan, T. (2012). Kirkpatrick's levels and education 'evidence'. *Medical Education, 46*(1), 97–106.

Chapter 18
Promoting Scholarship in Faculty Development: Relevant Research Paradigms and Methodologies

Patricia S. O'Sullivan and David M. Irby

18.1 Introduction

If you ask faculty members how they are using what they learned in a faculty development program, you might be surprised to hear how they have changed their teaching practices and discovered a new community of fellow teachers. However, if you tried to measure the impact of those faculty development programs using the traditional approach to research, you might be puzzled to discover 'no significant difference.' We (O'Sullivan and Irby 2011) struggled with this dilemma and found that most research on faculty development follows the positivist paradigm. A paradigm defines the prevailing model of exemplary practices for a community of researchers; it illuminates areas for investigation and obscures others. The positivist research paradigm assumes that reality is ordered, predictable and ultimately knowable through objective measures and rigorous application of the scientific method. Acting on these presumptions, researchers have postulated a mechanical or linear model of faculty development that begins with a faculty development activity where participants acquire new knowledge, skills and attitudes, which they then employ or convey to learners, who in turn ultimately provide improved patient care. Much of the published work on faculty development has followed this paradigm. See Fig. 18.1 for a visual model of this approach to the study of faculty development.

P.S. O'Sullivan, Ed.D. (✉) • D.M. Irby, Ph.D.
Department of Medicine and Office of Research and Development in Medical Education,
University of California San Francisco School of Medicine, San Francisco, CA, USA
e-mail: patricia.osullivan@ucsf.edu; david.irby@ucsf.edu

Y. Steinert (ed.), *Faculty Development in the Health Professions: A Focus on Research and Practice*, Innovation and Change in Professional Education 11, DOI 10.1007/978-94-007-7612-8_18, © Springer Science+Business Media Dordrecht 2014

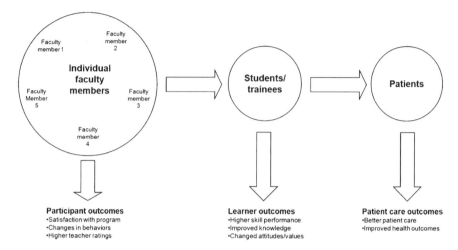

Fig. 18.1 The traditional, linear model of faculty development research assumes a causal chain of events, starting with a faculty development program, continuing through changes in actions of individual faculty participants to changes in the actions of learners, and culminating in changes to patient care (Adapted from O'Sullivan and Irby 2011, and used with permission of Academic Medicine)

We argue that in order for the field of faculty development to advance, we need to utilize other research paradigms and methodologies in addition to the positivist paradigm with its emphasis on empirically driven randomized controlled studies. We have divided this chapter into five sections. First, we review findings from prior reviews of the literature on faculty development programs, focusing on the research paradigms that the researchers chose for including or excluding studies in the review. By and large, we find that these reviews have been overly constrained by the predominance of the positivist paradigm. Second, we stress the importance of working from a conceptual framework for faculty development, which can enrich and broaden the inquiry process. Our framework for examining faculty development (O'Sullivan and Irby 2011) leads to a broader set of questions requiring a variety of research paradigms compared to the model in Fig. 18.1. Third, we explore how four paradigms and their accompanying research methodologies can expand the way in which we investigate faculty development programs, drawing on the positivist, post-positivist, interpretivist and critical theory paradigms. Fourth, we review three methodologies that are less frequently used in faculty development research to explore their potential to provide new directions for faculty development research: educational design research, success cases and sustainability narratives. Finally, we describe how this discovery-oriented research fits into the broader arena of scholarship, and how readers might begin to undertake scholarship in this exciting area of faculty development.

18.2 Prior Reviews of Faculty Development Research

Working within the positivistic paradigm, at least six systematic reviews of the teaching improvement and faculty development literature have focused on the effectiveness of faculty development practices (Amundsen and Wilson 2012; Levinson-Rose and Menges 1981; McLean et al. 2008; Steinert et al. 2006; Stes et al. 2010; Webster-Wright 2009). Most of these reviews sought to address the question: What are the features of faculty development that make it effective? All but the Amundsen and Wilson review (2012) grouped studies by format such as workshops and consultations, by level or type of learning examined such as self-report or observed behavior, and by individual variables such as duration of the activity. The authors of these reviews lamented the meager generalizations that could be gained from these studies. They also found it difficult to draw meaningful conclusions because of the limited number of studies that met the review criteria, which were highly influenced by the positivist paradigm. Adherence to such criteria inherently eliminates research from alternative paradigms (to be described below), thus restricting the usefulness and informative nature of such reviews.

Reading these reviews reminds us of watching a fly butting its head against a window trying to get out of the house. It continuously repeats the process of ramming the windowpane, but no matter how hard it tries, there is no way through it. Yet, just a few feet away, the door is open to the outside and the fly could proceed outside unimpeded if it would just switch course. Researchers studying faculty development programs are somewhat like the fly in that we predominantly use a limited set of research paradigms and research methodologies – attempting to answer all questions using the positivist paradigm and quantitative methodologies. We need to open the door and broaden our questions, paradigms and research methodologies.

Amundsen and Wilson (2012) examined the prior literature reviews that focused exclusively on effectiveness measures and reoriented their review of faculty development in higher education to address two additional questions: 'How are educational development practices designed?' and 'What is the thinking underpinning the design of educational development practices?' Based on their review, they found that studies could provide evidence for the following clusters of practice: a *skill focus* on the acquisition of teaching skills and techniques (e.g. voice projection), a *method focus* on mastery of a particular teaching method (e.g. problem-based learning), a *reflection focus* on change in individual teacher conceptions of teaching and learning, an *institutional focus* on institutional support for teaching improvement, a *disciplinary focus* on disciplinary understanding to develop pedagogical knowledge, and an *action research or inquiry focus* on individuals or groups of faculty investigating teaching and learning questions of interest to them. The authors argue that their review of the literature using clusters of practice resulted in an enhanced understanding of faculty development and the situated nature of teaching practice in the academic workplace, thereby overcoming the limitations of the prior reviews. See Chap. 17 for a broader description of the results of these reviews.

18.3   A Conceptual Framework for Faculty Development

After reviewing literature from faculty development, continuing medical education, teacher education, quality improvement and workplace learning, we proposed a conceptual framework for conducting faculty development research (O'Sullivan and Irby 2011). See Fig. 18.2 for a visual representation of this framework.

While our work preceded Amundsen and Wilson's review (2012), we are struck by the similarities of our conclusions. The core concept in our framework is about locating faculty development within two separate but related communities: (1) the faculty

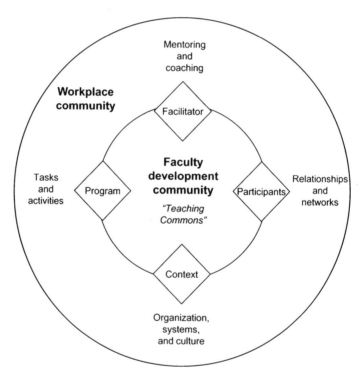

Fig. 18.2 The new model for faculty development research suggests that faculty development is embedded in two communities of practice (the faculty development community and the workplace community) and, to bring about desired change, requires the interaction of four primary components (facilitator, participants, context, and program) with their associated processes (mentoring and coaching; relationships and networks; organizations, systems, and cultures; and tasks and activities) – all in the workplace (Used with permission of Academic Medicine: O'Sullivan and Irby 2011)

development community and (2) the community of teaching practice in the workplace (Billett 2001; Lave and Wenger 1991). The faculty development community is often described as a 'teaching commons' (Huber and Hutchings 2005), which refers to the real and virtual environments where faculty members discuss their questions, concerns and challenges as educators, and learn new roles and new skills. The second community, the workplace, can be situated in classrooms and clinical settings where the teaching takes place. For the faculty development community located in the teaching commons, the four key components are the participants, the faculty development program, the facilitator, and the context in which the program occurs (e.g. classroom, clinic, and online). For the workplace community of teaching practice (i.e. the classroom and/or clinical setting), there are four associated components in the model. Participants have relationships and networks of associations with colleagues and learners in the work environment. The analogous component to the faculty development program in the workplace is the tasks and activities in the work setting. The parallel role of the facilitator is the mentoring that might be available to faculty in the workplace setting. Finally, context relates to the organization and culture of the workplace setting. Each of these components as well as their interactions within and across communities represents critical areas in need of further investigation.

To investigate all of the components in this framework, we need to ask an expanded set of questions employing a broader array of research methodologies that go well beyond those employed by the positivist paradigm. The conceptual framework broadens the purview of research opportunities beyond faculty development activities themselves in order to account for the powerful influences of the workplace environment on the faculty members' teaching practices. We encourage research on the overall framework, on each separate component, on associations among the components, and on how each component leads to a desired outcome. All of this will be required to offer policy guidance to those responsible for leading and funding faculty development programs.

18.4 Research Paradigms

Before describing the four research paradigms and associated research methodologies, we define the terms being employed. A *research paradigm* reflects the philosophical underpinnings of knowledge development. 'Paradigms are sets of beliefs and practices, shared by communities of researchers, which regulate inquiry within disciplines' (Bunniss and Kelly 2010, p. 360). An example is the positivist paradigm described above. The term *methodology* refers to the applied approach to the study of a particular issue. Research methodologies are nested within broader research paradigms or assumptions about the nature of the world, how we interact with it, and how we know it. Examples of methodologies include experimental design, surveys, correlational studies, ethnography, phenomenology and case studies. Finally, *tools* are the specific research methods used to obtain information for a study, such as cognitive tests, observation forms, interviews and focus groups.

The four research paradigms we include are drawn from the Bunnis and Kelly (2010) review of research paradigms used in medical education research: positivism, post-positivism, interpretivism and critical theory. We summarize them succinctly here and elaborate on each more fully below. Positivism, the most prevalent paradigm, assumes that reality is knowable and measurable. It uses the scientific method to develop abstract laws in order to describe and predict patterns, and employs quantitative methodologies to test hypotheses. Post-positivism assumes that objective knowledge of the world is not fully possible or accessible and therefore seeks probable truths. In this paradigm, knowledge is developed through falsification of hypotheses. Post-positivists use quantitative *and* qualitative methodologies. Interpretivism asserts that reality is subjective and changing and therefore there is no ultimate truth. Meaning is socially constructed, resulting in multiple and diverse interpretations of reality. Interpretivism uses qualitative methodology to understand various interpretations of phenomenon. Finally, critical theory argues that reality may be objective but truth is continually contested by competing groups. Therefore, knowledge is co-constructed between individuals and groups, and mediated by power relationships. Scholars who adopt the critical theory paradigm utilize quantitative and qualitative methodologies to advocate for change. These four research paradigms, and their associated assumptions about the nature of the world, influence the choice of research methodologies and tools. In the following sections, we will briefly describe each paradigm and summarize its strengths and limitations. Then we will provide examples that illustrate how that paradigm has been applied to the study of faculty development. Finally, based on our conceptual framework for studying faculty development, we suggest questions that could be explored within each paradigm. See Table 18.1 for a summary of the paradigms, associated methodologies, defining characteristics, typical research questions, and their relationship to our framework of faculty development.

We acknowledge that there are a number of research methodologies that may be applicable to faculty development that we have not included. We chose to be selective rather than exhaustive. On the other hand, there are methodologies not frequently used in faculty development research that could provide informative answers. Consequently, our review of the research paradigms will be brief to concentrate on some lesser-known methodologies that include: educational design research, success cases and sustainability narratives.

18.4.1   Positivist Paradigm

While we argue for the importance of alternative paradigms, we believe that the positivist paradigm can be an appropriate and important paradigm to answer a given research question. The positivist paradigm is designed to discover what exists through prediction and control, and is characterized by the scientific method (Bunniss and Kelly 2010). This paradigm has framed educational research for over

Table 18.1 Research paradigms, associated research methodologies and their defining characteristics along with illustrative questions associated with faculty development and related connections to the O'Sullivan and Irby conceptual framework for research on faculty development (2011)

Research paradigms	Research methodologies	Defining characteristics of methodologies	Illustrative questions for faculty development	Components of O'Sullivan and Irby's (2011) conceptual framework
Positivism	Experimental and Quasi-experimental	Explores cause and effect relationships where causes can be manipulated to produce different kinds of effects. Assumes random assignment of subjects and random assignment to groups. Uses quantitative methods	Do structured reflection exercises within workshops work better than unstructured reflection? Does training on feedback skills improve participant feedback to residents?	Program Tasks and activities in the workplace
	Survey	Describes and explains using many subjects and questionnaires. Explores causal relationships and, where possible, uses randomization. Employs quantitative methods	How satisfied are participants with faculty development programs? What pedagogical strategies do faculty developers utilize?	Program Facilitator
Post positivism	Correlational	Explores relationships to make predictions. Examines one set of subjects with two or more variables for each. Uses quantitative and qualitative methods	Does it make a difference if participants in faculty development programs come as individuals or as members of workplace teams?	Organizations, systems and culture in the workplace; Relationships and networks in the workplace
	Case-control/ prospective/ retrospective	Explores cause and effect relationships where causes already exist and cannot be manipulated. Examines programs that already exist and looks backward to explain why components or programs work. Uses quantitative and qualitative methods	Does participation in a longitudinal faculty development program accelerate academic promotions? Does having an instructional coach in the workplace improve implementation of teaching skills?	Organization, systems and culture in the workplace Mentoring and coaching in the workplace

(continued)

Table 18.1 (continued)

Research paradigms	Research methodologies	Defining characteristics of methodologies	Illustrative questions for faculty development	Components of O'Sullivan and Irby's (2011) conceptual framework
Interpretivism	Qualitative methods including ethnography, case study, observation, interviews, focus groups, document review	Employs direct observation, interviews and document review to give a complete snapshot of a case that is being studied. Uses qualitative methods	What relationships develop during and after participating in faculty development activities? What is the developmental trajectory of faculty members involved in faculty development?	Participants; Relationships and networks in the workplace Participants; Organization, systems and culture in the workplace
	Educational design research (mixed methods)	Involves an iterative process of small experiments using formative assessment to test and refine educational designs based on principles from previous research. Uses quantitative and qualitative methods	What is the consequence of altering a component of a faculty development program on how participants utilize the component in their practice?	Program; Relationships and networks in the workplace; Organization, systems and culture in the workplace
	Success cases	Detects impact of activities by identifying successful and unsuccessful implementations. Surveys most and least successful cases and then conducts in-depth analyses of selected success cases. Uses quantitative and qualitative methods	What components of faculty development produce the greatest impact on the participants' learners?	Program; Tasks and activities in the workplace

Critical theory	Mixed methods	Seeks to envision and advocate for a better future. Uses philosophical analysis and other methods of inquiry to make a narrative case for empowerment and emancipation	How does serving as a faculty developer affect one's professional identity and change relationships with colleagues? Who is advantaged by faculty development and who is marginalized?	Participants; Relationships and networks in the workplace; Mentoring and coaching in the workplace; Relationships and networks in the workplace
Sustainability narratives		Engages experts and stakeholders in creating alternative scenarios of the future. Involves analyses of each scenario using existing and new data. Creates scenarios and recommendations based on analysis. Uses quantitative and qualitative methods	What would be needed to create a sustainable future for faculty development in the clinical workplace?	Whole model; Organization, systems and culture in the workplace; Tasks and activities in the workplace

a half century, with its focus on experimental research design, use of randomization, quantitative measures (Cronbach 1957), and the presumption that the researcher is objective and removed from the object being studied.

Over the last decade, there have been repeated calls for more rigorous educational research, which typically means using experimental design in the positivist paradigm (Feuer et al. 2002). True-experimental, pre-experimental, and quasi-experimental research designs, as described by Campbell and Stanley (1963), seek to maximize internal and external validity so that the results of a study can be assumed to be causal and generalizable (Campbell and Stanley 1963). Since the medical sciences hold the randomized-controlled trial (RCT) as the study design with the highest rigor and quality (Hulley et al. 2007), there has been increasing expectation that RCTs be part of health professions educational research. While RCTs cannot always be conducted, researchers have embraced a number of quasi-experimental designs that allow for elements of control from either historic or delayed intervention groups.

The strength of the positivist paradigm is the emphasis on internal and external validity. Yet, this emphasis causes an inherent weakness. Creating studies with strong internal validity means that many elements of the design of the study are controlled. This limits the external validity since it makes it harder to generalize to other settings, interventions or tools. However, given these trade-offs, internal validity is considered most important. Maximizing internal validity includes reducing biases in interventions, participants, tools and researchers. This is accomplished chiefly by randomizing participants, pre and post intervention testing, and including control groups and tools with good psychometric characteristics. Implementing such controls often precludes studying what happens in the natural settings of classrooms and clinics. Additionally, such designs may actually eliminate the very elements that characterize what happens in educational interventions (Berliner 2002; Norman 2008). For an excellent summary of the methodologies associated with the positivist paradigm, see Norman and Eva's (2010) article. They include experimental, epidemiologic, psychometric and correlational designs as well as reviews and meta- analyses as part of this tradition.

The positivist paradigm and experimental designs have been applied to the study of faculty development programs, including programs for residents as teachers. For example, Morrison et al. (2003) reported on a randomized, controlled trial of a longitudinal residents-as-teachers curriculum. They provided a 13 h program on teaching to 13 out of 23 residents in the program, and pre- and post-tested the residents using a 3.5 h, eight-station objective structured teaching examination (OSTE). While the intervention and control groups had equivalent entering characteristics and pre-OSTE performance, the intervention group residents significantly improved their pre-to-post OSTE teaching scores while the control group residents did not. In another study, Furney et al. (2001) randomly assigned residents, who act as teachers to students, to an intervention and control group. One group received training in the use of the One Minute Preceptor model of clinical teaching and the other did not. They assessed both groups before and after by measuring student ratings of their teaching and by measuring residents' self-perceptions of their teaching abilities. Residents in the intervention group reported greater use of One Minute Preceptor skills compared to control group residents, which was confirmed by student ratings of the specific skills.

Using a quasi-experimental design, Hewson et al. (2001) used a retrospective self-report along with trainee ratings in a time-series design to demonstrate the effectiveness of a faculty development program. Both self and trainee ratings showed improvement post faculty development. Another quasi-experimental design used participants compared to non-participants (e.g. Corchon et al. 2011), although this is a challenging design to implement because participation in faculty development is voluntary and it is difficult to identify and recruit equivalent faculty who did not participate in faculty development for a control group.

Considering our model, we could imagine using the positivist paradigm to address a question about the interaction between the faculty development program and the organization/culture within which the participants work. A research question might be: 'Could the outcomes of a faculty development program be improved by giving participants materials to evaluate their work environment?' Using the One Minute Preceptor example by Furney et al. (2001) mentioned above, we might repeat the pre and post measures used in that study, but randomly give half of the workshop participants a tool to assess their workplace for resources and people that would enable them to use the One Minute Preceptor model. Our hypothesis is that by giving a checklist indicating potential ways to overcome barriers and gain support, participants with the checklist will do better at implementing the micro-skills of the One Minute Preceptor model in their workplace than those without such a checklist.

18.4.2 Post-Positivist Paradigm

The post-positivist paradigm seeks to maintain the positivist focus on objective truth and the importance of experimental research methodologies but recognizes that truth can only be imperfectly and probabilistically known. Researchers are not objective observers, as the positivists believe, but rather are actors who bring their own biases to what they observe, analyze and report. Post-positivists seek objectivity by recognizing and seeking to minimize the effects of biases, and by seeking falsification instead of verification as the positivists do. Post-positivists also do not exclude data obtained from qualitative methods, thus rejecting the dichotomy between quantitative and qualitative methodologies (Clark 1998). Clark (1998) argues that this shift is partly due to recognizing that there are human elements operating even in an electron microscope, thus questioning if any data are truly 'objective'.

The post-positivists, like the positivists, adhere to strong research methodologies and prefer experimental and quasi-experimental designs. However, they also use tools such as surveys, interviews and focus groups, and therefore attend to issues of bias more than the positivists. The strength of the post-positivist paradigm is the acceptance of qualitative research methods while maintaining the focus on generalizability and prediction, and the willingness to incorporate the natural context into the research. The major limitation of the post-positivist paradigm, like that of the next two paradigms (interpretivist and critical theory), is the inability to control external variables that are part of the complexities of natural events, which in turn threatens validity and reduces claims about generalizability. Unlike the interpretivist and critical theory paradigms, the post-positivists are still focused on seeking objective truth.

An example of post-positivist research that fits our conceptual framework for faculty development research includes a study by Moses et al. (2009). In order to characterize the impact of a longitudinal faculty development program, the authors examined two outcomes: (1) networks of education colleagues using pre-to-post social network mapping, and (2) educational scholarship of participants employing structured interviews. They found increased educational networks with participation in the program but showed little effect on scholarly productivity. In another study, Burdick et al. (2010) used a combination of pre and post surveys and interviews to identify the utility and impact of an international educational leadership fellowship program. They found that participants were actively engaged in applying the knowledge and skills gained in the fellowship program to their home institutions.

Thinking as post-positivist researchers, we became interested in how to develop mentors in the workplace, an important component of our conceptual framework. We thought that we might use a quasi-experimental design to investigate how mentoring influences team management skills in the workplace. Team members from multiple work groups would be surveyed to determine the level of mentoring they receive and the quality of team management skills they report in the workplace prior to the intervention. All teams would then participate in a faculty development activity on team management skills. One third of the teams would designate some-one within their work group to serve as their coach or mentor upon return to the workplace, one third of the teams would periodically receive coaching from an outsider who is skilled in team management and mentoring, and the final third of the teams would receive no mentoring in the workplace. The team members would be resurveyed about mentoring and team management skills 3 and 6 months following the intervention.

This proposed investigation and the other studies referred to above reflect the components of our faculty development framework that relate to the application of knowledge, skills and attitudes learned in the faculty development program to actual practice in the workplace – including subsequent teamwork, scholarship and educational networks. Applying the post-positivist paradigm to our model would add to our understanding of participants' practices once they return to the workplace.

18.4.3   Interpretivist Paradigm

The interpretivist paradigm posits that meaning is a socially constructed reality and therefore there is no objective truth. Qualitative research methods are used to illuminate the multiple and diverse perspectives or interpretations of reality held by individuals and groups. The purpose of this paradigm is to describe, understand and interpret human thought, interactions and discourse, including the reasons for such actions. The basic method is inductive, beginning with the thoughts of specific individuals or groups and building up to general themes and conclusions about their thoughts, values and actions. It tends to be holistic, deeply contextual, and typically an in-depth study of a few number of cases. Drawing on the disciplines of anthropology, sociology and linguistics, qualitative research represents a cluster of rigorous and diverse research methods, including ethnography, discourse analysis, and case studies. Unlike positivist research that is driven by a hypothesis that is being tested, qualitative analytic methods can take one of two different approaches: (1) analysis that is driven by a theoretical position or (2) analysis that is inductively built up from the data, known as grounded theory (Glaser and Strauss 1967; Strauss and Corbin 1998).

Qualitative researchers gather information through observations, field notes, reflective journals, interviews, focus groups and analyses of documents and materials. Data are coded into themes and subthemes that iteratively lead to meaningful generalizations (Braun and Clarke 2006). To validate the themes and interpretations, researchers often have multiple investigators code the data and corroborate findings, and they conduct member checking to ensure that those who were interviewed concur with the reports of their thinking, perceptions and beliefs (Lincoln and Guba 1985). The strength of such research is the ability to uncover hidden perspectives on a wide variety of issues, develop and confirm socially constructed theories, and anticipate changes in future beliefs and actions of individuals and groups. The limitations derive from the situated nature of the findings that raise questions about generalizability.

One example of a study of faculty development that used the interpretivist research paradigm is reported by Steinert et al. (2010) who sought to understand why some clinical teachers regularly attend faculty development activities and others do not. They conducted focus groups with 23 clinical teachers who attended their workshops. Using thematic analysis of focus group transcripts, the team discovered that regular participants perceived that workshops facilitated their personal and professional growth; the topics were viewed as relevant to their needs as teachers; and participation in the program generated a new and supportive network of colleagues. Participants also valued learning and self-improvement. Barriers against participation were also identified along with suggestions for increasing participation. The results were used to design future workshops, based upon the recognition that motivation, values and social dimensions are important components of faculty development.

Using our framework for research on faculty development, investigators using the interpretivist paradigm might conduct a qualitative study to examine those who actually conduct faculty development, specifically identifying their background preparation, pedagogical content knowledge (i.e. transformations of subject-matter knowledge into instructionally powerful teaching scripts that facilitate student learning (Shulman 1986)), beliefs about teaching and learning, reflective practices, improvement strategies, identity formation and career trajectories as faculty developers. Specific research questions might include: How do faculty developers describe their identity and its formation? How does being a faculty developer affect their everyday work? What impact does the role of being a faculty developer have on them, the faculty development teaching commons and the larger community of teaching practice? The tools employed could include interviews, focus groups, debriefs from observations and reviews of recordings of teaching practices, reviews of workshop materials, and examination of curriculum vitae.

18.4.4   Critical Theory

Critical theory is a school of thought that draws on the social sciences to examine, critique and advocate for change in culture and society. The most common meaning of critical theory arises from sociologists who have used philosophies such as Marxism, idealism and post-colonial theory to challenge social injustices; a less common meaning of critical theory comes from literary criticism. The social critical theory model confronts positivist assumptions along with any accompanying forms of authority, hegemony and injustice. The focus is on the use of language, symbolism, communication and meaning to empower human beings and to challenge established power and authority. Research methods include the use of linguistics, rhetoric and most of all philosophical analysis. This narrative form of scholarship can examine and critique individual, group and organizational relationships of power and privilege, opening up for scrutiny commonly accepted dimensions of culture and values. However, this paradigm is held hostage to the conceptual framework that shapes the critique (e.g. Marxism, idealism, post-colonial theory), the limited generalizability of the recommendations advocated based on that theory, and the challenges to the findings coming from alternative theories. Critical theory is a rhetorical, narrative vehicle for advocating and achieving social justice.

This paradigm is infrequently used in research on faculty development but offers some interesting perspectives on these activities. Bleakley et al. (2008) and Bleakley (2011) have written extensively using this paradigm, examining such topics as the democratizing force of medical education research; post-colonial dilemmas in global medical education; and power, identity and location in medical education.

When considering the critical theory paradigm and our framework of faculty development, we could pose questions such as: How are faculty members empowered to become excellent teachers through faculty development? Who is advantaged by faculty development and who is marginalized? What does this do to the power relationships and the culture of the institution? How are institutional resources differentially allocated to support faculty in their roles as teachers, researchers and clinicians? What are the power differentials in academic departments and promotions committees between researchers and educators? Critical theory examines, describes, exposes and challenges inequities at all levels and can be a powerful voice for change.

18.5   Alternative Research Methods

In addition to the research paradigms describe above, we will describe some additional promising research methodologies, often involving mixed methods, to address questions posed from our faculty development framework. Mixed methods represent a methodology that can be used within multiple research paradigms and can move faculty development research forward. We describe three promising methodologies with accompanying faculty development examples: design research, success cases and sustainability narratives.

18.5.1   Design Research

Design research is a methodology that has evolved over the last 30 years and is nested under the post-positivist and intepretivist paradigms. The goal of design research is to develop formative experiments to test and refine educational designs based on principles derived from previous research and to address theory and practice simultaneously (Collins et al. 2004). As a methodology, it serves to address theoretical questions in the real world recognizing the need to generate research findings from formative evaluation. Collins et al. (2004) developed the approach as a means of determining what was implemented versus what was intended. They wanted to examine a range of outcomes that exceeded the ones commonly focused on in educational research. In general, the approach is to make theoretically driven design changes and to test them in a practical environment in order to determine their impact in a formative manner. Thus, it is an iterative process of examining prototypes.

For faculty development, an example might be to study a workshop where teaching scripts are shared and discussed to improve feedback skills. This could be followed by a survey of skill use, which, after careful reflection on the theoretical and empirical guidelines for improving feedback, might lead to another workshop that includes role-plays to practice feedback scripts. A subsequent survey might find need for additional tips on giving feedback to learners experiencing difficulty. Next, an email reminder with feedback tips related to micro-skills might be sent as follow-up. These rapid cycles could use small samples of participants to quickly revise program components following theory-based guidelines.

Educational design research follows a series of interventions over an extended period of time using multiple methods. Bereiter (2002) asserts that design research can help to sustain an innovation and focuses the research on the future instead of the past. In the case of an innovation, the researcher must be a close collaborator with the designer and be an interventionist vs. an objective observer (Bereiter 2002; McKenney and Reeves 2012).

To report a design experiment, a researcher would include goals and elements of the design, a description of the settings where implemented, description of each phase implemented, outcomes found and lessons learned (Collins et al. 2004). Dolmans and Tigelaar (2012) provide a useful guide for design-based research in medical education.

Educational design research is pertinent to faculty development because it allows for the examination of evolving program innovations. Using educational design research, we would start a series of micro-cycles, which involves performing the steps of the research with small samples of participants and short time lines as we illustrated with the feedback workshop example above (McKenney and Reeves 2012). In the analysis and exploration stage, we would identify and diagnose the problem to be addressed, primarily by exploring relevant literature and data that we may have from previous offerings or participants' subsequent performance related to the specific skill. In the example above, this stage was captured by the components added to the faculty development program. Performance reported by participants indicated a gap and thinking about this gap from a theoretical perspective resulted in incorporating skill practice. This analysis would be followed by the design and construction phase where we would carefully document how we arrive at the solution to the problem and then construct the prototype using principles we had identified from the literature. In this case, we would add an in-workshop simulation to practice the skill, and get and receive feedback. The third phase in the micro-cycle is evaluation and reflection. As the goal was to improve the use of feedback skills, the follow-up reminder of micro-skills represented a theoretically justified intervention. Did it work? Why or why not? All of this information would then be used to reject, refute and/or refine the design principles. From this, the prototype is redesigned and the micro-cycle repeated. Using such a series of micro-cycles, faculty developers would be in a position to argue for the best way to do faculty development to teach a specific skill. This approach links nicely to knowledge translation, which is discussed in Chap. 19.

18.5.2 Success Cases

A method that could be employed even within an educational research design methodology is called the success case method, which seems well aligned with studying faculty development. This method fits within the interpretivist paradigm. Brinkerhoff and Dressler (2003) describe the success case method as the analysis of extreme groups using case study and storytelling. The core purpose is to discover how well an initiative is working and to identify the contextual factors that support successful implementation.

As Brinkerhoff (2005) notes, there is more to achieving the desired effects of training than putting on a good training program. He points out the problem of relying on the Kirkpatrick framework (Kirkpatrick 1994) that does not include inquiry beyond the training event itself and fails to account for the larger performance environment. Kirkpatrick proposed four levels of training program evaluation: participant reaction, learning, behavior change, and results. Faculty developers may refine an offering to perfection, but a participant's work environment may restrict implementation of the instructional strategy in their own workplace. To make faculty development successful, we need to analyze what happens once participants return to their workplaces. The success case method is designed for this type of inquiry.

This method has two major components: (1) a brief self-report survey that identifies levels of success in implementing an innovation, which is based on the conceptual model used to design the intervention; and (2) a sample of the most and least successful participants, who are randomly selected to receive an in-depth interview to ascertain what, when and how they used the intervention; what results were achieved; how valuable were the results; and what factors enabled success. The summary report would include the initial quantitative survey results and the in-depth qualitative analysis of the cases.

Olson et al. (2011) provide a detailed description of how the success case method was used to identify ways in which continuing medical education activities, closely related to faculty development, contributed to implementation of tobacco cessation practice guidelines in outpatient practices. In this study, Olson et al. (2011) used clinical outcome data to identify success cases (i.e. clinical practices). For the in-depth interviews, they sought input only from participants who had implemented the guidelines successfully; believing that there was little benefit in interviewing unsuccessful cases where people might not be as forthright about describing why they failed to implement the program. At each selected site, up to three persons were interviewed to obtain multiple perspectives. The authors concluded that even though they only studied success cases, it did provide valuable insights that generated hypotheses for future testing.

Recently, a faculty developer asked us which of our workshops was most highly rated by participants. The question prompted a thought about studying this question employing the success case method. Using existing workshop ratings, we could select the highest rated and lowest rated workshops, selecting one or two from each category. Then, through in-depth interviews with selected participants who attended those workshops, we could identify specific features of the workshops that made for success or failure. In addition, the success case method could also allow us to explore barriers and supports for faculty development, such as networks of relationships, institutional structures, personal commitments, and intellectual and personal characteristics (Caffarella and Zinn 1999).

18.5.3 Sustainability Narrative

Sustainability narrative is a research methodology that resides outside the normal modes of inquiry for the education community. This methodology explores the development of a society through the lens of human and environmental systems (Swart et al. 2004) and imagines what the future would be like if people's lives were improved, without compromising the economic systems on which they depend (Kemp-Benedict 2006). For example, closing a factory to improve the quality of air would not lead to sustainability if people no longer have a place to work. Translated into faculty development, sustainability narrative could be used to imagine future programs, examine different scenarios for their growth and deployment, and create strong support for such programs without compromising resources or interfering with workplace practices.

An example of a sustainability narrative arose at our university from a desire to develop a cadre of faculty members both at UCSF and at international institutions who could lead faculty development workshops on an occasional, part-time basis.

From a sustainability narrative approach, we would develop scenarios asking how this program might look in the future to be sustainable given economic concerns and key stakeholder expectations. Scenarios might answer questions that are faculty centered such as: how promotion and tenure criteria might change to sustain these faculty developers; how compensation might be altered to support these faculty developers; and how recognition can be enhanced for faculty developers. Other scenarios could describe the future providers who were the recipients of teaching from those who participated in faculty development. There could be scenarios depicting sustained hospital/clinic-based faculty development groups that improve patient care. Thinking about all of these aspects to craft a narrative would change the kind of research that would be undertaken and would be quite different from a traditional faculty development evaluation depicted in Fig. 18.1.

The sustainability research process involves having experts and stakeholders develop narratives (Kemp-Benedict 2006) that address the future, explore alternative scenarios, and provide plausible stories that include issues such as resources as well as the resilience and incentives of the system (Swart et al. 2004). From the example above, the scenario could be quite complex if we explore how to expand faculty development to other sites and countries or it could be very narrow if we focus on a single campus-level faculty development center. Decisions about the scope of the scenario drive the selection of a research design. However, the designs will not be simple because they will need to address a number of issues (Swart et al. 2004) such as: does the way we study our scenario address local issues or more global issues? How are the financial impacts addressed? Where does this research and emphasis on sustainability fit with institutional priorities? The research methodology integrates both a quantitative approach by developing a quantitative model of variables that can be measured in the scenario and a qualitative approach to analyze other aspects of the scenario. Additionally, there is a major focus on addressing marginalized groups. Thus, this method fits within the critical theory paradigm.

Various authors have suggested different steps (Alcamo 2001; Swart et al. 2004) to the sustainability narrative process, but overall the process includes:

1. Bringing together a sufficiently large and diverse group of experts and stakeholders to generate ideas about the future; they call this developing the storyline, which includes making assumptions visible. A writing team transforms the generated input and scenarios into a narrative.
2. Using rigorous research methods, based on the narrative, decide what should be incorporated in the analysis and what data should be collected as baseline.
3. Developing a model that can be tested quantitatively and/or use the scenarios developed to guide a qualitative investigation. The qualitative analysis involves exploring the possibilities of surprise as well as the steps toward change.
4. Writing the final product as a coherent and engaging story about options for the future.

A way of employing this process for faculty development would be to ask experts and stakeholders to describe the future of faculty development. In Table 18.2, we offer sample questions (Sarriot et al. 2008). By responding to these questions, experts

Table 18.2 Questions for experts and key stakeholders for developing a sustainability scenario

Experts and key stakeholders	Possible questions
Providers	What services are most critical for faculty development in medical education? What capacities will individuals need to deliver these services?
Health care units	How does the local clinical or hospital organization function? What affordances and hindrances do they provide for faculty development?
Local supports	How will the university be mobilized to ensure that the necessary faculty development occurs? What are the local units that can be used?
Communities	What are the communities and how are they organized? How will the community create demand for faculty development? What will be their expectations?
Outside actors	What do accrediting organizations for students, residents and employees expect? What should faculty development do to ensure that improvements are made? What resources are needed?

and stakeholders would provide the researcher with information to develop scenarios that could be crafted into a sustainability narrative pertinent to faculty development.

Armed with the narrative, the next step would be to complete a baseline assessment of relevant components of the faculty development program. The data collection likely would use a combination of methods including survey, focus group, and review of existing data. This step can precede or happen in conjunction with the model-building step. The model of what should be happening in the future is derived from the narrative. Then, using existing data, the model would be tested using a variety of research methods. The last step is to iteratively collect data, refine the model, and write the 'story', based on the narrative, describing a reasonable expectation of what could happen next.

For faculty development programs, it may not be essential to follow all of these steps, but the initial one opens new kinds of questions that can be studied. Some might see the first step as akin to a needs assessment, but the focus is on the future. Also, coming from the critical theory paradigm, the experts and stakeholders may represent groups whose voices have not been heard in the past. The narrative developed could address relationships of power, such as the clinic director's willingness to allow providers to participate in faculty development and/or implement an innovation promoted in the faculty development program within his or her clinic. We think this method would be applicable to the study of each component of our model of faculty development as well as the model as a whole.

18.6   Faculty Development Researchers

While educators are encouraged to conduct research on faculty development, they may lack adequate training and resources to do so. Some medical schools have invested heavily in educational research and faculty development, and in the process have created strong cultures of educational scholarship while others have not. In either case, faculty members interested in conducting educational research are encouraged to either seek educational research consultation and/or training through participation in faculty development programs or graduate programs in education or medical education. Educational researchers in offices of medical education can be helpful in framing the research from a learning theory perspective, identifying relevant literature, honing a researchable question, designing and conducting a study, and analyzing and reporting the results. Another strategy is to find colleagues who share a common interest in educational research and work collaboratively on a research project. Often these colleagues can be found in academies of medical educators (Irby et al. 2004; Searle et al. 2010), longitudinal faculty development programs (Gruppen et al. 2006), education committees, and educational leadership positions. Collaborative research not only overcomes a sense of isolation but also offers one of the best ways to advance the work, ensure completion of tasks, and disseminate the results. Such collaborations can be established locally or can be created with colleagues within and across specialties beyond the institution. Regardless of research strategy adopted, rigorous research on faculty development is difficult to do well. Using our conceptual framework for research on faculty development along with the paradigms and methodologies described in this chapter, we hope that those interested in advancing understanding of faculty development will find important questions and appropriate research methods in this chapter.

We have focused largely on the scholarship of discovery, which creates new knowledge about faculty development. Boyer (1990), however, argues that there are other important forms of scholarship beyond *discovery*. These include: *integration* of knowledge as in a review of the literature or an integrative conceptual framework; *application* of knowledge as in connecting theory to practice; and *teaching* as in transforming and extending knowledge for the benefit of learners. Others have elaborated on the scholarship of teaching and learning to offer guidelines for its description and assessment (Glassick et al. 1997). Finally, the criteria for evaluating educators for academic advancement have been defined for the roles of direct teaching, curriculum development, advising and mentoring, educational leadership, learner assessment, and educational research (Simpson et al. 2007). We recommend these resources to our readers.

18.7 Conclusion

In this chapter, we have described four paradigms and their associated methodologies that can be deployed to investigate faculty development programs, and we have advocated for an expanded set of questions derived from our conceptual framework for research on faculty development. Most of the research on faculty development to date has been related to the community created during faculty development activities, or within the teaching commons. Much less research has addressed the workplace community of teaching practice. As our examples of hypothetical research studies on faculty development describe, there are many areas where further research is needed. Such research could help guide decisions about the most effective strategies to adopt in order to change teaching practices in the workplace.

We have asserted that the assumptions of the positivist paradigm and to a lesser extent post-positivist paradigm are unduly restricting the publication, funding and research on faculty development. We have offered alternative ways of looking at faculty development by offering an expanded set of paradigms and research methodologies. However, we acknowledge two important factors that may hinder the use of alternative paradigms, methodologies and tools. First is the dominant use of positivist and post-positivist paradigms by reviewers in journals. Reviewers may apply positivist and post-positivist paradigms to their critiques of studies conducted in the interpretivist and critical theory paradigms and thus reject them for publication. Therefore, it behooves authors of such research on faculty development to write clearly about their paradigms, methodologies and tools in order to provide strong evidence for the rigor of the methodologies. Second, researchers in this field are often expected to demonstrate positive outcomes of educational interventions on the improvement of patient care. This challenge will be more difficult to overcome but is still worth confronting.

We generated our model, in part, to illustrate the multiple relationships among faculty development and workplace communities. The workplace environment often mediates the individual's ability to implement the skills acquired. Thus, the connection to improved patient care must be studied through this mediated lens. Researchers using alternative paradigms and associated research methods and a newer faculty development model will be better equipped to describe the effects of faculty development on the participants, their learners, and where possible on the patients that they serve. This will expand the current focus on the faculty development participants toward examining the impact on workplace settings where teaching takes place.

We hope that this chapter inspires others to be willing to ask diverse questions about faculty development and apply less well-known paradigms and methodologies to inquiry on faculty development. In addition, we encourage readers to join the large community of researchers who are willing to engage in sustained programs of study on faculty development programs over time. There is much to explore in faculty development and many ways of doing so.

18.8   Key Messages

- Research on faculty development has been overly constrained by adherence to the positivist research paradigm and its associated use of randomization, control groups, and quantitative methods.

- The O'Sullivan and Irby (2011) conceptual framework for research on faculty development expands the areas of inquiry by proposing two distinct but overlapping communities: the community created by faculty development activities, referred to as the teaching commons, and the community of practice in the workplace where teaching occurs (in classrooms, clinics and online).
- To investigate these two different communities, four research paradigms will need to be used: positivist, post-positivist, interpretivist and critical theory. Each of these paradigms has associated research methodologies and tools.
- Three additional research methods offer promise for illuminating various aspects of the faculty development framework: educational design research, success cases and sustainability narrative.
- Engaging in research on faculty development requires establishing a network and taking advantage of local and national resources.

References

Alcamo, J. (2001). *Environmental issue report No. 24: Scenarios as tools for international environmental assessments*. European Environment Agency. Luxembourg: Office for Official Publications of the European Communities. Available from: http://www.eea.europa.eu/publications/environmental_issue_report_2001_24

Amundsen, C. & Wilson, M. (2012). Are we asking the right questions? A conceptual review of the educational development literature in higher education. *Review of Educational Research, 82*(1), 90–126.

Bereiter, C. (2002). Design research for sustained innovation. *Cognitive Studies, Bulletin of the Japanese Cognitive Science Society, 9*(3), 321–327.

Berliner, D. C. (2002). Comment: Educational research: The hardest science of all. *Educational Researcher, 31*(8), 18–20.

Billett, S. (2001). *Learning in the workplace: Strategies for effective practice*. Crows Nest, NSW: Allen & Unwin.

Bleakley, A. (2011). Professing medical identities in the liquid world of teams. *Medical Education, 45*(12), 1171–1173.

Bleakley, A., Brice, J., & Bligh, J. (2008). Thinking the post-colonial in medical education. *Medical Education, 42*(3), 266–270.

Boyer, E. L. (1990). *Scholarship reconsidered: Priorities of the professoriate*. Princeton, NJ: Carnegie Foundation for the Advancement of Teaching.

Braun, V. & Clarke, V. (2006). Using thematic analysis in psychology. *Qualitative Research in Psychology, 3*(2), 77–101.

Brinkerhoff, R. O. (2005). The success case method: A strategic evaluation approach to increasing the value and effect of training. *Advances in Developing Human Resources, 7*(1), 86–101.

Brinkerhoff, R. O. & Dressler, D. E. (2003). Using the success case impact evaluation method to enhance training value & impact. San Diego, CA: American Society for Training and Development International Conference and Exhibition. Available from: http://www.blanchardtraining.com/img/pub/newsletter_brinkerhoff.pdf

Bunniss, S. & Kelly, D. R. (2010). Research paradigms in medical education research. *Medical Education, 44*(4), 358–366.

Burdick, W. P., Diserens, D., Friedman, S. R., Morahan, P. S., Kalishman, S., Eklund, M. A., et al. (2010). Measuring the effects of an international health professions faculty development fellowship: The FAIMER Institute. *Medical Teacher, 32*(5), 414–421.

Caffarella, R. S. & Zinn, L. F. (1999). Professional development for faculty: A conceptual framework of barriers and supports. *Innovative Higher Education, 23*(4), 241–254.

Campbell, D. T. & Stanley, J. C. (1963). *Experimental and quasi-experimental designs for research*. Boston, MA: Houghton Mifflin.

Clark, A. M. (1998). The qualitative-quantitative debate: Moving from positivism and confrontation to post-positivism and reconciliation. *Journal of Advanced Nursing, 27*(6), 1242–1249.

Collins, A., Joseph, D., & Bielaczyc, K. (2004). Design research: Theoretical and methodological issues. *Journal of the Learning Sciences, 13*(1), 15–42.

Corchon, S., Portillo, M. C., Watson, R., & Saracíbar, M. (2011). Nursing research capacity building in a Spanish hospital: An intervention study. *Journal of Clinical Nursing, 20*(17–18), 2479–2489.

Cronbach, L. J. (1957). The two disciplines of scientific psychology. *American Psychologist, 12*(11), 671–684.

Dolmans, D. H. & Tigelaar, D. (2012). Building bridges between theory and practice in medical education using a design-based research approach: AMEE Guide No. 60. *Medical Teacher, 34*(1), 1–10.

Feuer, M. J., Towne, L., & Shavelson, R. J. (2002). Scientific culture and educational research. *Educational Researcher, 31*(8), 4–14.

Furney, S. L., Orsini, A. N., Orsetti, K. E., Stern, D. T., Gruppen, L. D., & Irby, D. M. (2001). Teaching the one-minute preceptor: A randomized controlled trial. *Journal of General Internal Medicine, 16*(9), 620–624.

Glaser, B. G. & Strauss, A. L. (1967). *The discovery of grounded theory: Strategies for qualitative research* (1st Ed.). Chicago, IL: Aldine Publishing Company.

Glassick, C. E., Huber, M. T., Maeroff, G. I., & Boyer, E. (1997). *Scholarship assessed: Evaluation of the professorate*. San Francisco, CA: Jossey-Bass.

Gruppen, L. D., Simpson, D., Searle, N. S., Robins, L., Irby, D. M., & Mullan, P. B. (2006). Educational fellowship programs: Common themes and overarching issues. *Academic Medicine, 81*(11), 990–994.

Hewson, M. G., Copeland, H. L., & Fishleder, A. J. (2001). What's the use of faculty development? Program evaluation using retrospective self-assessments and independent performance ratings. *Teaching and Learning in Medicine, 13*(3), 153–160.

Huber, M. T. & Hutchings, P. (2005). *The advancement of learning: Building the teaching commons*. San Francisco, CA: Jossey-Bass.

Hulley, S. B., Cummings, S. R., Browner, W. S., Grady, D. G., & Newman, T. B. (2007). *Designing clinical research* (3rd Ed.). Philadelphia, PA: Lippincott Williams & Wilkins.

Irby, D. M., Cooke, M., Lowenstein, D., & Richards, B. (2004). The academy movement: A structural approach to reinvigorating the educational mission. *Academic Medicine, 79*(8), 729–736.

Kemp-Benedict, E. (2006). Narrative-led and indicator-driven scenario development: A methodology for constructing scenarios. Available from: http://www.kb-creative.net/research/NLIDD.pdf

Kirkpatrick, D. (1994). *Evaluating training programs: The four levels*. New York, NY: McGraw-Hill.

Lave, J. & Wenger, E. (1991). *Situated learning: Legitimate peripheral participation*. Cambridge, UK: Cambridge University Press.

Levinson-Rose, J. & Menges, R. J. (1981). Improving college teaching: A critical review of research. *Review of Educational Research, 51*(3), 403–434.

Lincoln, Y. S., & Guba, E. G. (1985). *Naturalistic inquiry*. Beverly Hills, CA: Sage Publications.

McKenney, S. E. & Reeves, T. C. (2012). *Conducting educational design research* (1st Ed.). New York, NY: Routledge.

McLean, M., Cilliers, F., & Van Wyk, J. M. (2008). Faculty development: Yesterday, today and tomorrow. *Medical Teacher, 30*(6), 555–584.

Morrison, E. H., Rucker, L., Boker, J. R., Hollingshead, J., Hitchcock, M. A., Prislin, M. D., et al. (2003). A pilot randomized, controlled trial of a longitudinal residents-as-teachers curriculum. *Academic Medicine, 78*(7), 722–729.

Moses, A. S., Skinner, D. H., Hicks, E., & O'Sullivan, P. S. (2009). Developing an educator network: The effect of a teaching scholars program in the health professions on networking and productivity. *Teaching and Learning in Medicine, 21*(3), 175–179.

Norman, G. (2008). The end of educational science? *Advances in Health Sciences Education, 13*(4), 385–389.

Norman, G. & Eva, K. W. (2010). Quantitative research methods in medical education. In T. Swanwick (Ed.), *Understanding medical education: Evidence, theory and practice,* (pp. 301–322). Oxford, UK: Wiley-Blackwell.

Olson, C. A., Shershneva, M. B., & Brownstein, M. H. (2011). Peering inside the clock: Using success case method to determine how and why practice-based educational interventions succeed. *The Journal of Continuing Education in the Health Professions, 31*(Suppl. 1), S50–S59.

O'Sullivan, P. S. & Irby, D. M. (2011). Reframing research on faculty development. *Academic Medicine, 86*(4), 421–428.

Sarriot, E. G., Ricca, J. G., Yourkavitch, J. M., & Ryan, L. J.; Sustained Health Outcomes (SHOUT) Group. (2008). *Taking the long view: A practical guide to sustainability planning and measurement in community-oriented health programming.* Calverton, MD: Macro International Inc.

Searle, N. S., Thompson, B. M., Friedland, J. A., Lomax, J. W., Drutz, J. E., Coburn, M., et al. (2010). The prevalence and practice of academies of medical educators: A survey of U.S. medical schools. *Academic Medicine, 85*(1), 48–56.

Shulman, L. S. (1986). Those who understand: Knowledge growth in teaching. *Educational Researcher, 15*(2), 4–14.

Simpson, D., Fincher, R. M., Hafler, J. P., Irby, D. M., Richards, B. F., Rosenfeld, G. C., et al. (2007). Advancing educators and education by defining the components and evidence associated with educational scholarship. *Medical Education, 41*(10), 1002–1009.

Steinert, Y., Macdonald, M. E., Boillat, M., Elizov, M., Meterissian, S., Razack, S., et al. (2010). Faculty development: If you build it, they will come. *Medical Education, 44*(9), 900–907.

Steinert, Y., Mann, K., Centeno, A., Dolmans, D., Spencer, J., Gelula, M., et al. (2006). A systematic review of faculty development initiatives designed to improve teaching effectiveness in medical education: BEME Guide No. 8. *Medical Teacher, 28*(6), 497–526.

Stes, A., Min-Leliveld, M., Gijbels, D., & Van Petegem, P. (2010). The impact of instructional development in higher education: The state-of-the-art of the research. *Educational Research Review, 5*(1), 25–49.

Strauss, A. L., & Corbin, J. M. (1998). *Basics of qualitative research: Grounded theory procedures and techniques (2nd Ed.).* Thousand Oaks, CA: Sage Public.

Swart, R. J., Raskin, P., & Robinson, J. (2004). The problem of the future: Sustainability science and scenario analysis. *Global Environmental Change, 14*(2), 137–146.

Webster-Wright, A. (2009). Reframing professional development through understanding authentic professional learning. *Review of Educational Research, 79*(2), 702–739.

Chapter 19
Knowledge Translation and Faculty Development: From Theory to Practice

Aliki Thomas and Yvonne Steinert

19.1 Introduction

Faculty developers are expected to support faculty members through state-of-the-art learning activities, including courses and workshops, and to ensure that new learning is integrated into practice and sustained over time. They must also make sure that the design, implementation and evaluation of faculty development activities are informed by the most up-to-date research in the field. Knowledge translation (KT) is a process that has the potential to meet these expectations.

KT is increasing in importance in fields such as public health, medicine and rehabilitation research (Canadian Institutes of Health Research 2012; Davis et al. 2003; Glasgow et al. 2003). It also has important implications for medical education and faculty development, although this link has not been fully explored to date. KT is a term used to describe a process designed to address a longstanding issue: the underutilization of available scientific findings and evidence-based research in systems of care (Davis et al. 2003; Grol and Grimshaw 2003; Grol and Jones 2000). KT is considered an interactive, non-linear and interdisciplinary process used to move knowledge into practice and includes all the steps between the creation of new knowledge and its application. That is, KT aims to bridge the research-practice

A. Thomas, Ph.D., OT (c), erg (✉)
Occupational Therapy Program, School of Physical and Occupational Therapy and Centre for Medical Education, Faculty of Medicine, McGill University, Montreal, QC, Canada
e-mail: aliki.thomas@mcgill.ca

Y. Steinert, Ph.D.
Centre for Medical Education and Department of Family Medicine,
Faculty of Medicine, McGill University, Montreal, QC, Canada
e-mail: yvonne.steinert@mcgill.ca

Y. Steinert (ed.), *Faculty Development in the Health Professions: A Focus on Research and Practice*, Innovation and Change in Professional Education 11, DOI 10.1007/978-94-007-7612-8_19, © Springer Science+Business Media Dordrecht 2014

gap by promoting the *integration* and *exchange* of research and evidence-based knowledge into clinical practice in order to improve outcomes for consumers, students and patients (Canadian Institutes of Health Research 2012; Landry et al. 2003; Nutley et al. 2003). Furthermore, KT requires ongoing collaborations and exchange among all relevant stakeholders, including researchers within and across disciplines, health care providers, educators and patients (Sudsawad 2007).

The concepts underlying KT and the term itself are not new to the field of continuing medical education (Akl et al. 2009; Farmer et al. 2011; Flodgren et al. 2011; Forsetlund et al. 2009; Grimshaw et al. 2003; Horsley et al. 2010; Salerno et al. 2002; Skeff et al. 1992). In this context, the KT focus is on transferring new scientific evidence regarding developments in diagnostic measures and new treatment approaches into the clinical setting in order to improve practice and optimize patient care.

The application of KT to faculty development has not been explored as extensively. However, the implications of knowledge translation for faculty development can include: (1) basing faculty development programs on the best available knowledge and/or scientific evidence; (2) using educational and other knowledge translation strategies that are known to be effective; (3) recognizing that, in the absence of scientific evidence to support faculty development activities or when scientific knowledge is not congruent with existing practices or values, alternative sources of knowledge are needed; and (4) conceptualizing faculty development activities as knowledge translation interventions in their own right.

This chapter, which focuses on the applications of KT in faculty development and on faculty development as a legitimate KT intervention, is divided in three sections. First, we define KT, discuss the key objectives of KT and examine the applications of KT and the KT process to faculty development. Second, we describe a framework for integrating knowledge into clinical practice: the knowledge-to-action (K2A) cycle. We conclude the chapter with an illustration of how KT concepts can be applied to faculty development, using an example of the K2A process for a faculty development intervention on 'giving effective feedback'.

KT is an essential component in the creation, exchange, synthesis and application of knowledge in health care and educational contexts. We hope that the chapter will be useful in helping the reader apply the principles and concepts of KT to the development, implementation and evaluation of faculty development programs.

19.2 Knowledge Translation: Definition and Objectives

19.2.1 What Is Knowledge Translation?

Many terms have been used to describe the process involved in transferring knowledge into action (McKibbon et al. 2010; Straus et al. 2009). For example, Graham et al. (2006) reviewed the terms and definitions used to describe the knowledge to action process (e.g. 'implementation science', 'dissemination', 'diffusion', 'knowledge transfer', 'uptake' and 'knowledge exchange'). The Canadian Institutes of Health Research (CIHR) define KT as:

> A dynamic and iterative process that includes synthesis, dissemination, exchange and ethically-sound application of knowledge to improve the health of Canadians, provide more effective health services and products and strengthen the health care system. This process takes place within a complex system of interactions between researchers and knowledge users which may vary in intensity, complexity and level of engagement depending on the nature of the research and the findings as well as the needs of the particular knowledge user (CIHR 2012).

Two important concepts are highlighted in this description. First, given that *knowledge creation* (knowledge from original research), *knowledge synthesis* (knowledge from systematic reviews and clinical practice guidelines) and *knowledge dissemination* (publications in peer-reviewed journals and presentations at scholarly conferences) are not sufficient to affect knowledge use and change practice (Straus et al. 2011), there is a shift from passive diffusion or simple dissemination of knowledge to active and conscious participation of both knowledge producers and knowledge users. Additionally, a collaborative interaction between researchers and knowledge users at every step of the KT process is believed to facilitate optimal use of research evidence and other forms of knowledge in clinical practice (Grimshaw et al. 2002; Lavis et al. 2003; Oborn et al. 2010). The second concept of importance in this definition is that of the 'knowledge user'. Knowledge users or 'end-users' can be anyone within the health care system, including clinicians, educators, multidisciplinary teams, patients and decision-makers. While the assumption is that knowledge users are those individuals who, for the most part, integrate the knowledge in their practice, knowledge users can be extensively involved in the knowledge creation and exchange processes. Indeed, the KT framework discussed in this chapter advocates for a participatory model whereby end users are involved in developing research questions and are actively involved in carrying out the research activities.

19.2.2   Why Is Knowledge Translation Important?

Despite the rise in available scientific research findings and the many advantages of using knowledge from research to inform clinical practice (Duncan et al. 2002; Grimshaw et al. 2006), numerous studies have found that health professionals do not readily integrate findings from scientific research into clinical decision-making (Cabana et al. 1999; Korner-Bitensky et al. 2006; McGlynn et al. 2003). Recognition of the gap between what is known to improve patient outcomes and what is used in daily practice has led to a burgeoning interest in KT across the health professions. Developing effective KT interventions that maximize clinicians' knowledge about best practices is an important step towards closing the knowledge-to-practice gap in the clinical setting as well as in the context of educational practice and faculty development.

19.3 Applications of Knowledge Translation to Faculty Development – and Faculty Development as a Knowledge Translation Intervention

The overriding goal of faculty development is to support the development of faculty members in their multiple roles (e.g. teachers, researchers, administrators) (McLean et al. 2008; Steinert 2000, 2011). Moreover, there are many possible outcomes for faculty members participating in faculty development activities, including changes in knowledge, skills and attitudes in teaching, research and leadership practices (Steinert et al. 2006, 2012), with the ultimate goal of improving student outcomes and patient care.

Consider the following example that can help illustrate one application of KT in faculty development: A faculty development team is interested in promoting the use of scoping study methodology in medical education. Scoping studies use a rigorous and systematic multistep process for identifying, reviewing and summarizing a broad body of literature, including published research, reports and consultations with experts. One objective of the faculty development activity could be as follows:

> At the end of the workshop, participants will identify the 6-step scoping review methodology as outlined in the Arksey and O'Malley (2005) framework and identify one question that could be addressed using this methodology.

Participants could use the knowledge gained from this faculty development activity to conduct a scoping review on a topic of interest in medical education or to develop a more focused research question.

At the same time, participants and faculty developers could ask a number of potential questions about a faculty development activity on *'the applications of scoping reviews in medical education'*. A clinician could ask: 'What will I learn?' 'Will I be able to apply what I learned?' 'Who can help me identify review topics that are most amenable to a scoping review?' Members of the faculty development team may ask: 'What is the educational evidence that would inform the best methods for teaching health professionals about a new literature review methodology (e.g. workshop, didactic presentation, academic detailing, audit with feedback). 'What knowledge and skills do participants need in order to carry out a scoping review? 'What educational methods should be used during the faculty development activity? 'What data should be gathered regarding the impact of the workshop on participants' ability to conduct a scoping study'?

All these questions encompass constructs linked to KT. Questions about the design, implementation and assessment of outcomes are undoubtedly of the utmost importance for faculty development teams, program evaluators, researchers and educators. These questions represent essential elements of best practice in faculty development and embody the many possible contributions that faculty development activities and research can make to faculty development practice and scholarship. A faculty development team will need to answer all these questions as they design, develop and evaluate the impact of a faculty development activity intended to promote the knowledge and skills needed to effectively conduct scoping reviews in medical education.

19.4   The Knowledge Translation Process: Using an Established Framework

How does knowledge creation and exchange occur? How is knowledge integrated in practice and how is it used in a sustainable and effective manner? These questions are currently at the heart of many KT researchers' agendae. Whether the focus is on creating and summarizing research findings and other forms of knowledge, on identifying the individual and organizational factors that will support or hinder research uptake in clinical settings (Estabrooks et al. 2003; Gravel et al. 2006) or on developing and evaluating the effectiveness of various KT interventions (Armstrong et al. 2011; Farmer et al. 2011; Gagliardi et al. 2011), there is no dearth of research activity in this area. Most KT scholars would agree that the field is at an important juncture as researchers, policy-makers, practitioners and educators strive to design and evaluate KT interventions that will lead to behavior change and improved practice outcomes.

Given the complexity of changing clinical and educational practice environments, and the multiple factors that can influence that change, several authors recommend that the implementation of research findings in practice be guided by conceptual models or frameworks (Graham et al. 2006; Sudsawad 2007). Frameworks can help to explain and predict the intended change and identify the multiple factors that can increase or decrease the likelihood that this change will occur (Graham et al. 2008). Furthermore, the use of a framework which considers the different stakeholders involved in knowledge creation, exchange and translation emphasizes the notion that all groups should focus their efforts on action plans that take into account the opinions and contributions of all those who will be involved in, and affected by, the proposed change (Graham et al. 2008).

A KT framework that would meet this expectation for a faculty development initiative would consider the needs, expectations and contributions of a faculty development team, participating clinicians and educators, and the organization that employs the health professionals. The framework would support the implementation of mechanisms that promote a collaborative approach to identifying the knowledge gaps, the feasibility of various interventions aimed at changing practice, and the primary outcomes of interest.

At the same time, we should note that although frameworks can assist stakeholders in their pursuit of best practices, no one framework can capture the complex interactions of knowledge creation and knowledge use in all practice settings. Due consideration must therefore be given to the limits of any one framework. The application of the various constructs embedded in many frameworks in any given area of practice, whether it is in healthcare, medical education or faculty development, is only possible insofar as there is available knowledge and evidence. Furthermore, the source, nature and relevance of the evidence used to inform practice must be acceptable to all stakeholders. We acknowledge that faculty development may not yet have a substantive body of published rigorous research to inform most decisions. We also recognize that there may be epistemological concerns regarding the various sources of evidence used to inform faculty development practices and some skepticism about what can and should be considered the gold standard in terms of 'evidence'. Moreover, we recognize that there may be limits to the applicability of empirical research in the day-to-day contexts of most faculty developers. For these reasons, we have chosen to discuss one framework, which we present as a guide rather than a gold standard to be used as a prescriptive tool, that crosses all contexts and addresses all practice issues in faculty development.

19.4.1 The Knowledge-to-Action Framework

Several models and frameworks have been developed to guide KT efforts and address individual users' perspectives as well as contextual factors. It is beyond the scope of this chapter to describe this body of literature in any detail; we invite the reader to consult the work by Estabrooks et al. (2006), Graham et al. (2007) and Sudsawad (2007) for more comprehensive discussions of these frameworks.

In this chapter, we discuss the 'knowledge-to-action' (K2A) framework developed by Graham et al. (2006). We favor this framework because of its conceptual clarity and ease of use, and also because of its applicability to faculty development, as will be illustrated later in the chapter.

The K2A framework falls within the social constructivist paradigm which 'privileges social interaction and adaptation of research evidence that takes local context and culture into account… and offers a holistic view of the KT phenomenon by integrating the concepts of knowledge creation and action' (Graham and Tetroe 2010). The framework is the result of a review of more than 31 planned action theories. Planned action theories, which fall under the larger umbrella of change theories (Tiffany and Lutjens 1998), are prescriptive theories used to predict how various stakeholders will respond to planned and/or anticipated change situations and support change agents in their attempts to influence the factors that will facilitate the change in practice (Graham et al. 2006). The significance of using planned action theories in the development of the K2A framework rests with the notion that the planning and implementation of change in practice can only be achieved with an in-depth understanding of the individual and organizational factors that describe behaviors and support or impede the implementation of change.

The cyclic nature of the K2A process and the important role of feedback loops are key concepts underpinning this framework (Graham et al. 2006). Of significance to both researchers and practitioners is the notion that the K2A framework considers various sources of information as knowledge, including knowledge from research findings as well as other forms of knowing such as experiential knowledge (Graham et al. 2006). Experiential knowledge refers to learning from colleagues and experience through reflection and is considered a requirement for integrating and making sense of the knowledge that emerges from scientific research (Rycroft-Malone et al. 2004).

19.4.2 Knowledge-to-Action Components

The K2A framework is comprised of two main components: (1) knowledge creation and (2) action. Each component contains several phases. The K2A considers knowledge creation and synthesis (knowledge cycle) and knowledge application (action cycle) as iterative processes that are constantly interacting and informing each other. The boundaries between knowledge creation and application are fluid, suggesting once again a bidirectional and dynamic relationship between the two major components of KT (Straus et al. 2010).

19.4.2.1 Knowledge Creation Funnel

At the center of the K2A conceptual framework lies the knowledge creation funnel. The funnel represents the creation of knowledge from research findings and outcome evaluations that will be translated to the knowledge users. Figure 19.1 shows that knowledge creation consists of three phases: knowledge inquiry, knowledge synthesis, and knowledge tools and products. The 'knowledge inquiry' stage consists of original research or 'first generation knowledge'. It constitutes the many primary studies that address a particular question. The 'knowledge synthesis' stage includes research summaries such as systematic reviews where the available research on a given question is appraised and summarized. 'Knowledge tools' consist of the best available research further synthesized into tools such as practice guidelines, decision-making algorithms, and educational modules intended to help end-users apply new knowledge. As we move down the funnel, the knowledge becomes more and more synthesized and potentially more useful to the end users (Tetroe 2011). Chapters 17 and 18 give a number of useful suggestions on how this research could be framed or conducted.

19.4.2.2 Action Cycle

Surrounding the funnel are the seven major action steps or stages that comprise the knowledge-to-action model derived from the review of the planned action theories discussed earlier. The action cycle is depicted by a circle with arrows, which

Fig. 19.1 The knowledge-to-action framework: A model for knowledge translation (Graham et al. 2006; Reproduced with permission from the lead author)

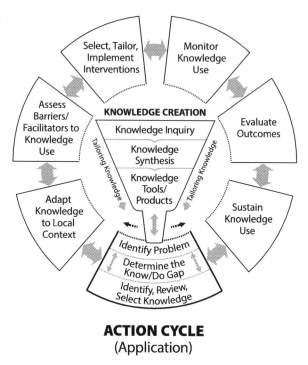

ACTION CYCLE
(Application)

suggests that the steps in the process need to be followed in sequence. The authors acknowledge that this is not always possible in real life contexts. In fact, they argue that KT interventions rarely take place in environments where the knowledge gaps are clearly defined and where the actions required for changing behaviors are readily implementable and sustainable (Tetroe 2012). Thus, the stages can occur simultaneously or sequentially, and the knowledge creation segment can impact upon a number of the stages at different points in time (Graham et al. 2006). For example, as new scientific evidence emerges, is synthesized and ready for dissemination, stakeholder groups responsible for translating the knowledge into practice must verify that the knowledge or new scientific evidence is adapted to the context. If the knowledge is not relevant or adapted in a manner that makes its use appropriate in a particular context, the target group is unlikely to use it.

The seven stages involved in moving knowledge into practice are: identifying a problem in practice or a gap in knowledge and identifying, reviewing, and selecting the knowledge to be implemented to address the gap; adapting or customizing the knowledge to the local context; evaluating the determinants of the knowledge use (barriers and facilitators); selecting, tailoring and implementing interventions to address the knowledge or practice gap; monitoring the knowledge use in practice; evaluating the outcomes or impact of using the new knowledge; and determining strategies for ensuring that the new knowledge is sustained (Graham et al. 2006).

19.5   Application of KT in Faculty Development: A Case Example

In this final section, we describe each stage of the K2A framework in detail, illustrating the application of the cycle by using an example of a faculty development intervention on 'giving effective feedback'. The following scenario will serve as the context for our faculty development initiative:

> You are a new member of a faculty development team housed in the Faculty of Medicine of a research-intensive university. You are contacted by a departmental leader at one of the local teaching hospitals to tell you that his staff could benefit from learning about how to give effective feedback to students. You spend a few minutes on the phone asking questions about 'the problem' and find out that students who come on rotation to this department have complained that the staff (including nurses, physicians and residents) give feedback at the wrong time and in front of patients, that the feedback is often very negative and degrading, and that there is very little feedback on how students can improve. You are now charged with the responsibility of designing a faculty development intervention that will address the needs or feedback 'problem' in this department.

We will now demonstrate how we can use the K2A cycle, including both the knowledge creation and action cycles, to design, implement and evaluate the outcomes of a faculty development activity as a KT strategy intended to help clinical teachers learn about giving effective feedback. We begin with the action cycle and move to the knowledge creation funnel as we discuss the fluid and permeable boundaries that exist between the two components.

19.5.1   Identifying the Knowledge-to-Action Gaps and Identifying, Reviewing and Selecting the Knowledge to Be Implemented

This stage consists of two steps: identifying an important problem in practice or a gap in knowledge and returning to the knowledge creation funnel to identify, review and select the knowledge needed to address the problem. In addition, this first step should consist of rigorous methods and consultations with key stakeholders. Needs assessments can be used to identify gaps in knowledge and practice.

Returning to our case example, the faculty development team must identify the nature of the problem by gathering all the relevant information regarding the feedback problem at the designated site. A discussion with the departmental leader will generate key information about the characteristics of the students (e.g. demographic information; level of training) as well as those of the teaching faculty (e.g. clinical experience, teaching experience, formal training in teaching, previous faculty development on giving effective feedback). The team can also ask for examples of situations where there was ineffective feedback. To promote collaboration and exchange among clinical teachers and leaders at this site, the team should collect clinical teachers' perspectives regarding the nature and delivery of feedback. This can be done with a face-to-face meeting or through a written needs assessment. Student perceptions of feedback at this site would also be helpful.

The second step consists of identifying, reviewing and selecting the appropriate knowledge and/or evidence needed to address the problem. There are two categories of knowledge or evidence that are needed in our case example. The first is evidence on 'feedback' as the central construct. For example, what evidence is available on the characteristics of effective feedback? What does the literature tell us about when and where to give feedback and about the types of feedback that should be given in different situations and with different levels of learners? (Bienstock et al. 2007; Hewson and Little 1998; Milan et al. 2006). The second type of evidence relates to the effectiveness of different interventions designed to address the identified need. For example, this would consist of evidence about how to plan, deliver and evaluate a faculty development activity on providing effective feedback (e.g. Brukner et al. 1999; Holmboe et al. 2001; Salerno et al. 2002; Skeff et al. 1992). This evidence can emerge from faculty development or educational research and might include preferred modes of delivery (e.g. workshop, short course, on site in-service), selection and training of workshop facilitators (e.g. peers, experts in the field), the use of educational materials (e.g. handouts, books, articles, online tutorials) and the duration of the intervention (e.g. half day, full day, blocks of time spread throughout an extended period). Should a workshop be considered the 'method of choice', evidence related to this format (e.g. interactive plenaries, small group discussions, mixed format), and participant evaluations of workshops (i.e. anonymous or not, multiple choice vs. open ended) should be reviewed.

A literature search for evidence on both types of knowledge, often in collaboration with an expert librarian, is also necessary. The identified literature should then be appraised for its quality and relevance to the identified problem, as is typically the case with scientific evidence used in clinical practice. All information that will be useful in the design, implementation and evaluation of a faculty development intervention on giving effective feedback should be retrieved and reviewed.

Although there is available evidence on the topic of giving effective feedback, it is still recommended that faculty development teams consider additional options in situations where there is no available evidence or research. In situations where there is a scarcity of rigorous faculty development research evidence, it is recommended that the team solicit the assistance of other faculty development colleagues at their institution, or at other institutions, for suggestions on how to design a specific workshop. Alternatively, the team can design the activity based on sound pedagogical principles of adult learning that may have been used to design other faculty development initiatives. In fact, this may be an ideal opportunity to conduct the first evaluation of this type of KT intervention and disseminate the results. Consulting the various stakeholders about their preferences regarding both the content and the modes of delivery is essential for providing a tailored program that will meet the needs and expectations of all.

19.5.2   Adapting or Customizing the Knowledge to the Local Context

In this second stage of the K2A process, the value, appropriateness and usefulness of the knowledge are considered in light of the needs of the particular practice setting. KT experts advocate for a participatory process whereby all relevant stakeholders and potential knowledge users are consulted to ensure that the knowledge is appropriate, relevant and useful.

Once the literature and other possible sources of knowledge have been reviewed, appropriate findings can be used to inform a preliminary design of a faculty development intervention (i.e. a workshop or other educational method). A meeting should be scheduled with the relevant stakeholders to discuss the proposed content, the preferred method for delivering the content, the length and format of the intervention, the materials to be used, and other design and implementation issues of importance.

'Customizing or adapting the knowledge' is key at this stage. Both sources of knowledge (feedback content and best methods for delivering the content) may need to be 'customized'. For example, if teachers in this example face similar challenges as those found by Kogan et al. (2012), the intervention should focus on both cognitive and affective factors, including the tension of balancing positive and negative feedback, perceived self-efficacy, and the teachers' perceptions of residents' insight, receptivity and skill. On the other hand, if the quality of feedback is poor (e.g. Kaprielian and Gradison 1998), the intervention might focus on specific feedback strategies and characteristics (Hewson and Little 1998). Given the research findings on the role of reflection and experiential learning in enhancing feedback processes (Hewson 2000), role-plays or simulations (Gelula and Yudkowsky 2003; Stone et al. 2003) may be considered a worthwhile instructional method. Suppose, however, that the participants are not interested in taking part in a role-play activity. An alternative to having them do a role-play is to have the facilitators participate in the role-play, as this can be less intimidating for participants. An additional way to customize the knowledge is to conduct the role-play (or simulation) privately in a room with a facilitator only, rather than in the presence of the larger group. Another aspect of the evidence-informed methods that can be modified or customized is the duration of the KT activity. Suppose that there is evidence that supports offering training on feedback over three short sessions (Hewson 2000) but that this is not realistic in this setting due to time constraints, the intervention can then be offered over two longer sessions or the sessions can be offered over a longer period of time. While this alternative is not evidence-based, it may be the only option for this site and may result in better attendance and reduced attrition over time.

19.5.3   Evaluating the Determinants of the Knowledge Use (Barriers and Facilitators)

This stage consists of assessing the barriers that can limit the uptake of the knowledge so that the barriers may be targeted by specific strategies. Barriers can be specific to the individual (e.g. lack of time, lack of experience in a given domain, lack of knowledge, lack of self-efficacy, negative attitudes) or related to the organizational environment (e.g. insufficient resources, lack of access to learning resources).

This is a challenging step in the K2A cycle as there are many possible facilitators and barriers that can have an impact on the design and implementation of the faculty development activity that has been designed. The barriers can be about the knowledge of feedback or about the implementation of the faculty development activity.

In our example, possible barriers at the individual level may include negative attitudes towards faculty development, lack of motivation, and lack of relevant experience. Results from a needs assessment may reveal that participants do not wish to attend faculty development activities, do not value group discussions or question the benefits of this type of professional development activity. Another possible barrier may be that the group is heterogeneous with participants of varying levels of experience, motivation and interest in the activity.

System-level or organizational barriers include lack of dedicated time to participate in professional development activities, heavy clinical caseloads, and an organizational culture that does not privilege professional development. The organization may, for example, agree to support participants to attend the activity but without remuneration. Or, it may encourage continuing medical education for best clinical practice, but may not support professional development activities related to teaching. Additionally, another common barrier to the uptake of health-related evidence in practice is individual and/or organizational attitudes towards the value of research versus the value of experience and the perceived legitimacy of each as sources of knowledge for clinical decision-making. Similarly, in the context of faculty development, there may be resistance to the new feedback 'practices' as some may be skeptical about the legitimacy of the research evidence, favoring experiential knowledge and expertise as superior forms of knowledge.

It is a critical part of the faculty development team's role to identify the potential supports and barriers as early as possible in the process and to discuss ways to address these without alienating either one of the stakeholder groups.

19.5.4 Selecting, Tailoring, Implementing and Monitoring the KT Interventions

In this stage, interventions to facilitate and promote awareness and implementation of the knowledge are selected, tailored and then executed. Interventions can target the individual, although, depending on the specific barriers that have been identified, they may also need to target the organization. KT interventions can be single or multi-component, and can include educational interventions such as courses, on-site workshops, audit and feedback, outreach visits, and reminders. KT interventions can also target policy and organizational changes aimed at promoting changes in culture and increasing support as well as funding for training.

In this case, the KT intervention (i.e. the faculty development activity on giving effective feedback) will be designed using the literature that was retrieved and appraised, the expert consultations, the information gathered from the stakeholders regarding the nature of the problem, as well as the knowledge of the barriers and facilitators to the implementation of the activity.

At this stage of the K2A cycle, it is useful to work with content experts (experts on giving effective feedback) as well as process experts or expert faculty development teams. When the activity has been designed, the unit leader should be consulted to confirm that it is suitable and that it meets the original identified needs.

The implementation phase of this step in the cycle consists of the delivery of the KT feedback intervention that has been planned for this site. As is the case with any faculty development activity, be it a workshop or online tutorial, contingencies can be built in to deal with unforeseen situations such as a different number of participants than expected, problems with technology, and lack of participation or interaction.

19.5.5 Monitoring Knowledge Use

In this stage, one must consider the type of knowledge that will be monitored (Straus et al. 2010). Several descriptions of knowledge use exist in the context of KT interventions. Nomenclature most frequently seen in the KT literature is instrumental, conceptual and persuasive use of knowledge (Alkin and Taut 2002; Dunn 1983). *Instrumental* use refers to a concrete application of the knowledge in practice. *Conceptual* use refers to changes in understanding or attitudes without any effect on actual behavior or change in practice. *Persuasive use* consists of using knowledge as a persuasion tool to convince others to support certain positions or opinions (Alkin and Taut 2002).

To assess the use of knowledge, appropriate indicators should be developed and different tools or measures assessing those indicators should be used. An important consideration in this stage is that the impact of the knowledge on the end user, whether it is a patient or a learner, must be evaluated. According to Straus et al. (2010), the monitoring stage should consist of rigorous evaluation methods including both qualitative and quantitative methods. The challenge of evaluating complex interventions is highlighted in Chap. 17.

In the feedback scenario, a number of different measures can be used. For conceptual use of knowledge, a scale assessing beliefs and attitudes can be used. It may also be useful to conduct a qualitative assessment through interviews or focus groups to ascertain whether there have been changes in attitudes and beliefs about the impact of a faculty development activity on participants' feedback practices. Changes in knowledge can be assessed with a short answer quiz or online survey. Measuring instrumental use of knowledge will be a greater challenge. Objective measures of behavior change are considered the gold standard; however, they are costly and challenging to implement. Chart audits, observation, video with simulated recall, and consultations with learners to inquire about the impact of teachers' feedback practices can be useful methods for measuring the impact of a workshop on actual feedback practices. In the absence of the necessary resources to conduct these types of evaluations, participants' perceptions of the impact of the KT intervention on their feedback practices can be obtained using self-report questionnaires and interviews.

19.5.6   Evaluating the Outcomes or Impact of Using the New Knowledge

This stage consists of evaluating the impact of the KT process in order to determine if implementation of the new knowledge was successful and worthwhile. It specifically consists of measuring desired changes in levels of knowledge and attitudes as well as changes in practice following the KT interventions.

In our example, a key outcome of the KT intervention on giving effective feedback is that participants will apply effective principles of feedback with learners. The two major knowledge outcomes that should be measured in this stage of the K2A are: (1) participants' knowledge about what giving constructive feedback entails, their attitudes about giving feedback, and their beliefs about the value of giving effective feedback (conceptual) and (2) participants' use of effective feedback strategies in practice (instrumental).

When planning the evaluation of effectiveness, both the purpose of the evaluation and the selection of the measures need to be carefully considered. The purpose may be to collect evidence that justifies the faculty development resources devoted to the design and implementation of the KT intervention on providing effective feedback, to demonstrate that the KT activities have an impact on knowledge and practice regarding giving effective feedback, or to evaluate specific features of the activity (e.g. the use of a particular educational strategy) if there is no evidence for that strategy in the literature. The outcomes of the activity should also be assessed with the objective of disseminating the findings and contributing to the body of literature on faculty development. Researchers or program evaluators can be consulted to assist with designing the outcome measures and evaluation process, measuring the outcomes, and analyzing the data. (See Chap. 18 for additional information on research paradigms and an alternative framework for exploring the impact of a faculty development activity.)

With regard to the type of measure or evaluation tool, this depends upon whether there are existing measures for the outcome of interest (e.g. Sender Liberman et al. 2005; Stone et al. 2003). Identification of available measures is typically done at the planning stage of the K2A cycle, during the literature review. Measures with strong psychometric properties should be used when available. If there are no existing measures on the impact of faculty development interventions on effective feedback practices, a new measure can be developed, but it will need to be validated and pilot tested prior to its use.

19.5.7 Sustaining Knowledge Use

The final stage of the action cycle consists of planning and managing changes to implementation strategies in the face of evolving contextual factors and/or barriers by cycling back through the action cycle. According to the K2A cycle, 'sustained knowledge use refers to the continued implementation of innovation over time and depends on the ability of the knowledge users and the organization to adapt to change' (Davies and Edwards 2009, p. 165). Although this stage is later in the K2A cycle, KT experts advocate for considering this stage as early as possible in the implementation process.

For our feedback example, the faculty development team can schedule a follow-up phone call or administer an online survey to assess the continued impact of the KT intervention on conceptual and instrumental use of the feedback knowledge. Site visits and the use of reminders are useful strategies for discussions of sustainability and changes in the practice setting (Bloom 2005). They can also serve as incentives for uptake of new knowledge. Whichever method is selected as part of an assessment of sustainability, it should be *evidence-based, feasible* and *acceptable* to the relevant stakeholders.

Evidence-based strategies include strategies that are known to be effective and efficient for monitoring knowledge use. The literature may, for example, suggest that online surveys yield a higher response rate than mail surveys and are more effective than focus groups for identifying some of the sustainability issues (Dillman 2000). Teachers (i.e. the participants) and managers should be consulted at different times and confidentially in order to allow them to disclose their opinions freely. Essentially, three important questions should be addressed at this stage: (1) How is the knowledge about giving effective feedback being used? (2) If it is not being applied, what are the main reasons? (3) What next steps can be taken to support educators and the organization in implementing effective feedback strategies?

It is essential that the monitoring plan be feasible. Ambitious and resource demanding strategies may yield less than optimal outcomes. New measurement tools take time to develop and validate, making it challenging to move forward in a timely manner. Consider what resources are available and will yield the best information regarding sustainability of the knowledge use.

Acceptability is another important factor in this stage of the K2A cycle. For example, participants may not accept to be interviewed, and individuals at the managerial level may not support a monitoring phase. The teachers' and managers' ability to sustain the change, that is to continue to implement effective feedback strategies, must be considered at this stage. Ability can be influenced by affordances in the environment (e.g. having enough learners to practice with, having a manageable workload) and by individual factors such as motivation, external recognition of changes in behavior, and confirmation or validation that changes in the behavior (feedback practices) improve learners' experiences.

19.6   Conclusion

As valued members of faculty development teams and potential contributors to the broader scholarship of faculty development and knowledge translation, we urge the reader to consider his or her role in this important enterprise.

The K2A is a framework that offers a useful structure for conceptualizing and organizing KT activities and evaluating their impact on desired outcomes. The framework presents the boundaries between knowledge creation and action as open and fluid. This suggests that faculty development activities can and should be conceptualized as important KT interventions that are grounded in scientific research as well as in other accepted and valued sources of knowledge. These interventions must be assessed and disseminated widely in an effort to add to the knowledge creation component of the KT process. Implementation studies that describe the processes used to transfer new knowledge in practice will yield results that could equally inform the action cycle. Results from original research, or from syntheses of available research, should in turn be used to promote best practices in faculty development activities. It is vital for both faculty development practice and scholarship that the results of the evaluation and/or research be integrated back into the knowledge creation component.

Faculty development teams should be encouraged to disseminate all aspects of their interventions (planning and development, evaluation, successes, challenges), and when appropriate, present their research findings at scholarly conferences or submit manuscripts for publication in relevant journals. They should also be encouraged to find ways to disseminate their results to the important stakeholder groups that were involved in the various stages of the K2A process. The different groups should find ways to collectively discuss the results from implementation studies, explore the applications of the new knowledge in practice, and discuss what processes need to be put in place to ensure that new knowledge is embraced, used and sustained in practice.

Knowledge dissemination will not only help other faculty development teams in the future as they plan and implement their own faculty development activities/KT interventions, but it will add to the body of literature on faculty development research. As with any field of study, the scientific evidence that emerges from this research can improve teaching practices, strengthen the field, increase the body of knowledge, and support continued scholarship.

19.7   Key Messages

- Faculty development activities should be conceptualized as KT interventions intended to improve medical education and faculty development practices.
- The design of faculty development activities as KT strategies should be informed by the best available research in the field.

- Rigorous methods for assessing the impact of faculty development (KT) activities on practice are needed.
- Dissemination of knowledge obtained from assessments of effectiveness and outcome measures of the faculty development interventions as KT strategies are essential for building a body of research and practice in the field.

References

Akl, E. A., Mustafa, R., Wilson, M. C., Symons, A., Moheet, A., Rosenthal, T., et al. (2009). Curricula for teaching the content of clinical practice guidelines to family medicine and internal medicine residents in the US: A survey study. *Implementation Science, 4*, 59.

Alkin, M. C. & Taut, S. M. (2002). Unbundling evaluation use. *Studies in Educational Evaluation, 29*(1), 1–12.

Arksey, H. & O'Malley, L. (2005). Scoping studies: Towards a methodological framework. *International Journal of Social Research Methodology, 8*(1), 19–32.

Armstrong, R., Waters, E., Dobbins, M., Lavis, J. N., Petticrew, M., & Christensen, R. (2011). Knowledge translation strategies for facilitating evidence-informed public health decision-making among managers and policy-makers. *Cochrane Database of Systematic Reviews,* (6).

Bienstock, J. L., Katz, N. T., Cox, S. M., Hueppchen, N., Erickson, S., & Puscheck, E. E. (2007). To the point: Medical education reviews-providing feedback. *American Journal of Obstetrics and Gynecology, 196*(6), 508–513.

Bloom, B. S. (2005). Effects of continuing medical education on improving physician clinical care and patient health: A review of systematic reviews. *International Journal of Technology Assessment in Health Care, 21*(3), 380–385.

Brukner, H., Altkorn, D. L., Cook, S., Quinn, M. T., & McNabb, W. L. (1999). Giving effective feedback to medical students: A workshop for faculty and house staff. *Medical Teacher, 21*(2), 161–165.

Cabana, M. D., Rand, C. S., Powe, N. R., Wu, A. W., Wilson, M. H., Abboud, P. A. C., et al. (1999). Why don't physicians follow clinical practice guidelines? A framework for improvement. *JAMA, 282*(15), 1458–1465.

Canadian Institutes of Health Research. (2012). *More about knowledge translation at CIHR: Knowledge translation – Definition.* Available from: http://www.cihr-irsc.gc.ca/e/39033.html

Davies, B. & Edwards, N. (2009). The knowledge-to-action cycle: Sustaining knowledge use. In S. Straus, J. Tetroe & I. D. Graham (Eds.), *Knowledge translation in health care: Moving from evidence to practice,* (pp. 165–173). Oxford, UK: Wiley-Blackwell and BMJ.

Davis, D., Evans, M., Jadad, A., Perrier, L., Rath, D., Ryan, D., et al. (2003). The case for knowledge translation: Shortening the journey from evidence to effect. *BMJ, 327*(7405), 33–35.

Dillman, D. A. (2000). *Mail and internet surveys: The tailored design method (2nd Ed.).* New York, NY: John Wiley and Sons.

Duncan, P. W., Horner, R. D., Reker, D. M., Samsa, G. P., Hoenig, H., Hamilton, B., et al. (2002). Adherence to post-acute rehabilitation guidelines is associated with functional recovery in stroke. *Stroke, 33*(1), 167–177.

Dunn, W. N. (1983). Measuring knowledge use. *Knowledge: Creation, diffusion, utilization, 5*(1), 120–133.

Estabrooks, C. A., Floyd, J. A., Scott-Findlay, S., O'Leary, K. A., & Gushta, M. (2003). Individual determinants of research utilization: A systematic review. *Journal of Advanced Nursing, 43*(5), 506–520.

Estabrooks, C. A., Thompson, D. S., Lovely, J. J., & Hofmeyer, A. (2006). A guide to knowledge translation theory. *Journal of Continuing Education in the Health Professions, 26*(1), 25–36.

Farmer, A. P., Légaré, F., Turcot, L., Grimshaw, J., Harvey, E., McGowan, J., et al. (2011). Printed educational materials: Effects on professional practice and health care outcomes. *Cochrane Database of Systematic Reviews*, (7).

Flodgren, G., Parmelli, E., Doumit, G., Gattellari, M., O'Brien, M. A., Grimshaw, J., et al. (2011). Local opinion leaders: Effects on professional practice and health care outcomes. *Cochrane Database of Systematic Reviews*, (8).

Forsetlund, L., Bjørndal, A., Rashidian, A., Jamtvedt, G., O'Brien, M. A., Wolf, F., et al. (2009). Continuing education meetings and workshops: Effects on professional practice and health care outcomes. *Cochrane Database of Systematic Reviews*, (2).

Gagliardi, A. R., Légaré, F., Brouwers, M. C., Webster, F., Wiljer, D., Badley, E., et al. (2011). Protocol: Developing a conceptual framework of patient mediated knowledge translation, systematic review using a realist approach. *Implementation Science, 6*, 25.

Gelula, M. H. & Yudkowsky, R. (2003). Using standardised students in faculty development workshops to improve clinical teaching skills. *Medical Education, 37*(7), 621–629.

Glasgow, R. E., Lichtenstein, E., & Marcus, A. C. (2003). Why don't we see more translation of health promotion research to practice? Rethinking the efficacy-to-effectiveness transition. *American Journal of Public Health, 93*(8), 1261–1267.

Graham, I. D., Logan, J., Harrison, M. B., Straus, S. E., Tetroe, J., Caswell, W., et al. (2006). Lost in knowledge translation: Time for a map? *Journal of Continuing Education in the Health Professions, 26*(1), 13–24.

Graham, I. D., Logan, J., Tetroe, J., Robinson, N., & Harrison, M. B. (2008). Models of implementation in nursing. In N. Cullum, D. Ciliska, R. B. Haynes, & S. Marks (Eds.), *Evidence-based nursing*, (pp. 231–243). Oxford, UK: Blackwell Publishing Ltd.

Graham, I. D., Tetroe, J. & the KT Theories Group. (2007). Some theoretical underpinnings of knowledge translation. *Academic Emergency Medicine, 14*(11), 936–941.

Graham, I. D. & Tetroe, J. (2010). The knowledge to action framework. In J. Rycroft-Malone & T. Bucknell (Eds.), *Models and frameworks for implementing evidence-based practice: Linking evidence to action*, (pp. 207–222). Oxford, UK: Wiley-Blackwell

Gravel, K., Légaré, F., & Graham, I. D. (2006). Barriers and facilitators to implementing shared decision-making in clinical practice: A systematic review of health professionals' perceptions. *Implementation Science, 1*, 16.

Grimshaw J. M., Eccles, M., Thomas, R., MacLennan, G., Ramsay, C., Fraser, C., et al. (2006). Toward evidence-based quality improvement. Evidence (and its limitations) of the effectiveness of guideline dissemination and implementation strategies 1966–1998. *Journal of General Internal Medicine, 21*(Suppl. 2), S14–S20.

Grimshaw, J. M., Eccles, M. P., Walker, A. E., & Thomas, R. E. (2002). Changing physicians' behavior: What works and thoughts on getting more things to work. *Journal of Continuing Education in the Health Professions, 22*(4), 237–243.

Grimshaw, J. M., McAuley, L., Bero, L., Grilli, R., Oxman, A., Ramsay, C., et al. (2003). Systematic reviews of the effectiveness of quality improvement strategies and programmes. *Quality and Safety in Health Care, 12*(4), 298–303.

Grol, R. & Grimshaw, J. (2003). From best evidence to best practice: Effective implementation of change in patients' care. *Lancet, 362*(9391), 1225–1230.

Grol, R. & Jones, R. (2000). Twenty years of implementation research. *Family Practice, 17* (Suppl. 1), S32–S35.

Hewson, M. G. (2000). A theory-based faculty development program for clinician-educators. *Academic Medicine, 75*(5), 498–501.

Hewson, M. G. & Little, M. L. (1998). Giving feedback in medical education: Verification of recommended techniques. *Journal of General Internal Medicine, 13*(2), 111–116.

Holmboe, E. S., Fiebach, N. H., Galaty, L. A., & Huot, S. (2001). Effectiveness of a focused educational intervention on resident evaluations from faculty: A randomized controlled trial. *Journal of General Internal Medicine, 16*(7), 427–434.

Horsley, T., O'Neill, J., McGowan, J., Perrier, L., Kane, G., & Campbell, C. (2010). Interventions to improve question formulation in professional practice and self-directed learning. *Cochrane Database of Systematic Reviews*, (5).

Kaprielian, V. S. & Gradison, M. (1998). Effective use of feedback. *Family Medicine, 30*(6), 406–407.

Kogan, J. R., Conforti, L. N., Bernabeo, E. C., Durning, S. J., Hauer, K. E., & Holmboe, E. S. (2012). Faculty staff perceptions of feedback to residents after direct observation of clinical skills. *Medical Education, 46*(2), 201–215.

Korner-Bitensky, N., Wood-Dauphinee, S., Teasell, R., Desrosiers, J., Malouin, F., Thomas, A., et al. (2006). Best versus actual practices in stroke rehabilitation: Results of the Canadian National Survey. *Stroke, 37*(2), 631.

Landry, R., Lamari, M., & Amara, N. (2003). The extent and determinants of the utilization of university research in government agencies. *Public Administration Review, 63*(2), 192–205.

Lavis, J. N., Robertson, D., Woodside, J. M., McLeod, C. B., & Abelson, J. (2003). How can research organizations more effectively transfer research knowledge to decision makers? *The Milbank Quarterly, 81*(2), 221–248.

McGlynn, E. A., Asch, S. M., Adams, J., Keesey, J., Hicks, J., DeCristofaro, A., et al. (2003). The quality of health care delivered to adults in the United States. *New England Journal of Medicine, 348*(26), 2635–2645.

McKibbon, K. A., Lokker, C., Wilczynski, N. L., Ciliska, D., Dobbins, M., Davis, D. A., et al. (2010). A cross-sectional study of the number and frequency of terms used to refer to knowledge translation in a body of health literature in 2006: A Tower of Babel? *Implementation Science, 5*, 16.

McLean, M., Cilliers, F., & Van Wyk, J. M. (2008). Faculty development: Yesterday, today and tomorrow. *Medical Teacher, 30*(6) 555–584.

Milan, F. B., Parish, S. J., & Reichgott, M. J. (2006). A model for educational feedback based on clinical communication skills strategies: Beyond the 'feedback sandwich'. *Teaching and Learning in Medicine, 18*(1), 42–47.

Nutley, S., Walter, I., & Davies, H. T. O. (2003). From knowing to doing: A framework for understanding the evidence-into-practice agenda. *Evaluation, 9*(2), 125–148.

Oborn, E., Barrett, M., & Racko, G. (2010). *Knowledge translation in health care: A review of the literature.* Cambridge, UK: Cambridge Judge Business School Working Paper Series.

Rycroft-Malone, J., Seers, K., Titchen, A., Harvey, G., Kitson, A., & McCormack, B. (2004). What counts as evidence in evidence-based practice? *Journal of Advanced Nursing, 47*(1), 81–90.

Salerno, S. M., O'Malley, P. G., Pangaro, L. N., Wheeler, G. A., Moores, L. K., & Jackson, J. L. (2002). Faculty development seminars based on the one-minute preceptor improve feedback in the ambulatory setting. *Journal of General Internal Medicine, 17*(10), 779–787.

Sender Liberman, A., Liberman, M., Steinert, Y., McLeod, P., & Meterissian, S. (2005). Surgery residents and attending surgeons have different perceptions of feedback. *Medical Teacher, 27*(5), 470–472.

Skeff, K. M., Stratos, G. A., & Bergen, M. R. (1992). Evaluation of a medical faculty development program: A comparison of traditional pre/post and retrospective pre/post self-assessment ratings. *Evaluation and the Health Professions, 15*(3), 350–366.

Steinert, Y. (2000). Faculty development in the new millennium: Key challenges and future directions. *Medical Teacher, 22*(1), 44–50.

Steinert, Y. (2011). Commentary: Faculty development: The road less traveled. *Academic Medicine, 86*(4), 409–411.

Steinert, Y., Mann, K., Centeno, A., Dolmans, D., Spencer, J., Gelula, M., et al. (2006). A systematic review of faculty development initiatives designed to improve teaching effectiveness in medical education: BEME Guide No. 8. *Medical Teacher, 28*(6), 497–526.

Steinert, Y., Naismith, L., & Mann, K. (2012). Faculty development initiatives designed to promote leadership in medical education. A BEME systematic review: BEME Guide No. 19. *Medical Teacher, 34*(6), 483–503.

Stone, S., Mazor, K., Devaney-O'Neil, S., Starr, S., Ferguson, W., Wellman, S., et al. (2003). Development and implementation of an Objective Structured Teaching Exercise (OSTE) to evaluate improvement in feedback skills following a faculty development workshop. *Teaching and Learning in Medicine, 15*(1), 7–13.

Straus, S. E., Tetroe, J., & Graham, I. D. (2009). Defining knowledge translation. *CMAJ, 181*(3–4), 165–168.

Straus, S. E., Tetroe, J., & Graham, I. D. (2011). Knowledge translation is the use of knowledge in health care decision making. *Journal of Clinical Epidemiology, 64*(1), 6–10.

Straus, S. E., Tetroe, J., Graham, I. D., Zwarenstein, M., Bhattacharyya, O., & Shepperd, S. (2010). Monitoring use of knowledge and evaluating outcomes. *CMAJ, 182*(2), E94–E98.

Sudsawad, P. (2007). *Knowledge translation: Introduction to models, strategies, and measures.* Austin, TX: Southwest Educational Development Laboratory, National Center for the Dissemination of Disability Research.

Tetroe, J. (2011). The knowledge-to-action cycle. Retrieved August 15th, 2011, from http://pram. mcgill.ca/i/Tetroe-FMED604-KT-CIHR-march2011.pdf

Tiffany, C. R. & Lutjens, L. R. J. (1998). *Planned change theories for nursing: Review, analysis, and implications.* Thousand Oaks, CA: Sage.

Part VI
Conclusion

Chapter 20
Faculty Development: Future Directions

Yvonne Steinert

20.1 Introduction

The chapters in this book have addressed the scope of faculty development, common approaches to the professional development of faculty members, practical applications, and the central role that research, scholarship, and knowledge translation can play in creating evidence-informed faculty development. In this chapter, we will build on lessons learned and chart a number of future directions as faculty development in the health professions moves forward. These directions include: moving away from the notion of one-time development to ongoing learning, and in the process, shifting our emphasis from the workshop to the workplace; attending equally to all faculty roles and expanding our focus from the individual to the organization; building on available evidence and previous success in the design and delivery of formal faculty development programs; introducing faculty development early in the careers of students at all levels of the educational continuum; mapping a research agenda for faculty development that includes new paradigms, methods of inquiry, and foci for investigation; and learning from each other.

20.2 Moving from the Workshop to the Workplace

As stated in Chap. 1, faculty development has historically been viewed as a planned program, something that is 'done to' faculty members, rather than an activity in which they engage on an ongoing basis. In many ways, it is time to alter our thinking about faculty development and embrace a broader view that moves us away from the notion

Y. Steinert, Ph.D. (✉)
Centre for Medical Education and Department of Family Medicine,
Faculty of Medicine, McGill University, Montreal, QC, Canada
e-mail: yvonne.steinert@mcgill.ca

Y. Steinert (ed.), *Faculty Development in the Health Professions: A Focus on Research and Practice*, Innovation and Change in Professional Education 11, DOI 10.1007/978-94-007-7612-8_20, © Springer Science+Business Media Dordrecht 2014

of *development* to *learning*, from *one-time* training to *ongoing* professional development, and from the classroom (or workshop) to the workplace.

The plea to move from one-time development to ongoing professional learning has been made by a number of educators in the field of higher education (e.g. Clarke and Hollingsworth 2002; Knight 2002). As Webster-Wright (2009) noted, professionals learn from a range of activities that include formal programs, interactions with colleagues, and learning on the job. Several authors in this volume have also underscored the importance of learning from experience (O'Sullivan and Irby Chap. 18; Swanwick and McKimm Chap. 3; Steinert Chap. 7), which includes role modeling and reflective practice (Mann Chap. 12) as well as peer coaching and mentorship (Boillat and Elizov Chap. 8). However, despite an increasing awareness of the role of informal learning in the professional development of health professionals (Eraut 2004), we must ask ourselves what has prevented us from recognizing workplace learning as a legitimate form of faculty development to date. Is it that we take experiential, workplace learning for granted? Or is it that such learning lacks 'visibility', credibility, and accountability? Irrespective of the underlying reasons, research and dialogue about how faculty members develop, in both formal and informal settings, are imperative. Moreover, although the importance of workplace learning may appear self-evident, we need to find innovative ways to render informal learning more 'visible'.

Building on the work of Billett (1996) and Eraut (2004), Chap. 7 describes the role of workplace learning in faculty development. Although we will undoubtedly continue to promote formal (structured) faculty development initiatives, we must value learning in the workplace, promote strategies that reinforce transfer to the workplace, and reach health professionals who do not attend formal faculty development activities. We should also examine cultural differences in workplace learning and contemplate whether workplace learning is, in fact, a cultural practice.

20.2.1   Valuing Learning in the Workplace

As outlined in Chap. 7, we need to recognize and validate learning in the workplace. We should also heed lessons learned in other fields and deliberately use the workplace as an environment for learning, attempting to facilitate engagement, make expert guidance more intentional, and strengthen affordances while diminishing organizational barriers. Billett (2002) has said that engagement is a fundamental pre-requisite for learning in the workplace. As faculty members and faculty developers, what can we do to heighten engagement? If possible, we should also try to decrease the perceived distinction between working and learning (DuFour 2004), promote the notion of learning *for* and *in* the workplace, and remember that enhancing individual learning in the workplace can strengthen organizational capacity (Bierema 1996). The literature suggests that postgraduate medical education is characterized as 'a process of learning from experience' (Teunissen et al. 2007, p. 763). Would it not be possible to characterize faculty development in a similar fashion?

20.2.2   Enhancing 'Transfer of Learning' to the Workplace

In discussing the transfer of knowledge from educational settings to the workplace, (Eraut 2004) describes five inter-related stages:

> ...the extraction of potentially relevant knowledge from the context of its acquisition and previous use; understanding the new situation (a process that often depends on informal social learning); recognizing what knowledge and skills are relevant; transforming this [knowledge and skill] to fit the new situation; and integrating [new competencies] with other knowledge and skills in order to behave differently in the new situation (p. 256).

As faculty members and faculty developers, we should carefully consider this complex process and the strategies that can facilitate transfer in the design and delivery of formal faculty development programs and activities.

In discussing workshops and seminars, de Grave et al. (Chap. 9) highlight the need for us to pay more attention to the transfer of learning to the workplace and stress the following key characteristics, adapted from Grossman and Salas (2011): learner attributes (including cognitive ability, self-efficacy, motivation to learn); the design of the faculty development event (including behavioral modeling and realistic training environments); and the nature of the work environment (including support and the availability of follow-up). Clearly, we should acknowledge these factors in the design of our activities and work to ensure careful monitoring and follow-up. In our own setting, participants have valued 'booster sessions', often 3–6 months after a formal activity, as well as the availability of post-workshop consultations. Embedding new knowledge and skills in the workplace is a key challenge for all of us.

20.2.3   Bringing 'Formal' Faculty Development Activities to the Workplace

It would also be beneficial to bring formal faculty development activities *to* the workplace. In describing attendance at formal activities, it has been said that 'those who need faculty development the most, attend the least' (Steinert et al. 2009, p. 42). It is interesting to note that most faculty development activities have traditionally been conducted away from the workplace, requiring faculty members to take their 'lessons learned' back to their own contexts (Steinert 2012). Perhaps it is time to reverse this trend and think about how we can penetrate the work environment and integrate formal activities into the natural setting in which health professionals work. In a study on why faculty members participate in faculty development (Steinert et al. 2010b), participants specifically requested 'outreach activities', described as formal professional development in their place of work. As one participant commented, 'I would like to see faculty development come out of the medical school [building], and go into the hospitals...' (p. 905). It is clearly more difficult to 'stay away' from faculty development if it is conducted onsite, with the chair or unit director in attendance.

20.2.4 Developing Communities of Practice

The development of a community of practice as an outcome of faculty development has been discussed in a number of chapters in this volume (e.g. Anderson et al. Chap. 14; Cook Chap. 11; Gruppen Chap. 10; O'Sullivan and Irby Chap. 18). That a community of practice can facilitate faculty development has also been shown (Steinert et al. 2010a). The challenge is to build on Wenger et al.'s (2002) design principles (e.g. design for evolution; open a dialogue between inside and outside perspectives; invite different levels of participation; create a rhythm for the community), outlined in Chaps. 7 and 14, and help faculty members to find a common purpose and shared language, opportunities for dialogue and meaningful exchange of information, and joint activities and practices. By working together and participating in a larger community, health professionals can build new knowledge and understanding, develop approaches to problems faced in the multiple facets of their diverse roles, and achieve a sense of belonging (Steinert 2010). Describing and evaluating this trajectory is an additional direction for future inquiry.

20.3 Expanding the Focus of Faculty Development

As noted in Chap. 1, faculty development should address *all* faculty roles, including that of teacher and educator, leader and manager, and researcher and scholar. Professional development in this area should also aim to enhance career development and organizational change. A similar argument has been made by Drummond-Young et al. (2010) who state that a comprehensive faculty development program in nursing should include instructional development, professional development, leadership development, and organizational development.

20.3.1 Addressing all Faculty Roles

Although faculty members and faculty developers might all agree with expanding the focus of faculty development, as discussed at the 1st International Conference on Faculty Development (2011), the literature and many of the authors in this book continue to emphasize the educational role of faculty members. Why is this? Is it that faculty members are least prepared for this role? Is it because early efforts in faculty development primarily focused on teaching improvement (as outlined in Chap. 2)? Although the answer to this question is not obvious, the sociocultural and economic contexts in which faculty development initiatives unfold may play a role. For example, faculty development offerings are often designed in response to 'urgent' educational needs, and 'service' to the community may be the first priority.

This observation might partially help to explain the emphasis on teaching improvement and the apparent focus on the individual. So might the recent emphasis on the professionalization of teaching (Eitel et al. 2000; Purcell and Lloyd-Jones 2003), though the development of standards for all faculty roles may well be forthcoming. At the same time, funding for educational development may be more readily available than resources for career development (which may be perceived as a 'luxury'), and leadership development and research capacity building may not be seen to require formal development. In fact, some might even believe that leadership is a 'mystical and ethereal' process that is not amenable to change (Kouzes and Posner 1995). Despite these possible reasons, however, it would be worthwhile for us to become more mindful of how we invest in faculty development and how we can systematically address *all* faculty roles, many of which overlap and are often carried out simultaneously. Health professionals in all settings (including the university, the hospital, and the community) need to be prepared for complex and demanding roles that go well beyond teaching, and a broader focus would benefit both individual faculty members and the organizations in which they work.

20.3.2 Shifting from an Individual to an Organizational Focus

As highlighted by Jolly (Chap. 6), faculty development initiatives need to explicitly try to influence the organizational culture. Such efforts are needed to support the individual faculty member's growth and development as well as the institutional environment in which education, leadership, and research takes place. Hafler et al. (2011) describe a 'hidden curriculum' that affects faculty members in multiple ways. As these authors observe:

> …efforts to improve the instructional value, impact, and/or relevance of formal faculty development programs will be dictated in part by the broader array of cultural messages that faculty members encounter as they go about learning what being a 'good faculty member' means (Hafler et al. 2011, p. 442).

This observation is an additional call for faculty development efforts to address the organizational culture, sustain individual change, recognize faculty members' accomplishments, and facilitate effective participatory practices. So is the observation by Hodges (Chap. 4) and Goldszmidt et al. (2008) that, despite participation in formal activities designed to foster research, many faculty members may not actually conduct more (or better) research because of organizational factors that include a lack of research support, 'protected time', and a community of practice committed to scholarship. Awareness of the organization's values and goals is also essential in order to embed faculty development in the organization, as is attention to those elements that foster ongoing change and development (e.g. Snell Chap. 13). In diverse ways, expanding our focus from the individual to the organization will help to increase capacity, foster and sustain innovation, and reward excellence.

20.4   Building on Evidence and Previous Success

Thomas and Steinert (Chap. 19) describe the role of evidence in the design and delivery of faculty development initiatives. Although the evidence base in faculty development is not as firmly established as in other fields, we should strive to develop programs based on what we know – from both empirical studies and from our collective experiences. Moreover, despite the suggestion of a renewed emphasis on professional learning in informal settings, formal (structured) faculty development programs are here to stay. The literature to date has provided us with important information about what works in the design and delivery of formal initiatives (Spencer Chap. 17), including the use of a range of instructional methods (e.g. small group discussions, interactive exercises, role plays or simulations), the promotion of experiential learning and reflective practice, the provision of feedback and effective peer relationships, and the enhancement of relevance and application through project work. We should incorporate these elements into our program design and build on 'key features' that appear to be associated with positive outcomes (Steinert et al. 2006, 2012).

20.4.1   Creating Comprehensive, Stage-Specific Programs

Silver (Chap. 16) suggests that we consider the design and delivery of *comprehensive* faculty development programs that can 'serve the multiple needs of teachers, educators, researchers and administrators'. This recommendation encourages us to think programmatically and move away from 'one-time events', even though the latter have the advantage of enticing new participants (Steinert et al. 2010b). In describing faculty development to enhance teaching effectiveness, Hodgson and Wilkerson (Chap. 2) suggest that we should build comprehensive programs that are developmental in nature (Dreyfus and Dreyfus 1986) and that can demonstrate that faculty members have achieved varying levels of competency. Using a competency framework (e.g. Academy of Medical Educators 2012; Milner et al. 2011; Molenaar et al. 2009; Srinivasan et al. 2011), as suggested by Hodgson and Wilkerson (Chap. 2), can help to monitor the achievement of faculty milestones and progress over time. In a similar vein, and describing the role of faculty development in building research capacity, Hodges (Chap. 4) proposes that it would be worthwhile to create developmental, articulated programs that progress from short courses to longer programs, fellowships, and graduate degrees, as the interests, skills, and needs of faculty members evolve. Leslie (Chap. 5) also describes stage-specific faculty development activities, depending on the career stage of a faculty member. For example, early career faculty may have different needs than mid-career faculty; they may also prefer different ways of meeting those needs.

Regardless of the scope of the faculty development endeavor, the common denominator rests on the value of a comprehensive program that is responsive to the needs and priorities of faculty members and the organizations in which they work. The literature also demonstrates increasing evidence regarding the merit of programs that extend over time (Gruppen Chap. 10; Hodges Chap. 4; Steinert et al. 2006), suggesting that longitudinal programs yield more lasting results. In line with this observation, de Grave et al. (Chap. 9) recommend that we reconsider the role of workshops and seminars in the repertoire of faculty development initiatives and explore how they can be integrated into longitudinal programs, allowing for cumulative learning and practice.

20.4.2 Choosing a Conceptual Framework to Guide Program Design and Delivery

As suggested in a systematic review of faculty development to promote leadership, faculty development should be grounded in both theory and empirical evidence (Steinert et al. 2012). Models and principles of teaching and learning (Mann 2002) should inform the planning and development of interventions, and relevant theoretical frameworks should guide the choice of content and process. In a review of 55 community leadership development programs, Russon and Reinelt (2004) observed that programs did not articulate a program theory or 'theory of change' to describe 'how and why a set of activities are expected to lead to outcomes and impacts' (p. 105). As highlighted by de Grave et al. (Chap. 9) and Silver (Chap. 16), there is a clear need to identify and describe the conceptual frameworks that underpin our work.

At the same time, no single theory can explain how faculty members develop their skills and expertise in a variety of domains. As a result, we should choose a conceptual approach that can guide program design and delivery. For example, if we choose to view faculty development through the lens of expectancy-value theory (Eccles and Wigfield 2002; Heckhausen 1991), also described by Silver (Chap. 16), we might want to examine how our professional development activities can trigger faculty members' expectancies and values. According to this theoretical framework, we orient ourselves to the world according to our expectations and values (Steinert et al. 2009). Eccles and Wigfield (2002) have defined expectancies as 'beliefs about how one will do on certain tasks or activities' and values as the 'incentives or reasons for doing the activity'. In most faculty development activities, at least two expectancies (Heckhausen 1991) come into play: (1) the subjective probability of attaining an outcome in a specific situation and (2) the subjective probability of an outcome to be associated with specific consequences. For example, if health professionals believe that faculty development activities (be they formal or informal) can enable personal and professional growth, and that they are relevant to their needs, they may be more likely to participate. Awareness of these motivational factors (and their theoretical foundations) can also influence the design and delivery of most faculty development initiatives.

Alternatively, and as suggested in Chap. 1, situated learning theory can guide the design and development of a faculty development program or activity. Situated learning is based on the notion that knowledge is *contextually situated* and fundamentally influenced by the *activity*, *context*, and *culture* in which it is used (Brown et al. 1989). This view of knowledge, as situated in authentic contexts, and its key components of cognitive apprenticeship, collaborative learning, reflection, practice, and articulation of learning skills (McLellan 1996), has important implications for our understanding of faculty development. In a similar fashion, workplace learning (Billett 1996; Eraut 2004) and communities of practice (Wenger 1998), as outlined in Chap. 7, can guide our work in this area. Clearly, we need to heed the advice of de Grave et al. (Chap. 9) and articulate the theoretical (or conceptual) approaches that inform our faculty development practices.

20.4.3 Integrating Alternative Approaches

Part III describes a number of faculty development approaches that are used less frequently: peer coaching and mentorship (Boillat and Elizov Chap. 8) and online learning (Cook Chap. 11). How could these approaches be integrated more frequently into faculty development programs and activities? How can we capitalize on the benefits of peer-assisted learning and multiple mentoring in both formal and informal settings, and how we can promote enhanced online learning opportunities? In addition, how can we utilize simulation and other advanced technologies for faculty development? The Objective Structured Teaching Encounter (OSTE) is one example of how simulated practice can be used to facilitate professional learning (Boillat et al. 2012; Stone et al. 2003). However, the range of possibilities for using simulation to promote faculty development for all faculty roles is infinite (Ellen et al. 1994; Johnson et al. 1999; Krautscheid et al. 2008), and in many ways, the principles described by Cook (Chap. 11), that include a needs analysis, adherence to principles of instructional design, and careful planning and evaluation, apply in this context as well.

20.4.4 Promoting Reflection and Reflective Practice

In examining key features of effective faculty development programs, the role of reflection – and reflective practice – emerges as a critical ingredient to professional learning. As Raelin (1997) has said, 'reflection constitutes the ability to uncover and make explicit to oneself what one has planned, observed or achieved in practice' (p. 567). This author also postulates that reflection is as important to learning as experience, for without contemplation, 'lessons to be learned' may be overlooked. However, despite this observation, and those of other authors (e.g. Lachman and Pawlina 2006; Schön 1983), very little is known about how the process of reflection unfolds. In addition, few authors have explicitly described the reflective process in structured faculty development initiatives (e.g. Branch et al. 2009). As Mann

(Chap. 12) has stated, the role of reflection in faculty development will warrant more attention in the future and we will need to carefully examine ways in which to stimulate and nurture critical thinking in the development of health professionals as educators, leaders, and researchers.

20.4.5 Encouraging Interprofessional Faculty Development

The role and importance of interprofessional education and practice has been widely acknowledged. A number of interprofessional faculty development initiatives have also been described in the literature (e.g. Brashers et al. 2012; Silver and Leslie 2009), all of which have the potential of achieving identified goals and overcoming barriers to interprofessional collaboration and practice (Steinert 2005). Anderson et al. (Chap. 14) describe how faculty development can promote interprofessional education and practice. It is our belief that one of the most powerful ways to break down perceived barriers (or silos) and to enhance mutual respect and collaboration is by working together to meet common goals. Interprofessional faculty development can achieve this goal, by modeling the way and helping to create interprofessional communities of practice.

20.5 Starting Early in the Careers of Future Faculty Members

Although the primary focus of this book has been the development of faculty members, many authors across the health professions have expressed the view that faculty development should start early, often at entry to university (Busari and Scherpbier 2004; Dandavino et al. 2007; Gonzalez et al. 2003; Zsohar and Smith 2010). Undergraduate, graduate, and postgraduate students in the health professions teach in a variety of settings. In fact, in one study, it was estimated that postgraduate students spend as much as 25 % of their time in teaching activities, including the supervision, instruction, and evaluation of students and more junior trainees (Seely 1999). At the same time, learners across the educational continuum have identified teaching as an important part of their responsibilities and have expressed interest and enthusiasm in learning about their educational roles (Bing-You and Sproul 1992; Busari et al. 2002).

In examining medical education in particular, Dandavino et al. (2007) outline a number of reasons why undergraduate students should learn about teaching. As they suggest, students will become future faculty members and many of them will take on significant teaching roles. In addition, education is a core component of the doctor-patient relationship and it is anticipated that students will become more efficient communicators as a consequence of learning about teaching. It is also hoped that they will become better learners as a result of increased knowledge about teaching and learning. Similar observations have been made about graduate and postgraduate students. For example, studies have shown that postgraduate students contribute significantly to the education of students (Edwards et al. 2002) and that students perceive them as playing a critical role in their training (Sternszus et al. 2012; Walton and Patel 2008).

In many ways, the content of faculty development for undergraduate, graduate, and postgraduate students mirrors what we encounter in faculty development for practicing health professionals (Busari et al. 2006; Pasquinelli and Greenberg 2008; Soriano et al. 2010; Wamsley et al. 2004; Zsohar and Smith 2010), with a primary emphasis on teaching improvement. Program modalities are also similar and include workshops and seminars (e.g. Bardach et al. 2003; Nestel and Kidd 2002), student- or resident-as-teacher programs (Edwards et al. 2002; Pasquinelli and Greenberg 2008), and elective activities in medical education (Craig and Page 1987). Not surprisingly, the majority of teaching improvement programs are rated positively by learners, who value the experiential nature of activities, the role of feedback, and the learning that occurs 'on the job'.

At the same time, although most of the relevant literature focuses on students (at all levels of the continuum) as teachers, the need to prepare learners for leadership and management roles has been highlighted by some authors (Berkenbosch et al. 2012; Blumenthal et al. 2012; Gonzalez et al. 2003), and as Ackerly et al. (2011) have stated, 'the active cultivation of future leaders is [urgently] required' (p. 575). It should also be noted that leadership (or management) and research (or scholarship) are included as core competencies in different educational frameworks, as outlined by Snell (Chap. 13), and as a result, training in this area aligns well with both curricular expectations and health care priorities. As is the case with faculty members, faculty development in this area must address the multiple roles that future faculty members can play.

20.6   Mapping a Research Agenda for Faculty Development

As stated in Chap. 1 and summarized by Spencer (Chap. 17), research on the impact of formal (structured) faculty development activities has shown that overall satisfaction with programs is high and that participants recommend these activities to their colleagues. Faculty members also tend to report a positive change in attitudes, knowledge, skills, and behaviors following a particular program or activity; impact on learners or colleagues is less frequently observed, as is change at the organizational level. The literature to date has also helped to identify 'key features' of successful faculty development programs, though less is known about 'how' or 'why' change occurs.

From a methodological point of view, studies in this field have been limited by a number of challenges that characterize much of medical education research (Spencer Chap. 17), making conclusive statements and generalizations to other settings difficult. For example, the majority of studies in this area use descriptive, single-group designs to examine outcomes. These designs confound the ability to attribute outcomes directly to the intervention (Steinert et al. 2012) and make appraisal difficult. In addition, a number of studies either rely entirely on post-intervention measures or collect data several years after the intervention took place (Steinert et al. 2006, 2012), making the 'attribution of change' equally challenging. Researchers have also under-utilized qualitative methodologies which, in many ways, can more easily capture the process of change. In addition, and as outlined by O'Sullivan and Irby (Chap. 18), there has been an over-emphasis on a positivist paradigm.

However, the need for research in this field has never been greater, as we try to promote scholarship and academic inquiry, inform 'best' practices, and remain responsive to organizational needs and priorities. The timing is also opportune, as we have witnessed a world-wide increase in departments and centers dedicated to medical education research and scholarship (Steinert 2012).

20.6.1 Considering Alternative Research Paradigms, Methodologies and Methods

Recommendations for moving the faculty development research agenda forward are described in detail in Chaps. 17 and 18. In this section, we will only highlight some of the suggestions made.

20.6.1.1 Moving Beyond a Positivist Paradigm

O'Sullivan and Irby (Chap. 18) have wisely suggested that we consider moving away from a positivist tradition and conduct research framed by post-positivist, interpretivist, and critical theory research paradigms, using associated methodologies to enrich our understanding of faculty development. As these authors have stated, 'a paradigm defines the prevailing model of exemplary practices for a community of researchers; it illuminates areas for investigation and obscures others' (O'Sullivan and Irby Chap. 18). Changing paradigms would enable new perspectives and encourage us to consider innovative conceptual approaches and methodologies.

20.6.1.2 Ensuring That Research Is Informed by a Conceptual Framework

We stated earlier that faculty development programming should be informed by theoretical models and approaches; so should research and scholarship. With this in mind, O'Sullivan and Irby (2011, Chap. 18) suggest that we use a new conceptual framework that incorporates the notion of a faculty development community and a workplace community to conduct research in this area. In particular, these authors propose that we study the relationship between these two communities, their power and influence, and the impact of both on the culture and practices of the institutions in which they evolve. Using this framework can also lead to a broader set of questions (described in Chap. 18) and reinforces the value of examining workplace learning and communities of practice (as highlighted in Chap. 7). Additional theoretical frameworks are also summarized by Silver (Chap. 16) and other authors (e.g. de Grave et al. Chap. 9). Irrespective of which conceptual approach we adopt, we should strive to utilize theory in the design of our research and in the interpretation of our results.

20.6.1.3 Acknowledging the Complexity of Faculty Development Interventions

Spencer (Chap. 17) discusses the challenge of evaluating complex interventions and reminds us that the boundaries between research and evaluation are fluid. He also reinforces the perception that faculty development is a complex process. As outlined in Chap. 17, complex interventions are usually based on several working theories, some more well defined or evidence-based than others; they involve a wide range of participants (which in this case would include faculty developers, administrators, course participants, learners, and colleagues); and they are embedded in multiple social systems. In addition, the process is usually non-linear, with multiple pathways and feedback loops, and success is dependent upon a cumulative chain of events. These characteristics clearly describe formal (structured) faculty development activities, where many intervening, mediating variables (e.g. personal attributes, individual status, and responsibilities) interact with uncontrollable, extraneous factors. They also imply that we should select methodologies that can capture the complexity of faculty development interventions as well as the process of change.

20.6.1.4 Incorporating New Methodologies and Methods

As suggested above, we need to move away from an over-reliance on experimental and quasi-experimental designs and consider qualitative designs, using phenomenology, ethnography, case studies, and mixed methods (Drescher et al. 2004; O'Sullivan and Irby Chap. 18; Steinert et al. 2012). In many ways, qualitative methodologies would allow us to tease apart the process of change, corroborate anecdotal observations, and capture faculty members' stories. We should also consider using the methodologies suggested by O'Sullivan and Irby (Chap. 18). Educational design research is pertinent to faculty development because it allows for the examination of evolving program innovations. The researcher attends to program goals and design, a description of how the intervention unfolds, achieved outcomes, and lessons learned (Collins et al. 2004). Success cases, which can be used concurrently with design research, fit within an interpretivist paradigm. Success cases aim to reveal how well an initiative is working and try to identify the contextual factors that support successful implementation (Brinkerhoff and Dressler 2003). This methodology aligns well with the perceived need to examine the role of contextual factors in faculty development. Sustainability narratives are considered by O'Sullivan and Irby (Chap. 18) to be a research methodology that lies 'outside the normal modes of inquiry for the education community' as it explores the development of a society through the lens of human and environmental systems and imagines what the future would be like if people's lives were improved (Swart et al. 2004). However, the use of both this methodology and that of narrative research (Lieblich et al. 1998) would enable a rich understanding of the faculty development process as well as individual and organizational change.

Much has been written about the need to improve the research methods used in this field of inquiry (Steinert et al. 2006, 2012). Suffice it to say that we should use validated outcome measures, including newer methods of behavioral or performance-based measures of change. As well, we should utilize multiple methods and data sources to assess process and outcome. To date, we have witnessed an over-reliance on self-assessment methods and survey questionnaires to assess change. Moving forward, we should consider the use of alternative data sources and try to ascertain as many stakeholder perspectives (e.g. students; colleagues) as possible. Lastly, irrespective of the methodologies chosen, we should ensure congruence between study design, research questions, and data collection methods.

20.6.2   Exploring New Areas of Inquiry

In different ways, each chapter in this book suggests a new focus of inquiry. In this section, we will highlight only a few areas for further investigation that cut across a number of the authors' recommendations. We also invite the reader to contribute to the suggested research agenda.

20.6.2.1   Analyzing the Process of 'Formal' Faculty Development Programs and Activities

Although the need to assess faculty development outcomes and impact remains a priority, we should carry out process-oriented studies to better understand how change occurs as a result of formal (structured) interventions. As an example, we should consider expanding the focus of outcome-oriented studies to compare how different faculty development interventions promote change in faculty members' competence and performance (Steinert et al. 2012). That is, it would be worthwhile to compare different faculty development approaches (e.g. workshops, seminar series, longitudinal programs) and the methods used in these formats (e.g. role plays or simulations; peer feedback or reflection) to enable an understanding of which faculty development 'features' contribute to changes in faculty members' performance (Steinert et al. 2006). In discussing research capacity, Hodges (Chap. 4) suggests that we should examine the relationship between different types of faculty development programs and long-term success in research. Similarly, Friedman et al. (Chap. 15) recommend that we look at success factors in existing international partnerships, with specific attention to relationship factors. It would also be worthwhile to tease apart ingredients of success within specific programs (e.g. peer-peer interaction; project work; online follow-up). For example, Mann (Chap. 12) describes how current programs designed to promote reflective practice appear to be effective but time-consuming. Assessing the differential contributions of key features would help us to determine the design of relevant and feasible initiatives that best meet faculty members' needs and realities. Cook et al. (2008) suggest that we should pursue 'clarification' studies (in addition to 'description' and 'justification' studies) to deepen our understanding and 'advance the art and science of medical education' (p. 128). This recommendation, to understand 'why' or 'how' something works, is particularly relevant in this context.

The assessment of change, within the individual (e.g. how did faculty members' attitudes and values change) and over time (including the 'durability of change' and factors which help to sustain change) would also be worthwhile. Russon and Reinelt (2004) make an interesting distinction between *outcomes* (i.e. changes in attitudes, behavior, knowledge, and skills) and *impact* (i.e. the long-term future social change that a program works to create). Given health professionals' roles in creating educational, social, and health care change, assessment over time is critical. In addition, many of the outcomes anticipated in a planned faculty development program take time to emerge. This serves as a further reason to promote longitudinal assessment and follow-up.

Knight (2002) asks whether professional learning happens 'in ways assumed by delivery models which concentrate on provision of courses, workshops and other events…' (p. 230). We clearly need to explore this question in more depth, examine the impact of alternative approaches such as peer coaching and mentorship (Boillat and Elizov Chap. 8), and online learning (Cook Chap. 11), and begin to compare 'formal' and 'informal' ways of learning.

20.6.2.2 Understanding How People Learn in the Workplace

As highlighted in Chaps. 1 and 7, health professionals learn about their faculty roles in both formal and informal ways. However, although 'there are strong indicators that a great deal of learning takes place in the workplace, relatively little appears to be known about how people learn informally or about the relative value of different types of learning experiences' (Cheetham and Chivers 2001, p. 269). Even less is known about how health professionals learn in the workplace, and we should try to build on lessons learned in postgraduate medical education (Teunissen et al. 2007), clinical medicine, and dentistry (Cook 2009), using qualitative research methodologies to try to better understand this process. Clarke and Hollingsworth (2002) have argued that it is time to shift our thinking away from programs that 'change teachers' to viewing faculty members as 'active learners shaping their own professional growth through reflective participation in professional development programs and practice' (p. 948). This perspective, together with that suggested by O'Sullivan and Irby (Chap. 18), provides a research agenda for the future. It also underscores the need to understand the role of role modeling, reflection, and engagement in workplace learning.

A number of authors in this book (e.g. Anderson et al. Chap. 14; Mann Chap. 12; O'Sullivan and Irby Chap. 18) have suggested that future research in this area should incorporate current understandings of communities of practice, with attention to how they evolve, how they function, and how they can lead to individual and organizational growth and development. Such research would also be helpful in illuminating how communities of health professionals can be developed and sustained. At the same time, we need to think about how workplace learning and communities of practice can lead to enhanced learning for leadership and research. Not surprisingly, most of the work in this area has focused on the role of the teacher and educator.

20.6.2.3 Examining the Process of Becoming a Faculty Member

Although this volume has underscored the importance of looking at both formal and informal approaches to faculty development, little is known about the ongoing formation of faculty members. In a previously described study, Steinert (2012) explored the process of becoming a medical educator as seen through the eyes of 12 medical educators. A number of themes emerged in this study, including the notion of volition, on-the-job-learning, mentorship and role modeling, and belonging to a community of experts. It would now be interesting to study how health professionals learn to become faculty members and fulfill their responsibilities as leaders and researchers.

Leslie (in Chap. 5) and other authors (Lieff et al. 2012; Starr et al. 2003) have highlighted how we need to further understand the development of an academic identity, examining how it is developed within the health professions context, how it evolves over time, and how it can inform professional learning and practice. Leslie also points out that examining the formation of academic identity in association with networks of colleagues who have similar identities might allow us to learn more about collaborative scholarship and how faculty development can play a role in enhancing identity. Exploring faculty members' beliefs would also be beneficial, as core beliefs are likely to be a primary determinant of faculty members' behaviors (Williams and Klamen 2006). Interestingly, we often provide faculty development in a vacuum, paying little attention to identity or beliefs. In addition, the research that has looked at this area has primarily focused on the educational role of health professionals, examining faculty members' conceptions of learning (Swanwick and Morris 2010; Young 2008), beliefs about teaching (Light and Calkins 2008), and the role of disruption and transformation in faculty development (Kumagai 2010). Clearly, personal beliefs, values and conceptions are pivotal elements in all faculty roles and merit exploration.

20.6.2.4 Evaluating Context and Organizational Change

As stated at the outset (and in many of the book's chapters), professional development (be it formal or informal) occurs in a complex environment in which many unforeseen and unpredictable variables play a role. As a result, we should try to conduct more studies in which the interaction between different factors is investigated, highlighting 'under what conditions and why an intervention might be successful or not' (Steinert et al. 2006, p. 522). Jolly (Chap. 6) and Billett (1996) identify a number of ways in which the organization (or institution) can influence the process of faculty development. Systematic and sustained research on the organizational (and contextual) factors that both promote and hinder the professional development and learning of faculty members is indicated. So is the need to assess the impact of faculty development on the organization.

In various chapters, we have said that faculty development can – and should – enhance organizational capacity. However, we need to move beyond anecdotal observations and aspirations and verify whether this assertion is, in fact, true. The dearth of research assessing the impact of faculty development on the organization is surprising (Steinert et al. 2006, 2012). Is this because organizational change is difficult to measure? Is it because of medicine's historical focus on the individual (Bleakley 2006)? Whatever the reason, there is a clear need to assess outcomes and impact at the organizational and systems level. Research in this area will also provide valuable insights that can help to guide future policies and practices.

20.6.3 Ensuring That Research Informs Practice

No discussion of research on faculty development in the health professions (knowledge creation) would be complete without talking about how work in this area can inform our practice (knowledge-to-action). As outlined by Thomas and Steinert (Chap. 19), there are seven stages in moving knowledge into practice that include: identifying a problem in practice, or a gap in knowledge, and identifying, reviewing, and selecting the knowledge to be implemented to address the gap; adapting or customizing the knowledge to the local context; evaluating the determinants of the knowledge use; selecting, tailoring and implementing interventions to address the knowledge or practice gap; monitoring the knowledge use in practice; evaluating the outcomes or impact of using the new knowledge; and determining strategies for ensuring that the new knowledge is sustained (Graham et al. 2006).

As faculty members, researchers and faculty developers, we would be wise to consider the fluid nature of this process and ensure that our faculty development practices are informed by the 'best' available evidence.

20.7   Learning from Each Other

Nora (2010) points out that 'No medical school can accomplish its mission independent of other organizations' (p. S46). This is clearly true in the area of faculty development as well. Based on our collective experience (e.g. 1st International Conference on Faculty Development 2011) and the findings in this volume, there is mutual benefit in collaborating with universities and teaching hospitals, community hospitals and ambulatory sites, research institutes, and regional, national, and international organizations dedicated to the advancement of health professions education, leadership, and research. Although partnerships require time and attention, collaboration can help us to achieve goals that any one individual or organization may not.

In a similar vein, it would be beneficial to learn from, and collaborate with, colleagues outside of medicine. For example, as many authors in this book suggest, we can learn important lessons from colleagues in education (e.g. Clarke and Hollingsworth 2002; Webster-Wright 2009; Wenger 1998) and management (e.g. Kotter 1996; Nonaka and Takeuchi 2011), to name but a few. Moreover, by working together, we can enhance educational capacity, promote leadership and organizational growth, and develop a rigorous research agenda and network.

At the same time, the globalization of health professions education, research, and practice is evolving (Bleakley et al. 2008; Hodges et al. 2009; Marchal and Kegels 2003), and it will remain important to situate faculty development in a global context. Friedman et al. (Chap. 15) describe a number of successful international partnerships that benefit individuals, organizations, and society. They also highlight some of the elements that are key to building successful partnerships, including the partners themselves, available human, financial, and material resources, and a sense of engagement. Additionally, they identify factors leading to successful (and sustainable) partnerships that encompass frequent bilateral communication, a clear agenda and mutual goal-setting, adequate resources, and cultural competence. Cognizance of these factors, as well as the cultural 'positions' and attitudes that underlie our work (Bleakley et al. 2008), would enhance our ability to move forward in this area. Over 20 years ago, Boelen (1992) addressed the need for global action in medical education reform and detailed an agenda that included quality education, strategies for change management, and the monitoring of progress made. These priorities remain equally important today and faculty development has a critical role to play in making these changes happen (Steinert 2011). More recently, Silver (Chap. 16) has suggested that it is time to build and sustain an international faculty development community. In multiple ways, it would be worthwhile to explore an international agenda for faculty development and find ways to share accumulated 'know how' and build on our collective expertise.

20.8 Conclusion

'The changing roles of faculty members will continue to drive the changing nature of faculty development practices, as will the evolution of the organizations in which we work' (Steinert 2000, p. 49). Future directions for faculty development research and practice include: moving away from the notion of one-time development to ongoing learning, expanding the focus of faculty development, building on available evidence and previous success, introducing faculty development early in the careers of future health professionals, mapping a rigorous and meaningful research agenda for faculty development, and learning from each other. As stated at the outset, faculty development is an investment in the social capital of the organizations (or institutions) in which we work and an 'outward sign of the inner faith that institutions have in their workforce' (Bligh 2005, p. 120). Leslie (Chap. 5) suggests that being part of a culture that embodies a 'spirit of inquiry, discovery and innovation' is important to health professionals. We would add that faculty members are equally motivated by a sense of curiosity, creativity, and commitment, wishing to excel in all that they do. Faculty development is a way in which to foster this pursuit of excellence.

20.9 Key Messages

- Moving forward, we must find ways to recognize the role of workplace learning in faculty development and bring 'formal' activities to the workplace.
- Expanding the focus of faculty development to include *all* faculty roles as well as an emphasis on the organization will enhance both individual and organizational capacity.
- Promoting faculty development 'early' in the careers of undergraduate, graduate, and postgraduate students will help to prepare future faculty members.
- Creating a research agenda for faculty development involves the use of new paradigms, methodologies, and methods as well as areas of inquiry that promote an understanding of the process of formal programs, how people learn in the workplace, and how health professionals become faculty members.
- Learning from each other will enable the sharing of resources and expertise and help to create new partnerships and communities of practice that support ongoing professional development.

References

1st International Conference on Faculty Development in the Health Professions. (2011). Retrieved November 27th, 2012, from http://www.facultydevelopment2011.com

Academy of Medical Educators. (2012). *Professional standards*. London, UK: Academy of Medical Educators. Available from: http://www.medicaleducators.org/index.cfm/linkservid/180C46A6-B0E9-B09B-02599E43F9C2FDA9/showMeta/0/

Ackerly, D. C., Sangvai, D. G., Udayakumar, K., Shah, B. R., Kalman, N. S., Cho, A. H., et al. (2011). Training the next generation of physician-executives: An innovative residency pathway in management and leadership. *Academic Medicine, 86*(5), 575–579.

Bardach, N. S., Vedanthan, R., & Haber, R. J. (2003). 'Teaching to teach': Enhancing fourth year medical students' teaching skills. *Medical Education, 37*(11), 1031–1032.

Berkenbosch, L., Bax, M., Scherpbier, A., Heyligers, I., Muijtjens, A. M., & Busari, J. O. (2012). How Dutch medical specialists perceive the competencies and training needs of medical residents in healthcare management. *Medical Teacher, 35*(4), e1090–e1102.

Bierema, L. L. (1996). Development of the individual leads to more productive workplaces. *New Directions for Adult and Continuing Education, 1996*(72), 21–28.

Billett, S. (1996). Towards a model of workplace learning: The learning curriculum. *Studies in Continuing Education, 18*(1), 43–58.

Billett, S. (2002). Toward a workplace pedagogy: Guidance, participation, and engagement. *Adult Education Quarterly, 53*(1), 27–43.

Bing-You, R. G. & Sproul, M. S. (1992). Medical students' perceptions of themselves and residents as teachers. *Medical Teacher, 14*(2–3), 133–138.

Bleakley, A. (2006). Broadening conceptions of learning in medical education: The message from teamworking. *Medical Education, 40*(2), 150–157.

Bleakley, A., Brice, J., & Bligh, J. (2008). Thinking the post-colonial in medical education. *Medical Education, 42*(3), 266–270.

Bligh, J. (2005). Faculty development. *Medical Education, 39*(2), 120–121.

Blumenthal, D. M., Bernard, K., Bohnen, J., & Bohmer, R. (2012). Addressing the leadership gap in medicine: Residents' need for systematic leadership development training. *Academic Medicine, 87*(4), 513–522.

Boelen, C. (1992). Medical education reform: The need for global action. *Academic Medicine, 67*(11), 745–749.

Boillat, M., Bethune, C., Ohle, E., Razack, S., & Steinert, Y. (2012). Twelve tips for using the objective structured teaching exercise for faculty development. *Medical Teacher, 34*(4), 269–273.

Branch, W. T. Jr., Frankel, R., Gracey, C. F., Haidet, P. M., Weissmann, P. F., Cantey, P., et al. (2009). A good clinician and a caring person: Longitudinal faculty development and the enhancement of the human dimensions of care. *Academic Medicine, 84*(1), 117–125.

Brashers, V., Peterson, C., Tullmann, D., & Schmitt, M. (2012). The University of Virginia interprofessional education initiative: An approach to integrating competencies into medical and nursing education. *Journal of Interprofessional Care, 26*(1), 73–75.

Brinkerhoff, R. O. & Dressler, D. E. (2003). *Using the success case impact evaluation method to enhance training value & impact*. San Diego, CA: American Society for Training and Development International Conference and Exhibition. Available from: http://www.blanchardtraining.com/img/pub/newsletter_brinkerhoff.pdf

Brown, J. S., Collins, A., & Duguid, P. (1989). Situated cognition and the culture of learning. *Educational Researcher, 18*(1), 32–42.

Busari, J. O., Prince, K. J., Scherpbier, A. J., van der Vleuten, C. P., & Essed, G. G. (2002). How residents perceive their teaching role in the clinical setting: A qualitative study. *Medical Teacher, 24*(1), 57–61.

Busari, J. O. & Scherpbier, A. J. (2004). Why residents should teach: A literature review. *Journal of Postgraduate Medicine, 50*(3), 205–210.

Busari, J. O., Scherpbier, A. J., van der Vleuten, C. P., & Essed, G. G. (2006). A two-day teacher-training programme for medical residents: Investigating the impact on teaching ability. *Advances in Health Sciences Education, 11*(2), 133–144.

Clarke, D. & Hollingsworth, H. (2002). Elaborating a model of teacher professional growth. *Teaching and Teacher Education, 18*(8), 947–967.

Cheetham, G. & Chivers, G. (2001). How professionals learn in practice: An investigation of informal learning amongst people working in professions. *Journal of European Industrial Training, 25*(5), 247–292.

Collins, A., Joseph, D., & Bielaczyc, K. (2004). Design research: Theoretical and methodological issues. *Journal of the Learning Sciences, 13*(1), 15–42.

Cook, D. A., Bordage, G., & Schmidt, H. G. (2008). Description, justification and clarification: A framework for classifying the purposes of research in medical education. *Medical Education, 42*(2), 128–133.

Cook, V. (2009). Mapping the work-based learning of novice teachers: Charting some rich terrain. *Medical Teacher, 31*(12), e608–e614.

Craig, J. L. & Page, G. (1987). Teaching in medicine: An elective course for third-year students. *Medical Education, 21*(5), 386–390.

Dandavino, M., Snell, L., & Wiseman, J. (2007). Why medical students should learn how to teach. *Medical Teacher, 29*(6), 558–565.

Drescher, U., Warren, F., & Norton, K. (2004). Towards evidence-based practice in medical training: Making evaluations more meaningful. *Medical Education, 38*(12), 1288–1294.

Dreyfus, H. L. & Dreyfus, S. E. (1986). *Mind over machine: The power of human intuition and expertise in the era of the computer.* New York, NY: Free Press.

Drummond-Young, M., Brown, B., Noesgaard, C., Lunyk-Child, O., Matthew-Maich, N., Mines, C., et al. (2010). A comprehensive faculty development model for nursing education. *Journal of Professional Nursing, 26*(3), 152–161.

DuFour, R. (2004). Leading edge: The best staff development is in the workplace, not in a workshop. *Journal of Staff Development, 25*(2), 63–64.

Eccles, J. S. & Wigfield, A. (2002). Motivational beliefs, values, and goals. *Annual Review of Psychology, 53*, 109–132.

Edwards, J. C., Friedland, J. A., & Bing-You, R. (2002). *Residents' teaching skills.* New York, NY: Springer.

Eitel, F., Kanz, K. G., & Tesche, A. (2000). Training and certification of teachers and trainers: The professionalization of medical education. *Medical Teacher, 22*(5), 517–526.

Ellen, J., Giardino, A. P., Edinburgh, K., & Ende, J. (1994). Simulated students: A new method for studying clinical precepting. *Teaching and Learning in Medicine, 6*(2), 132–135.

Eraut, M. (2004). Informal learning in the workplace. *Studies in Continuing Education, 26*(2), 247–273.

Goldszmidt, M. A., Zibrowski, E. M., & Weston, W. W. (2008). Education scholarship: It's not just a question of 'degree'. *Medical Teacher, 30*(1), 34–39.

Gonzalez, L. S., Stewart, S. R., & Robinson, T. C. (2003). Growing leaders for tomorrow: The University of Kentucky administrative internship program. *Journal of Allied Health, 32*(2), 126–130.

Graham, I. D., Logan, J., Harrison, M. B., Straus, S. E., Tetroe, J., Caswell, W., et al. (2006). Lost in knowledge translation: Time for a map? *Journal of Continuing Education in the Health Professions, 26*(1), 13–24.

Grossman, R. & Salas, E. (2011). The transfer of training: What really matters. *International Journal of Training and Development, 15*(2), 103–120.

Hafler, J. P., Ownby, A. R., Thompson, B. M., Fasser, C. E., Grigsby, K., Haidet, P., et al. (2011). Decoding the learning environment of medical education: A hidden curriculum perspective for faculty development. *Academic Medicine, 86*(4), 440–444.

Heckhausen, H. (1991). *Motivation and action.* Berlin, DE: Springer-Verlag.

Hodges, B. D., Maniate, J. M., Martimianakis, M. A., Alsuwaidan, M., & Segouin, C. (2009). Cracks and crevices: Globalization discourse and medical education. *Medical Teacher, 31*(10), 910–917.

Johnson, J. H., Zerwic, J. J., & Theis, S. L. (1999). Clinical simulation laboratory: An adjunct to clinical teaching. *Nurse Educator, 24*(5), 37–41.

Knight, P. (2002). A systemic approach to professional development: Learning as practice. *Teaching and Teacher Education, 18*(3), 229–241.

Kotter, J. P. (1996). *Leading change.* Boston, MA: Harvard Business School Press.

Kouzes, J. M. & Posner, B. Z. (1995). *The leadership challenge: How to keep getting extraordinary things done in organizations.* San Francisco, CA: Jossey-Bass.

Krautscheid, L., Kaakinen, J., & Warner, J. R. (2008). Clinical faculty development: Using simulation to demonstrate and practice clinical teaching. *The Journal of Nursing Education, 47*(9), 431–434.

Kumagai, A. K. (2010). Commentary: Forks in the road: Disruption and transformation in professional development. *Academic Medicine, 85*(12), 1819–1820.

Lachman, N. & Pawlina, W. (2006). Integrating professionalism in early medical education: The theory and application of reflective practice in the anatomy curriculum. *Clinical Anatomy, 19*(5), 456–460.

Lieblich, A., Tuval-Mashiach, R., & Zilber, T. (1998). *Narrative research: Reading, analysis, and interpretation.* Thousand Oaks, CA: Sage.

Lieff, S., Baker, L., Mori, B., Egan-Lee, E., Chin, K., & Reeves, S. (2012). Who am I? Key influences on the formation of academic identity within a faculty development program. *Medical Teacher, 34*(3), e208–e215.

Light, G. & Calkins, S. (2008). The experience of faculty development: Patterns of variation in conceptions of teaching. *International Journal for Academic Development, 13*(1), 27–40.

Mann, K. V. (2002). Thinking about learning: Implications for principle-based professional education. *Journal of Continuing Education in the Health Professions, 22*(2), 69–76.

Marchal, B. & Kegels, G. (2003). Health workforce imbalances in times of globalization: Brain drain or professional mobility? *The International Journal of Health Planning and Management, 18*(Suppl. 1), S89–S101.

McLellan, H. (1996). *Situated learning perspectives.* Englewood Cliffs, NJ: Educational Technology Publications.

Milner, R. J., Gusic, M. E., & Thorndyke, L. E. (2011). Perspective: Toward a competency framework for faculty. *Academic Medicine, 86*(10), 1204–1210.

Molenaar, W. M., Zanting, A., van Beukelen, P., de Grave, W., Baane, J. A., Bustraan, J. A., et al. (2009). A framework of teaching competencies across the medical education continuum. *Medical Teacher, 31*(5), 390–396.

Nestel, D. & Kidd, J. (2002). Evaluating a teaching skills workshop for medical students. *Medical Education, 36*(11), 1094–1095.

Nonaka, I. & Takeuchi, H. (2011). The wise leader. *Harvard Business Review, 89*(5), 58–67.

Nora, L. M. (2010). The 21st century faculty member in the educational process - What should be on the horizon? *Academic Medicine, 85*(9 Suppl.), S45–S55.

Pasquinelli, L. M. & Greenberg, L. W. (2008). A review of medical school programs that train medical students as teachers (MED-SATS). *Teaching and Learning in Medicine, 20*(1), 73–81.

Purcell, N. & Lloyd-Jones, G. (2003). Standards for medical educators. *Medical Education, 37*(2), 149–154.

Raelin, J. A. (1997). A model of work-based learning. *Organization Science, 8*(6), 563–578.

Russon, C. & Reinelt, C. (2004). The results of an evaluation scan of 55 leadership development programs. *Journal of Leadership & Organizational Studies, 10*(3), 104–107.

Schön, D. A. (1983). *The reflective practitioner: How professionals think in action.* New York, NY: Basic Books.

Seely, A. J. E. (1999). The teaching contributions of residents. *CMAJ, 161*(10), 1239–1241.

Silver, I. L. & Leslie, K. (2009). Faculty development for continuing interprofessional education and collaborative practice. *Journal of Continuing Education in the Health Professions, 29*(3), 172–177.

Soriano, R. P., Blatt, B., Coplit, L., CichoskiKelly, E., Kosowicz, L., Newman, L., et al. (2010). Teaching medical students how to teach: A national survey of students-as-teachers programs in U.S. medical schools. *Academic Medicine, 85*(11), 1725–1731.

Srinivasan, M., Li, S. T., Meyers, F. J., Pratt, D. D., Collins, J. B., Braddock, C., et al. (2011). 'Teaching as a competency': Competencies for medical educators. *Academic Medicine, 86*(10), 1211–1220.

Starr, S., Ferguson, W. J., Haley, H. L., & Quirk, M. (2003). Community preceptors' views of their identities as teachers. *Academic Medicine, 78*(8), 820–825.

Steinert, Y. (2000). Faculty development in the new millennium: Key challenges and future directions. *Medical Teacher, 22*(1), 44–50.

Steinert, Y. (2005). Learning together to teach together: Interprofessional education and faculty development. *Journal of Interprofessional Care, 19*(Suppl. 1), 60–75.

Steinert, Y. (2010). Developing medical educators: A journey, not a destination. In T. Swanwick (Ed.), *Understanding medical education: Evidence, theory and practice,* (pp. 403–418). Edinburgh, UK: Association for the Study of Medical Education.

Steinert, Y. (2011). Commentary: Faculty development: The road less traveled. *Academic Medicine, 86*(4), 409–411.

Steinert, Y. (2012). Perspectives on faculty development: Aiming for 6/6 by 2020. *Perspectives on Medical Education, 1*(1), 31–42.

Steinert, Y., Boudreau, J. D., Boillat, M., Slapcoff, B., Dawson, D., Briggs, A., et al. (2010a). The Osler Fellowship: An apprenticeship for medical educators. *Academic Medicine, 85*(7), 1242–1249.

Steinert, Y., Macdonald, M. E., Boillat, M., Elizov, M., Meterissian, S., Razack, S., et al. (2010b). Faculty development: If you build it, they will come. *Medical Education, 44*(9), 900–907.

Steinert, Y., Mann, K., Centeno, A., Dolmans, D., Spencer, J., Gelula, M., et al. (2006). A systematic review of faculty development initiatives designed to improve teaching effectiveness in medical education: BEME Guide No. 8. *Medical Teacher, 28*(6), 497–526.

Steinert, Y., McLeod, P. J., Boillat, M., Meterissian, S., Elizov, M., & Macdonald, M. E. (2009). Faculty development: A 'Field of Dreams'? *Medical Education, 43*(1), 42–49.

Steinert, Y., Naismith, L., & Mann, K. (2012). Faculty development initiatives designed to promote leadership in medical education. A BEME systematic review: BEME Guide No. 19. *Medical Teacher, 34*(6), 483–503.

Sternszus, R., Cruess, S. R., Cruess, R. L., Young, M., & Steinert, Y. (2012). Residents as role models: Impact on undergraduate trainees. *Academic Medicine, 87*(9), 1282–1287.

Stone, S., Mazor, K., Devaney-O'Neil, S., Starr, S., Ferguson, W., Wellman, S., et al. (2003). Development and implementation of an Objective Structured Teaching Exercise (OSTE) to evaluate improvement in feedback skills following a faculty development workshop. *Teaching and Learning in Medicine, 15*(1), 7–13.

Swanwick, T. & Morris, C. (2010). Shifting conceptions of learning in the workplace. *Medical Education, 44*(6), 538–539.

Swart, R. J., Raskin, P., & Robinson, J. (2004). The problem of the future: Sustainability science and scenario analysis. *Global Environmental Change, 14*(2), 137–146.

Teunissen, P. W., Scheele, F., Scherpbier, A. J. J. A., van der Vleuten, C. P. M., Boor, K., van Luijk, S. J., et al. (2007). How residents learn: Qualitative evidence for the pivotal role of clinical activities, *Medical Education, 41*(8), 763–770.

Walton, J. M. & Patel, H. (2008). Residents as teachers in Canadian paediatric training programs: A survey of program director and resident perspectives. *Paediatrics & Child Health, 13*(8), 675–679.

Wamsley, M. A., Julian, K. A., & Wipf, J. E. (2004). A literature review of 'Resident-as-Teacher' curricula: Do teaching courses make a difference? *Journal of General Internal Medicine, 19*(5 Pt. 2), 574–581.

Webster-Wright, A. (2009). Reframing professional development through understanding authentic professional learning. *Review of Educational Research, 79*(2), 702–739.

Wenger, E. (1998). *Communities of practice: Learning, meaning, and identity*. New York, NY: Cambridge University Press.

Wenger, E., McDermott, R., & Snyder, W. M. (2002). *Cultivating communities of practice*. Boston, MA: Harvard Business School Press.

Williams, R. G. & Klamen, D. L. (2006). See one, do one, teach one - Exploring the core teaching beliefs of medical school faculty. *Medical Teacher, 28*(5), 418–424.

Young, S. F. (2008). Theoretical frameworks and models of learning: Tools for developing conceptions of teaching and learning. *International Journal for Academic Development, 13*(1), 41–49.

Zsohar, H. & Smith, J. A. (2010). Graduate student seminars as a faculty development activity. *Journal of Nursing Education, 49*(3), 161–163.